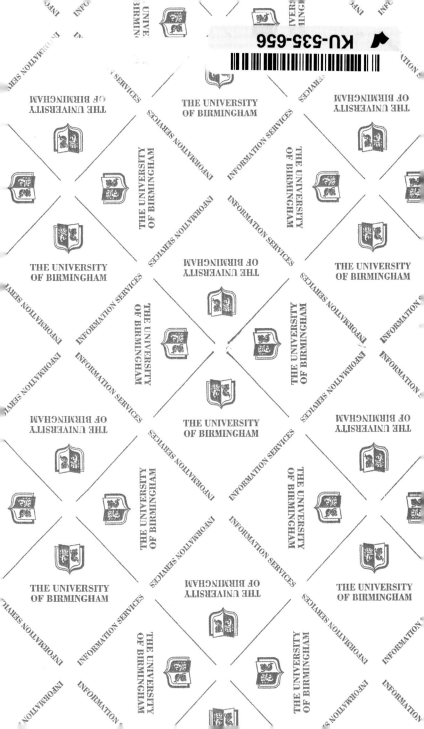

About the Author

Andrew Tyler is a freelance journalist who for
several years was a special correspondent for *New
Musical Express* on social and political issues. He
contributes to *Time Out*, *New Statesman*, *The
Observer*, *The Guardian* and others. He has
extensive experience as a youth worker. He is
married and lives in North London.

Street Drugs

Andrew Tyler

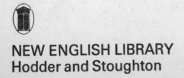

NEW ENGLISH LIBRARY
Hodder and Stoughton

For Sara, Davy, Oskie and
Penny

Copyright © 1986 by Andrew
Tyler

First published in Great Britain in
1986 by New English Library
Paperbacks, as a paperback
original

Second impression 1987
Revised and updated edition 1988

British Library C.I.P.

Tyler, Andrew
   Street drugs.
   1. Neuropharmacology
   2. Drug abuse
   I. Title
   615'.78   RM315

   ISBN 0-450-42273-9

Printed and bound in Great
Britain for Hodder and Stoughton
Paperbacks, a division of Hodder
and Stoughton Limited, Mill
Road, Dunton Green, Sevenoaks,
Kent TN13 2YA (Editorial Office:
47 Bedford Square, London
WC1B 3DP) by Richard Clay
Limited, Bungay, Suffolk.
Photoset by Rowland
Phototypesetting Limited,
Bury St Edmunds, Suffolk.

CONTENTS

ACKNOWLEDGEMENTS

MANY THANKS for generous help from all the following: John May (who fed me gems throughout), Richard Hartnoll and Roger Lewis at the Drug Indicators Project, John Witton, Mike Ashton and Harry Shapiro at the Institute for the Study of Drug Dependence, Dr Douglas Acres for looking over the drafts, Jane Goodsir at Release, Joan Jerome at Tranks, Giampi Alhadeff at City Roads, Mary Treacey at SCODA, Michelle Vincent at ASH, the Legalise Cannabis Campaign, Mick and Dean and Ed Glinert at Manchester's *City Life* magazine, Mark Steeles, the people at Tobacco Alliance, Stuart Gregory of the South West Training Unit, Don Aitken, Charlie Murray, Barney Hoskyns, Matthew Atha, Russ Hayton, Tony Bennett and my editors at NEL, Belinda Kirkin and Broo Doherty.

London, April 1988

INTRODUCTION TO SECOND EDITION

IN PREPARING this revised edition of *Street Drugs* I was faced with two options: either I could pick my way through the original text line by line, deleting, amending and updating where necessary; or leave the text alone and add a new self-contained section. I decided on the second course. The great majority of the original draft, in any case, has a long shelf life – dealing, as it does, with the history, pharmacology, health impact and sensations derived from the various drug substances. And even those passages which do describe the then contemporary scene (circa 1985) I believe were worth saving for the way they evoked a critical period in the evolution of the country's drug culture: namely, the period when heroin use became widespread and the nation took fright.

We now have a calamity of greater magnitude – the potentially lethal conjunction of injecting users (of whatever substance) and HIV infection. It's this development and all the scuttling of old medical and enforcement policies it threatens to provoke that gets much of the attention in the new chapters.

There are, at present, 15 officially sanctioned syringe exchange schemes across the country and 50-plus similar projects established through local initiatives. In March 1988 a government commissioned report[1] called for more of them, and urgently. Whatever inducements were needed to reel drug 'misusers' into treatment agencies then they should be introduced, said the report. Otherwise we would quickly reproduce throughout the country the HIV infection rates of the Edinburgh injectors. (This was quite ironic considering the authorities, including the medical establishment, had spent decades forcing drug users out onto society's margins where it was agreed they properly belonged.)

In response to the March 1988 report the government hedged. They needed time to consider the issues. From the Scottish Home and Health Department came a chillier reaction. They were to cease funding the two surviving Scottish syringe swap projects.

So here we are at the crossroads. Are we to continue our hypocritical double-dealing in response to drugs and drug takers, or do we begin playing straight?

If the authorities really believe that drug use equals degeneration which equals an increased risk of AIDS, then it must look to the hundreds of millions of prescriptions made out each year. Our culture is awash with dangerous pharmaceuticals, transfixed by the notion of the instant remedy. It's no wonder this catastrophic ideal reaches street level.

And the authorities have to look to their lucrative stake in tobacco and alcohol – two products that kill almost 110,000 people *every year*. Will AIDS ever exact such a toll? Up until December 1987 there were a total of 1,227 cases.

As well as the HIV issue, this new edition also looks at women on the scene, both users and dealers; policing patterns, trafficking and consumption trends, medical, policy and drug company developments. It provides an update on each substance individually, plus a thoroughly revised chapter on the law and a new list of useful addresses.

My thanks to anyone who lent a hand and who I may have neglected to include in the list of acknowledgements.

London, April 1988

Note

1 'AIDS and Drug Misuse, Part 1,' Report by the Advisory Council on the Misuse of Drugs, Department of Health and Social Security, HMSO, London, 1988

INTRODUCTION TO FIRST EDITION

IN ALL parts of the world legally prohibited drugs are being consumed by increasingly large numbers of people who would otherwise consider themselves entirely average. This book aims to chart that phenomenon together with the great range of attitudes and postures that have risen to meet it. I explore the political and historical background to the substances – for it is from these sources rather than any pharmacological reality that drugs get their reputations. I also examine the style and mode of their use, their likely physical and mental impact, and offer self-aid tips, a guide to the law, to current policy, trafficking trends and include a list of support groups, agencies and clinics.

The whole area is an extraordinary one, studded with myth and falsehood. My ambition has been to circumnavigate it in language that is approachable without being facile, for there have been too many volumes that don't let the general reader through their thickets of technical jargon, and others that get just a little too sticky with tales of blood and vomit.

So what is meant by the term 'street drugs'? I admit it is not an especially satisfactory one since the substances are not only or even mostly trafficked and consumed on the streets: most are controlled under the Misuse of Drugs Act and so require discreet handling. But I stick with the term to differentiate between those substances handed out by doctors as medicines, and those taken recreationally for a good time. Having indicated the demarcation point, however, it has to be said that on both sides of the fence the distinction keeps breaking down. Recreational drugs quite often result not in fun but misery, while the physician's medicine can provoke bigger problems than those they were set against. Perhaps it is not well appreciated that the majority of the substances we now consider vanquishers of youth were in the first place dispensed by the medical profession. In fact, so often does a drug follow the route from wonder cure to deadly fix that the rational person has to strain to avoid the conclusion that there is an amount of purposefulness to it all – if only by way of determined myopia.

No more powerful example exists than the case of the opiates. Modern medicine has always sought the safe, non-addictive painkiller-cum-sedative. Nature's own offering is the opium poppy (*Papaver somniferum*) and though not perfectly measuring up to the prescription, it is a plant of great utility. It was used in its simplest form in this country for some three hundred years before a combination of entrepreneurial activity and the fussing of a burgeoning medical lobby produced the first of a series of 'superior' alternatives. The first was morphine. Ten times more potent than opium, morphine was promoted not only as a more efficient painkiller, but as a 'cure' for those persons who, in the course of treatment, had become addicted to opium. How a substance actually derived from opium and so much more powerful could be expected to produce anything but a more vicious habit is to be wondered at; but the dislogic didn't end there. When it was finally recognised that morphine itself was leading to addiction, the newly-synthesised heroin began to be prescribed as an alternative that could both manage pain and overcome morphine addiction. But heroin is also largely derived from opium and is stronger still than morphine. Now that heroin has been unfrocked, a new substance called methadone is being issued by the state as a cure for the addiction heroin has brought about. Methadone is itself addictive and results in a withdrawal syndrome considered tougher and more protracted than heroin's.

Patterns of 'progress' like this have been repeated in other branches of the tree of psychoactive (mind-altering) medicines. For instance, the class of tranquillisers known chemically as the benzodiazepines (brand names Librium, Valium, etc.) are presently being touted as comparatively safe substitutes for their discredited predecessors, the barbiturates. And yet one authority[1] estimates that some quarter of a million people in the UK are dependent on them – a dependence every bit as gripping as heroin's.

We can see that such dispensing trends demolish the idea that the medical profession is imbued with any special wisdom in the matter of psychoactive drugs. And this is as true of the present as for the past. The trends also underline the point that whatever alternative supply sources may have latterly sprung up, the original fount of most street drugs, heroin included, is the medical profession.

But this book adds up to more than a club with which to beat Big Brother medical profession and Big Sister government. Ordinary people, without any help, are quite capable of injuring themselves with drugs, either because they don't know enough about them or – if I may be pardoned a philosophical aside – they don't know enough about themselves. If power derives from knowledge, then weakness and debilitation derive from ignorance. People who know about and respect the potency of the drugs they use are capable of enjoying them for many years – as long as the law doesn't intervene. Those who treat their bodies like a pharmaceutical spittoon (or allow the drugs traders to) will harm themselves as well as all those around them. Getting the game right involves, in the current jargon, good personal management. And this, I suggest, means absorbing five basic lessons:

1. It is possible to become dependent on any mind-altering drug.
2. The impact of a drug is not fixed. It depends on dose, expectations, the mental and physical condition of the user and the setting in which it is taken.
3. Highly processed and concentrated substances (pills, powders, etc.) require more cautious use than their plant equivalents.
4. Hazards are greatly increased when the body's sealed circulatory network is invaded by the hypodermic syringe.

5. Heavy, prolonged use is like heavy, prolonged borrowing from the bank. The benefits don't come free. They are on loan from finite stocks. This is illustrated by the sensations experienced during withdrawal – invariably exactly the opposite to those which were sought from the drug itself. Thus, tranquilliser withdrawal leads to agitation, amphetamine withdrawal brings on exhaustion, and barbiturates (anti-convulsants and sleepers) lead to seizures and restless, often nightmarish sleep.

The above lend a curious equality to the mind alterers, for though it might be impossible to utter irrevocable statements of fact about any of them, the big, important rules apply across the board. Looking at the way drugs have been perceived throughout history these straightforward formulae seem not to have been understood. In the pages that follow we will see how the status of a given substance has soared and plunged in line with the panics that were gripping society at the given moment. In the sixties, for instance, cannabis was seen as the comforter of an indolent, 'amotivational' breed of long-hairs. Yet three decades earlier in the United States it was linked with disaffected immigrant Mexicans who, it was believed, were made not indolent but violently mad by the drug. The reputation of cocaine has suffered even more extreme lurches. Though such movements have depended on society's topical panics, on a more fundamental level they have related to the climate created by powerful business and political interests. The opium wars prosecuted by Britain on the Chinese during the last century are an especially instructive case. So are the monumental manoeuvres down in South America with regard to the modern-day cocaine traffic.

If the generality of drugs tends towards a rough equivalence that has been unrecognised in history, then their specifics are also considerably different from what has been widely assumed. Right now we are seeing a stampede by 'concerned persons' in the direction of heroin. Yet the impact of the ever-popular amphetamine (speed) is being virtually overlooked: the problems incurred by speed's excessive use easily match those of heroin. Barbiturates are also underestimated.

A straw poll of experienced drug agency workers would probably produce the consensus that barbs are the most intrinsically hazardous of all substances – easy to overdose on, painful to withdraw from, and liable, when injected without care, to result in appalling physical damage such as gangrene.

Then there is alcohol. Along with tobacco and caffeine this is one of society's un-drug drugs. We not only refuse to get outraged by alcohol, we scarcely notice the thousands killed and maimed on the roads due to its effects, or the hundreds of thousands who suffer more surreptitious mental and physical harm. And yet there is nothing inherently dangerous about a bottle of whisky. Drunk in manageable portions it can charge the spirit and leaven the atmosphere – which can be said to be the case for virtually every other drug examined in this book.

It would be idiotic to dismiss the media coverage of the past two or three years for heroin as being without foundation. Heroin does carry with it hazards, and its use is increasing markedly among an age range from the early teens to the mid-forties. But it should also be appreciated that a large part of the problem with heroin lies in society's jittery reaction to it, and that such a reaction generates distortions and false-hoods about the drug's true nature which exacerbate existing dangers. A lot of first-time users hate the stuff and never return. For those who do persist, it generally takes several weeks of fairly diligent use before a habit develops. Many users adopt avoidance tactics – spreading out their hits over a period (although many kid themselves addiction isn't happening to them when it is). Nor is heroin *per se* a killer drug. Addicts can go on using for decades, even via a needle, and remain comparatively healthy, as long as they can acquire an unadulterated solution, administer it hygenically at a cost they can afford, and avoid contact with the law. Given the drug's present status these conditions are virtually impossible to meet.

The truth about the pattern of drug taking we are now witnessing is that heroin is simply one politically dangerous drug we take with us into an uncertain technochip future. The fact that its use has increased indicates that more people want to get painlessly numb (for that is its principal pharmacological effect) in a UK that for many feels run down, divided, fearful and out of work. There are other important factors to our drug 'epidemic', not least among them being availability. A whole range of exotic drugs, quite simply, can now be purchased at an appropriate price everywhere, whether through the surgery or from a friend. And while the total volume might not have increased (for example, the UK's overall consumption of alcohol is about 80 per cent down on 1900[2]) the variety has. The public, unable to be sated any more with the traditional offerings of booze, fags, tea and coffee, is demanding a variety of materials. The great pity is that society lacks the maturity to handle these new drugs (which is why I reject the 'libertarian' idea of freely prescribed heroin as simpleton). It also lacks the basic user-friendly information. The old cultural networks of a couple of decades ago have broken up. In the present climate we find drug information books being prosecuted under the Obscene Publications Act. Teachers and other professionals who dare to suggest cannabis is no more harmful than alcohol are being stripped of their jobs. Those who *know* drugs and might have something constructive to impart are forced on to the sidelines of the debate, as though they were extremists, which allows the air to get filled with the righteously ill-informed tut-tutting of those who know best; or else the language used to convey solid information is mordant and of no interest to those it is aimed at. This means young people (though not just the young) are coming to drugs knowing scarcely anything of them save what they have construed from the tabloid media. They will probably feel sordid, perhaps 'rebellious', and might well get a bad habit before they can set themselves right. For such people we must dispense with the fakery and the mystification and *inform* ourselves. Those who blame heroin for our damaged, rejected youth, for rising crime and poverty in already debased communities, are playing games of political evasion.

We must also create and properly fund a range of interconnecting services that don't over-concentrate on that dramatic ten-day Cold Turkey period. The struggle to regain self-respect and self-sufficiency goes on long afterwards and needs attending to. The disproportionate power in the hands of psychiatrists to decide and manage 'treatment' strategy should also be dissolved – a far bigger share going to the voluntary street agencies, to the mutual help groups and to the community services providing accommodation, education, job training and health care. It is with the help of these bodies that the problem user can discover that there is life without obsessive drug taking. And it is from them that s/he can receive the long-term bolstering that benefits us all. At the bottom line, though, there is just one person and his/her drugs. And that's where the determination lies.

London, April 1985

Notes

1 Malcolm Lader, 'The Rise of the Benzodiazepines', *MIMS Magazine*, 15.9.1983
2 *Beer Facts, 1983*, The Brewers' Society, Brewer Publications Ltd, London

1 INTO THE NINETIES: THE DRUG SCENE NOW

Mundane Horrors

THE UK drugs scene has become simultaneously more mundane and shocking since I completed the first edition of *Street Drugs* in January 1985. 'Substance abuse' is now assumed to be everywhere and where it is not then that is a cause for headlines; for instance, the double decker in the *Southern Evening Echo* dated 7 March 1986, which declared incredulously, 'Drugs Misuse Not A Major Problem', a reference to the findings of a nine-month study of the Southampton area by a local health and social services team.

The government, in its War On Drugs, seems to be dimly aware that it must adjust its gun-sights to account for the complex nature of the phenomenon. This is not a battle, some of its members have realised, that is conducive to non-stop rocket attacks on the enemy. It is not always easy to tell who or where the enemy is and, in any case, history demonstrates that showy war games might catch the eye but unless coupled with social/political remedies, they simply hype up the illicit market and engender increasingly ruthless responses from traffickers. But if elements within the government were beginning to understand, the will to act accordingly was still lacking.

Women on the Scene

That the scene has become an unshakeable fixture of British urban cultural life – as post-modern as City greed and

Saturday night yob-ism – struck home in October 1986. It was then that I was researching an article for *Time Out* magazine, and spent some time talking with a number of women heroin dealers and heard them discuss the routine horrors and drudgery of their lives. The events they described were often extraordinary and yet a 'logical' enough feature of the evolving culture in the more degenerate parts of major cities.

There was Laura, now retired, but at the time turning over several ounces a day. Being a dealer, she explained, was to be in a position of power, an unusual and dangerous niche for a woman to occupy, since there was no authority to turn to if things cut up rough. She was also a woman alone with a young child in a North London flat where she was visited by a constant traffic of strange, compulsive clients. One of them, perhaps resentful of her hold over his appetite, tipped off the gang that first called by in the summer of 1985.

One of her customers opened the door, she says, and they just came bursting in, claiming at first they were the police. 'All I could see were the gates of Holloway prison.' They took half an ounce of heroin, half an ounce of cocaine, £1,000 cash and emptied the pockets of her clients.

They were to come back many times. And in addition to their knives – transported in a blue zipper bag – they produced a shotgun, screwdrivers and bottles of acid. 'It got particularly appalling for my daughter,' says Laura, 'who became so well trained that as soon as she heard the knock on the door she'd dive under the bed and stay there till they'd gone.'

Like many women dealers with children – and there are plenty of them – Laura, middle-class, in her late twenties, says she was drawn to the trade because it promised both a regular personal fix and economic self-sufficiency. Her dealing began after an encounter with a long time woman friend who, with two young children to support, one handicapped, was trading from a house in Holloway. For a while they worked together, then Laura went solo, scoring initially from a gang of Turkish Cypriots who were organised by a wealthy man in his seventies. When the Cypriot connection failed she would resort to a rougher crowd in Dalston, north-east London, solid working-class British lads in their thirties and early forties. They charged her extra, made her wait and caused £10 notes to disappear up their sleeves. 'As a woman,' she told me, 'you really do have a hard time being taken seriously.' In many ways, she added, her status and function within the male-dominated drugs scene mirrored the way things were in the wider world.

Her own customers cut across the social spectrum, embracing a number of successful professional and arty types. Sometimes 20 of them would be thrown together in her front parlour waiting for their 'score'.

She said that the most bracing part was crossing London to take receipt from her supplier, sometimes concealing the contraband in her boots or knickers. The most depressing were the visits by the gang with the bag of knives who, it became clear, were making a specialty of menacing solitary London women.

Another of the victims, Chrissie, recalls how she was sitting in her kitchen one morning with three male acquaintances when the intercom sounded and two men came heaving up the stairs. She attempted to hide £350 in cash and seven grammes of heroin under a chair seat but the visitors, armed with a gun and screwdriver, managed to extract both from her. One of her male friends was kicked, another had the screwdriver stuck into his neck, while Chrissie was threatened with the gun at her head and was flung across the room. Throughout the episode her child remained in another room watching video cartoons.

The position of women like Laura and Chrissie (one of Chrissie's five brothers is a junkie on the rent scene; one of her four sisters is an addict and prostitute in Finsbury Park) rings bells with the advice and counselling agencies that are only now beginning to address themselves to the special predicament and function of women on the scene. Leah Davidson, practice co-ordinator with City Roads, a specialist in 'crisis intervention', has found 'women are far more reluctant to come forward and seek help. My experience,' she told me, 'is that they hold it together longer, keeping their homes running, looking after the kids and often supporting their men's habits. Because they don't get help until much further into their using careers, when they do come to us they're often a lot more screwed up.' This theme is repeated by other agencies, as was the persistent motif of female guilt. For a woman, simply being a junkie is bad marks. If she's also a prostitute, perhaps a prostitute with a child, then the shame and guilt are overpowering.

Baby-napping?

And so is the fear of having the child removed – prostitute or not – by the authorities. That fear becomes all the more real following an important ruling in December 1986 by the Law Lords, who had been asked by a welfare officer acting on behalf of an addict mother to overturn a care order placed by Berkshire County Council on her child. The infant had been born prematurely – weight 5 lbs – and then spent six weeks in intensive care before being fostered out. The Lords, in finding against the mother, decided that the council had been entitled to take into account the woman's treatment of the child while still in the womb; and that though heroin use, in itself, didn't amount to maltreatment, her use of the drug throughout the pregnancy was evidence of a continuum of neglect that would persist if the mother were to get custody. The mother called it 'legalised kidnapping', while various legal experts spoke portentously of the ruling's effect. If addict mothers could be held legally responsible for their unborn then it followed that any woman suspected of harming her baby through, for instance, drinking, smoking or skiing on dangerous slopes, could face not merely confiscation of the infant but a criminal prosecution by or on behalf of the child at a later date.

A precedent already exists in the US whereby a mother of a brain-damaged child, who died after birth, was charged with contributing to that death because she had taken amphetamines while pregnant.

Alarmed that the Lords ruling would inspire social services departments across the country to round up the offspring of user mothers, a group of social workers under the auspices of the Standing Conference on Drug Abuse, hammered out guidelines for their colleagues in the field. Drug use, they stressed, did not necessarily equate with child abuse or neglect, and by automatically registering it as such, parents would be deterred from approaching all professional help and thus any risks would be compounded. Subsequently, specialist working groups in different health regions also began drawing up guidelines for assessment and working with user parents.

Each family, they agreed, had to be assessed individually and certain basic information acquired relating to the pattern of use, the home environment, health risks and the family's social support system. Trust had to be generated if the interests of the family as well as society were to be served.

An example of the kind of overreaction that can occur is the case of the south London couple, both private patients of the president of the Association of Independent Doctors In Addiction, Ann Dally. Though acknowledged even by their social services department as 'very caring and loving parents' who had caused no harm to their 14-month-old-child, police were called in early in 1986, probably as a panic response to the Reading case, to affect a separation. Neither parent regarded themselves as chaotic 'junkies'. They were addicts, dependent on stable doses of methadone prescribed weekly by Dally. Neither had ever used heroin.

They were particularly bitter about the way police carried out the separation just as the family returned home from an afternoon in the park. Three patrol cars, two vans, three alsatians and more than 20 officers were involved in the operation, during which, the couple claimed, the child was wrenched from the mother's grasp and she clubbed over the head.

Junkie Babies

Dally underscores their argument that addicts, particularly when stabilised on their drug, are capable of making good parents. She also insists that the spectre of junkie babies is exaggerated. 'While such children can be very ill, I've never heard of one dying with or without medical supervision. Most overcome their troubles within a few weeks and grow up to be perfectly normal. It is the competence of parents that should be the criterion for deciding whether or not to take a child away, not the simple fact of drug abuse.'

The Dally Affair

But Dally had by now become immersed in a controversy even more central to the UK 'treatment' strategy: the question of how much and how often to prescribe to registered addicts. As president and co-founder of AIDA, she was an uninhibited advocate of what used to be known as the British System. This is where a doctor purges those s/he can of their 'vicious indulgence' while the rest s/he keeps stable on minimum daily doses for as long as is deemed necessary. The new British system, with which Dally has butted heads, is the Short Sharp Cure. This works on the assumption that if you abruptly deprive someone of what they most crave they will cease to crave it. It is usually operated through the special hospital drug clinics where, employing the heroin substitute methadone, it generally takes 6 to 12 weeks to reduce an addict from a daily dose of, say, one gramme, to absolute zero.

Proponents of this reduction method are often genuinely appalled by the idea of playing lifelong dope pusher to addicts and fearful of turning novice users into addicts. But Dally and co believe theirs is the humane, pragmatic response – increasingly so given the incidence of HIV infection among drug injectors. To abandon such people to the street when they could be kept stable and clean, is insane.

The irony of Dally's position is that it should arouse the emnity not of the Home Office, historically the scourge of liberal practitioners, but of her own General Medical Council that over the years has defended the physicians 'freedom to prescribe'. In January 1987, the GMC found Dally guilty of 'serious professional misconduct' in respect of her treatment of one patient. She is said to have failed to give an adequate initial physical examination, failed to monitor properly his progress or to arrange for ongoing medical care after discharging him. Though the Home Office participated in the prosecution, one of its inspectors told the hearing that he believed Dally was 'genuinely motivated' and had acted according to her belief about what was right for her patients. The guilty verdict meant a 14-month ban from possessing or prescribing controlled drugs, a decision upheld by the Privy Council.

Many in the field saw the GMC's action as vindictive and inept. Dally – despite misgivings about the way she'd financially profited through her prescribing – represented the most serious, articulate challenge to the clinic system with its rigid reduction regime. But instead of confronting her through debate, through comparison of results, her opponents sought to dispose of her as an irresponsible quack. In many ways the situation paralleled the gynaecological war games fought between establishment figures based at the London Hospital and the rogue consultant Wendy Savage, strongly backed by the majority of her patients, as well as grass roots health workers.

Just like Savage, Dally refused to button up. At the time of writing she was planning an appeal before the European Court of Human Rights and meanwhile she continued arguing that the attacks upon her, inspired by a coterie of powerful London consultant psychiatrists, were proof of the bankruptcy of the policies they had evolved.

Clinics in Crisis

Evidence of the failure of the clinic system has not been in short supply since I wrote the first draft. A number of surveys have revealed that a majority of users are unable to hack a regime that often involves several weeks delay for an appointment, demands a daily pick-up of drugs, compulsory psychotherapy and makes it almost impossible for patients to work or go on holiday. A study of a particularly stark case was published in the *British Medical Journal* (BMJ) in April

1986.[1] Based on the assessment of 183 Edinburgh drug users, it found that more than half were referred onto a clinic for help, and of these, only 60 started treatment. Out of the 60, 37 abandoned the two week detoxification programme after a few days and only four of the remaining 60 stayed heroin free after their treatment. The authors – who included the clinic's consultant psychiatrist – thought the results 'cast doubt' on the value of the clinic service offered at all 106 locations throughout the UK. They also referred to the 'lack of obvious success' of their own particular scheme 'reflected in the decline in the number of referrals since 1984 as practitioners and patients became progressively disillusioned with what was being offered.' The team's prescription was to shift to 'community services' which would be better organised and serviced by professionals and specialists.

Role of the GP

Even Dr Philip Connell, lynchpin of the London psychiatric mafia, chairman of the Home Office Advisory Council on the Misuse of Drugs, was forced to admit during a TV drugs debate, that 'there should be an in-depth review' of the treatment advice issued in 1984 by the DHSS (at his own committee's prompting). Those guidelines, he acknowledged, had been drawn up 'in a rush' to deal with over-prescribing by certain London GPs. The screws had been turned too tight, he seemed to be saying, on any physician attempting to deal with addiction outside the clinic set-up.

The addicts themselves had been making it plain enough that their own preference was to be administered to by ordinary GPs.

A national survey in mid 1985[2] revealed that one in five GPs in England and Wales attended an opiate user during the four week period of the study – a third of these patients being new to the practitioners.

Extrapolating nationally, the authors estimated that between 30,000 and 40,000 new drugs cases 'presented' to GPs in a year, confirming the importance of the ordinary practitioner in the national 'treatment' strategy. And yet the implicit message to those same GPs ever since the Brain Committee established the clinics in 1968 had been they were far too inexpert and corruptible to be trusted with addicts. This was a conclusion based on the behaviour of a handful of irresponsible London doctors. Confidence, not unexpectedly, waned. And, without training or other encouragement, the attitude of the practitioners themselves hardened towards addicts. They came to be seen as unmanageable, undeserving even of primary health care, something to be automatically referred on to the experts at the clinics. Now, however, not withstanding the spiteful attack on a prescient Ann Dally, GPs are suddenly being avidly courted.

Unveiling a new video training package at the end of 1987, junior health minister Ray Whitney said he thought the general practitioner belonged 'in the forefront' in the battle against drugs[3]; while Dr John Strang, principal advisor to the DHSS on drugs, and one of the video's stars, told *Doctor* magazine, 'The old image of drug abusers being difficult and troublesome patients is simply not true as many come from respectable middle-class backgrounds and hold down good jobs. Like it or not GPs need a better understanding of drug problems.'

Damage Limitation

How confusing then that so soon after this placatory message went out, the government should begin a new round in its anti-heroin advertising campaign, delivering up the old images of users as prostitutes, vomiting down toilets, stealing mum's housekeeping, brother John's ghetto blaster.

Clearly the authorities' treatment and prevention strategy was in a spin. And why? Because clean solutions were being sought to a problem that isn't amenable to such a fix. Our drugs malaise is the product of a culture awash with damaging though 'licit' drugs; a culture transfixed by the idea that there is a pill for every ill and that remedies have to be instant. The messenger of this false, catastrophic ideal is the medical-pharmaceutical lobby, abetted by ignorant governments hooked on tax revenues.

There can be no clearing of the ground to try out one pristine policy option against another because the ground is irredeemably polluted.

Grass roots workers as well as some politicians have instead moved towards the more mundane goal of damage limitation. For politicians this means quietening the most vociferous sectional interests – thus a host of street agencies and other ad hoc schemes are pump primed with just enough central government money to keep them alive but tethered; and Customs and Excise are given hundreds of new investigators. The general public, meanwhile, are dosed with a multi-million pound advertising campaign that breaks most of the ground rules on how to damp down rather than stoke up a drugs epidemic.

Penal Moves

Other exemplary acts include legislative changes that mean life sentences for major drug dealers and the confiscation of all assets assumed by the courts to have been acquired through drug sales. None of those innovations appears to have succeeded in achieving their publicly stated objective: the number of addicts continues to increase, record (although exaggerated) amounts of cocaine are making their way into the country, while the new asset confiscation measures (under the Drugs Trafficking Offences Act) have been criticised by the editors of the *Criminal Law Review* for reversing what were assumed to be three irrevocable principles of English criminal justice, including the presumption of innocence until proven guilty. Having made these legislative breaches in the war zone of drugs control, in which any draconian measure appears to be legitimate, the signs were that the tendency could spread. The Criminal Justice Bill before the House of Commons in 1988 provided for similar measures to be used against burglars and DHSS fraudsters.

Hitting Mr Small

The concern of experienced drug workers was not only with matters of judicial propriety, but the way the Drug Trafficking Offences Act was working in practice. Designed to punish the Big Hombres, such individuals invariably remained too slippery, too expert at international money laundering, according to Jane Goodsir of the legal advice agency Release, to answer for their acts. Instead, it was the five gramme user-dealers who were feeling the bite; in fact any regular user who was guilty of not declaring income (for example, from a market stall or prostitution) for tax purposes. Without receipts any such income could be assumed by the courts to have originated from drug sales. 'They could then be stripped,' said Goodsir, 'of most of their worldly goods.'

'It was these five gramme dealers,' she said, 'who were forming the bulk of the DTO convictions even though the authorities were pleased to depict them as major international gangsters.'

AIDS

But now to AIDS – the supernatural X factor that is the source of so much revisionist thinking among the policy makers. It was the high rate of HIV infection among drug injectors that inspired Philip Connell to consider 'flexible' options, and it is the reason why the Thatcher government, morally rigorous in its rhetoric but ultimately deeply pragmatic, should adopt some of the most innovative anti-AIDS measures to be found anywhere in the world. For so long as AIDS was assumed to be a gay plague or the haemophiliacs' curse, official action was torpid and restrained. But now that we have with us the infected injecting drug user, a clearer pathway is seen through to the heterosexual moral majority. Suddenly the posters and media ads are composed in plain-speak: 'It takes only one prick to give you AIDS'. But more than that, there are the needle exchange schemes, operated in 15 officially-sanctioned locations throughout the country and a further 50-plus as a result of local initiatives. The logic behind them is simple enough. The habit of sharing needles was leading to the rapid transmission of the AIDS virus. Sharing might be in part a product of comradely instincts and/or novice users receiving hands-on instruction from older users, but mostly it was because needles are in restricted supply. Increase the availability and you decrease the infection rate.

Reeling in the Addict

The argument against the swap schemes is that they, in effect, legitimise not just the consumption of controlled substances but their ingestion via the most dangerous route: via a syringe. How could the government justify, on the one hand, imprisoning people for using prohibited drugs while simultaneously supplying them with the works for that administration. The answer is: it cannot. Nor can the clinic system, directed in the main towards rapid detoxification and abstinence, be squared with the swap arrangements. The exigencies of AIDS control had exposed contradictions in the British System that had been present for 60 years, ever since a 'liberal' Lord Humphrey Rolleston, president of the Royal College of Physicians, had delivered his findings to the government.

Clean Works

It had long since become the habit to marginalise the junkie figure – to have him/her conveniently vanish at society's periphery. If the early '80s heroin boom made that more difficult (a lot of the new users looked uncomfortably like 'ordinary' people, the product of 'ordinary' parents) then the AIDS boom made it imperative to draw them back from the margins and inculcate in them good social habits. The health of the whole nation was at stake. No more cant and simplistic moralising. Now the message came in several equivocating parts. Don't use, but if you have to use, don't inject. But if you must inject, don't share your works. But if you do share your works, clean them properly.[4] There was even fresh advice from the DHSS on how to do this: not with bleach as previously dictated but as follows:

1. As soon as possible after use, an ordinary strength solution of washing up liquid in cold water (not hot because, like bleach this causes clotting of any residual bloody matter) should be prepared in a bowl. Draw this into the syringe, eject down the sink; (not back in the bowl), and repeat.
2. Now dismantle the works and immerse in boiling water for five minutes. Thirty minutes boiling is needed to kill off the more hardy hepatitis B virus.

Given that the chances of a strung-out user going through this palaver are not especially strong, the DHSS even set out the routine in 'an ascending order of efficacy', i.e. from minimum to maximum usefulness.

1. Flush repeatedly with cold water.
2. As above but with a mixture of washing up liquid and cold water.
3. Boil the dismantled works for five minutes.

There was also the option of the exchange schemes, an idea picked up in Amsterdam, where works are actually despatched to the user by bus as are supplies of methadone.

Needle Exchanges Evaluated

The UK schemes, after their first year, were showing broadly promising results but with far less success north of the border where restrictive Scottish Office guidelines and resistance from local health boards were causing ructions. Dundee (described by the Home Office Inspectorate[5] as having a 'considerable' drugs problem and where injecting is 'the norm' for both heroin and amphetamine users) was suffering the most. The city's first scheme, at the Royal Infirmary, closed in just two weeks due to lack of resources, which caused 'unacceptable levels of stress among the staff'. A second scheme, run by a GP for his drug dependent patients, also ended abruptly when other users showed up demanding needles. A third, at a drop-in day centre, also wound up after a month's business due to what the consultant psychiatrist in charge called 'repeated threatening and intimidating behaviour by addicts towards staff, one of whom was deliberately sprayed, by a known HIV positive individual, with blood from a syringe.'[6]

The tensions, he acknowledged, arose largely from serious staff shortages (is it really beyond the wit of the authorities to resource properly what must be one of the most demanding of all jobs?) together with unyielding ground rules. These declared that users couldn't get new needles without a dose of advice and counselling and that only three sets of equipment could be exchanged at any one time – and only on a one-for-one basis. Although these demands are superficially reasonable, the reality is that users are reluctant to be force-fed 'counselling' and that many are hitting up more than three times a day. Given the considerable distances some of them travelled – it being the only surviving scheme in town – they came to demand something more pragmatic.

Liverpool Rules

Liverpool told another story. Instead of trying to impose on their needle swap 'clients' the correct social attitudes and habits, the team that ran the Maryland Street scheme aimed first of all to make available 'a practical, non-judgmental resource'. Clients, on arrival, dropped their used equipment into a sharpsafe container in a room set aside especially and then made their selection from a range of barrels and needles. A maximum five barrels were usually handed out but this could be increased if the user was from far afield or was collecting for friends. Unlike the Dundee experience, there had been no tensions with staff and many of the users – some of whom were coming forward to an agency for the first time in their drug careers – ended up requesting advice on health and safer injecting techniques. By spring 1988 the HIV infection rate among those tested on this and other Liverpool projects was precisely zero.

'Drug users have used the scheme responsibly,' according to Maryland's co-ordinator, Allan Parry,[7] 'regarding it as a welcome change from the punitive, prejudiced attitude they normally associate with society's reaction to their drug use. The AIDS issue has caused great alarm in the injecting community, so many customers appreciate the scheme for what it is – a system that allows injecting drug users to minimise the harm of drug use to themselves and their friends, without harming others.'

The State As Pusher

All of which brings us back to the ultimate drug-related conundrum: is it wise or unwise for the state to act as supplier to addicts who say they cannot or won't quit, given that the risks of following either course are great? Joining Dr Ann Dally in the 'flexibility' camp is the consultant psychiatrist formerly in charge of Merseyside drug clinics, John Marks. 'We do not say to a chronic arthritic,' he notes, 'you will be cured in six months and even if you aren't your supply of analgesics will then be withdrawn. Yet we say precisely this to drug addicts. For a majority of drug users the choice now is not between using drugs or getting off them, but between clean drugs from a clinic or dirty drugs from the gangsters.'[8] Both Marks and Dally, it should be pointed out, are not *for* prescribing of methadone under any circumstance. They say they recognise that many users prefer and do better under a straight 'detox' or even quitting cold. Both favour longer term prescribing only where a habit appears deep-set and prescription seems the most pragmatic option.

Representing the anti-prescribing position is Crawley consultant psychiatrist, Raj Rathod, who believes that supplying methadone to addicts is to succumb to their blackmail. He believes users should be compelled to face the consequences of their addiction for therein lies the cure. 'Repeatedly shielding people from their responsibilities may be counterproductive as it promotes learnt helplessness.'[9]

Falling somewhere between the two is Edinburgh GP, Roy Robertson, whose early '80s survey of local injectors showed Edinburgh to be one of Europe's AIDS blackspots. While favouring exchange schemes for the sake of damage limitation, Robertson is firmly opposed to widespread methadone prescribing since he believes such a policy could easily run out of control. The extra resources required would inevitably be concentrated on medical establishments where the prescribing would take place, leading to a fatal neglect of the non-prescribing community agencies that have been 'maturing' since the early '80s.

John Marks of Merseyside would argue that in his former region the clinics are already run by multi-disciplinary 'community' teams, including nurses and social workers. 'The doctor is there only because he is legally required to sign the prescription. His function is to operate as an "intelligent layman".'

But there is a more obvious problem with Robertson's advocacy of needle swaps but not prescribing: What is the 'client' expected to do with his new needle other than fill it with criminally acquired substances that will be unsterile and contaminated? If that user is HIV positive his/her immune system will consequently be stressed, perhaps fatally.

The Big Think

Connell and his Advisory Council team sifted all these matters and in January 1988 informed the government that 'HIV is a greater danger to individual and public health than drug misuse. Accordingly, we believe that services which aim to minimise HIV risk behaviour by all available means should take precedence in development plans.' To this end they urged (in a report called 'AIDS And Drug Misuse Part 1'[10]) an extension to the syringe swap schemes, also the sale of syringes over the counter at high street chemists.

There had to be a loosening up on substitute prescribing, they urged, particularly by Scottish consultant psychiatrists who looked to be stand-offish and disinterested in their approach towards addicts. The clinics, in general, had to make themselves more friendly and cut down on waiting times. *All* GPs needed to be drafted in to provide care and advice for misusers. And there had to be a network of 'community-based' services in each health district which would provide advice and help, not just on drugs and HIV, but on housing, jobs, legal questions and primary health care.

The relevant specialists should make themselves available. For all services the priority was to attract and keep 'misusers', many of whom had never made contact with any agency and were deeply mistrustful. To achieve this, the customer – namely the misuser – had to be provided, in effect, with what s/he wanted. The location of each service needed to be nearby the user population and, if necessary, adopt a mobile role. Opening hours were to be tailored to the users' needs, including, perhaps, evening opening, since addicts were often late risers. The community-based schemes, in particular, had to be 'practical, non-judgemental and informal.' Free condoms and syringes should be provided, or the user directed to them. Nor was commitment to abstinence necessary. There was to be a whole 'hierarchy of goals' to which users might aspire, during which prescribing could take place. These started with the cessation of equipment sharing, onto quitting of the syringe altogether, then a decrease in the amount consumed, and, finally, abstinence.

For Crawley's Rathod and the Scottish psychiatrists, the message was plain. 'The value of substitute prescribing, undertaken with care, *must* (author's italics) be recognised.' Even the long-term prescribing of injectibles was sanctioned – although only in the 'most exceptional cases'.

There was an equivalent message to social service chiefs: 'If drug misusing parents were not to be deterred from seeking help, social service departments should work hard to ensure that drug misuse, per se, is never a reason or seen as such for separating parent and child. And to the prison department went the recommendation of free condoms for inmates – supplied in confidence.

In many respects the document is a humane, progressive piece of work. But there is also something almost comic about its feverish calls for 'flexibility' in order that the misuser might be reeled in. Whatever s/he wants – drugs, needles, jobs, a new flat – s/he should get. In the age of AIDS, the customer addict is king. S/he has something the rest of us don't want.

This comic turnabout also reveals the underlying contradictory drift of the British drug treatment policy. If abstinence, as the authors report, 'is now more important than ever . . . to contain the spread of AIDS,' why do they call for more prescribing – to the point where practitioners of the dry method (Rathod *et al.*) are to be conscripted into supplying drugs to their patients? A Cheshire GP, Jackie Chang, writing in the September 1987 edition of the specialist journal, *Druglink*, believed such an approach would 'subvert addiction treatment' since it sought to fuse the incompatible goals of abstinence and the curbing of HIV transmission. The goal of stabilising a user's intake and thus his/her behaviour might be squared with the spread of HIV infection, but abstinence is a separate endeavour. Her own suggestion was to provide 'a massive network of maintenance centres in which there would be no pretence at aiming for abstinence but which would be solely intended to prevent the spread of AIDS. Which drug is provided and how much will have to be left to the addict.' S/he could select heroin, even amphetamine, and rooms would be set aside for fixing – help in safe techniques being provided if required.

Such a policy, Chang believed, would not entirely solve the problem of illicit drugs, but because addicts would be getting what they wanted they would have no need to suck new users onto the scene as a way of paying for their fix. That should reduce the demand for illegal injectibles, and, as a result, minimise the potential for the spread of HIV and Hepatitis B.

The darkest side to Chang's scenario was, as she saw it, the necessity for 'a massive law enforcement effort . . . to effectively force addicts into the maintenance centres. Severe penalties would also be needed for anybody caught for offences such as importation or dealing and even possession of drugs for personal use.'

Is Chang's vision the product of demented thinking? Or has she seen the future?

As to the government, they 'welcomed' the Advisory Council's report but rejected two of the key recommendations: syringe swap schemes couldn't be urgently extended because they needed to be more fully evaluated. And condoms for prisoners was out since this would result in an increase in homosexual activity and, as a consequence, more risk of infection. Requests for additional funding also looked a no-go. Beyond that, they needed time to ponder.

The Scottish authorities went one better. On the very day the Council published its report, the Scottish Home and Health Department announced it was to cease funding the remaining two syringe swap schemes (in Glasgow and Edinburgh). Clearly they were trucking no interference from down south.

My own position hasn't changed since I completed the first edition of this book. It is that doctors, druggists and politicians are almost wholly responsible for the proliferation of drugs in our culture, heroin included, and that their efforts to retrieve the situation invariably make matters worse. I called then for the disproportionate power of the clinic psychiatrists to decide and manage treatment strategies to be dissolved – a far bigger share going to the community agencies and self-help groups. A central role for 'community-based' services *is* advocated by the Advisory Council's new report but its authors – four of whom are consultant psychiatrists – still can't dispose of their morbid deference for hospital-based shrinks – even though experience instructs them that these professionals have a good deal more to learn than teach about drug 'misusers' and their motivations.

In addition to the community projects suggested by the Council, another possible model for the future is the project a group of Ann Dally's former patients were attempting to formulate, called Drug Dependency Improvement Group. The plan was to establish their own clinic where minimum

stable doses would be administered by a doctor they themselves would hire. Similarly, there were moves to launch an
addicts' union along the lines of that operating in Holland
which, among other functions, dispenses maintenance doses
to users by bus.

Addict Self Defence

Addicts are constantly reporting that the most powerful
resource avilable to them are other users – so long as they are
constructively motivated. The need for addict self-help and
education will become even more imperative as the spread of
AIDS causes them further pain and stigmatisation. The gay
community has defended itself comparatively well in this
regard due to its organisational strengths. But 'junkies' have
no equivalent line of defence. They will badly need it, I
suspect, to meet attacks from the commercial, legal and
medical sectors, who will attempt everything from baby
snatching to forced HIV testing and quarantining.

As I write, things are comparatively calm. But then HIV
infection among injectors is still in the semi-hypothetical
phase. Fully developed AIDS cases are rare. Once they
develop the challenge will be widely felt, not least by the
under-funded, under-trained 'lay' drug workers. 'The advent
of AIDS,' wrote Paula Hendry, a Swansea worker,[11] 'means
we can no longer separate our work and personal lives as
sharply as we would probably prefer for our own comfort . . .
Even if we mobilise needle exchange and other measures
now, many of our clients will already have been infected. We
will find it difficult to counsel and advise them with the
necessary optimism and hope for the future, if the possibility
of their death is a fearsome, lurking spectre which we, as
counsellors, refuse to confront.'

The experience at the Whishart needle swap scheme in
Dundee already suggests that lay workers can't count on the
most basic support from the authorities as they undertake
their dismal, dangerous work, which, in turn, suggests they
too need to come together in common purpose.

Usage

The shape of the illicit drugs market has shown remarkably little change over the past two or three years, despite what amounted to a massive free advertising campaign on behalf of crack by the media and a sudden disinterest in the 'glue peril'. Crack has still to make serious inroads while another much-hyped drug that failed to make it was Angel Dust (PCP) – a combination stimulant/depressant/hallucinogen which produces at a low level, feelings of euphoric unworldliness, but at higher doses erratic, bizarre and sometimes powerfully violent behaviour. It is big on the American scene. Other UK non-starters were the various designer products concocted by taking an established drug and making minor alterations to its molecular structure. The idea is to evade the control laws, but loopholes are quickly closed as soon as a new 'analogue' shows signs of taking off. The UK government most recently slammed the door on derivatives of the opiods fentanyl (or phentanyl) and pethidine.

One vaunted new product of American origin that does seem to be taking off is Ecstasy, a speedy-hallucinogen that was first used as a psychiatric tool for warring marriage partners. It began gaining real currency in late 1987/early 1988 among super trendies in London's West End clubs where it inspired weird communal dance rituals, jerky and frenetic. The mood it generated was overwhelmingly peaceful, generous and cooperative (according to a young friend, a savant of the nightclub scene). From the West End it spread to coarser regions in the South East suburbs where an old maxim is sure to be borne out: it's not so much the drug itself that determines the experience but who takes it and in what setting.

Inevitably, attention was switched to amphetamine, a well-entrenched domestic product that was both cheap and potent and the main reason why coke had failed to get a grip. There had been talk of an international speed trafficking mafia and while this was surely hyperbole, something odd was happening with both the purity (sometimes down to 5 per cent) and the price (as low as £4 a gramme) of sulphate. The distortions could have been caused not so much by a massive new uptake of the product (it has been popular in the UK and other north European countries for more than 20 years) as by price wars played out against coke dealers.

Beyond these generalisations, the most striking feature of the domestic scene was the strong, apparently random, regional variations. In Liverpool, the proportion of heroin users resorting to fixing was considered fairly minimal, whereas in Gloucestershire and Staffordshire the rate could be as high as 75 per cent. This is according to the Home Office Drugs Inspectorate,[12] which gains its impressions from voluntary agencies, police, doctors and users themselves. In West Yorkshire, there was very little hard use of anything, while in Cheshire the growing speed and heroin injecting scene had led to a needle swap scheme in Warrington. Essex was smoking or snorting country – with the exception of Dagenham and Southend where more than half used the needle. As for London, the bohemian AC/DC north showed a far higher injecting and HIV infection rate than the south. This though was the picture in spring 1988. The scene was anything but static.

Enforcement

Just as the link between unemployment and destructive drug use is established to the satisfaction of most observers outside the Thatcher government, so the link between heroin use and crime is statistically clearer. A team at Liverpool University[13] decided after studying the criminal career of 300 16 to 34 year olds from the Wirral that there was now 'conclusive evidence' that heroin can accelerate or lead to acquisitive crime in young adults – typically burglary and theft.

The importance of the enforcement effort that has arisen to meet this challenge can be judged by the strenuous political warfare that has been taking place between police and Customs and Excise, each side anxious to catch the eye of their political bosses with the best end of year figures. Customs, by virtue of the pattern of international trafficking (bulk shipments across borders) inevitably continue making the biggest catches. But they would argue this is also because of 600 years of specialised experience and because they are less prone to corruption. Police forces like London's Metropolitan, by contrast, are constantly facing charges of 'verballing' defendants (planting words in their mouths) and hyping the importance of insignificant cases. Battle has focussed on the National Drug Intelligence Unit, a joint squad of police and Customs officers, formed in the summer of 1985. The issue that divides them more than any other is the question of who decides if and how far an identified drugs courier is allowed to 'run'. Customs maintain that it has been their historic right to decide whether or not to arrest a suspect at entry or tag him in order to snatch others in the network. The police believe that this should be their right and in the autumn of 1987 lobbied at cabinet level not just for that authority but to oversee the whole enforcement effort. They were turned down. The official word, subsequently, is that the two services have reached a concordat and are beginning to work smoothly together. But suspicions remain.

Though they lost the battle over couriers the police were sweetened by a considerable increase in specialist drug officers – a doubling to nearly 1150 between 1983 and 1987. Elaborate surveillance came to be much more commonplace, with the deployment of watching and listening equipment in, for instance, empty council property. And it became almost habitual for officers to dress up as deliverymen, labourers or train guards, before springing traps.

The then Metropolitan police commissioner, Kenneth Newman, pinpointed the new mode in February 1987 when he said that rather than indulging in random arrests of common users it was better to 'get to know local faces, observe and arrest the maximum number of suspects in disciplined and organised operations.'

Among the earliest examples was Operation Condor, the raid launched in July 1986 on the Afro-Caribbean Club in Brixton employing 1840 officers – a number of them bursting from a train – and including members of the D11 firearms

unit. The enterprise ended with 86 arrests; 31 were charged
with supply, 15 with possession, 2 of whom were additionally
accused of carrying offensive weapons.

Lambeth Council leader, Linda Bellos, attacked the scale
of the raid but was on the streets in its aftermath as part of the
effort to placate the crowds. In the event the night passed off
comparatively peacefully – but other police sorties have
produced less equable reactions.

In Bristol, Operation Delivery on 24 July 1987, resulted in
hours of violence as locals fought with 600 riot police. The
raid itself procured 2½lb of cannabis worth £4,000; 20 people
faced drugs charges. The ensuing violence, by contrast, resulted in twice as many court appearances and dozens of
injuries. Inevitably, cries went up for cannabis either to be
policed consistently or decriminalised altogether. These calls
came from the police themselves as well as the right wing
Economist magazine.

The Guardian's Ian Aitken decided that 'the outright legalisation of marijuana would be the single most effective move
towards restoring the rule of law in our cities.'

Whatever minimal impact such raids might have on the
supply network, police forces like the Met clearly believed
they had important public relations value; a way of informing
the public that they were mounting a suitably epic response to
what Home Secretary Douglas Hurd called 'the single most
threatening form of crime facing the capital'. To amplify the
message, the press, more and more, came to be invited along
on the hunt – from briefing, right through to the raid itself.
And even if such operations should go drastically wrong, the
poor results could always be blamed on bad luck or the super
cunning of impossibly well-organised traffickers. An example
was Operation Butterfly, a raid by 100 officers on south
London council flats, whose occupants had turned the district
into a 'drugs supermarket'. After months of planning, just four
people were arrested with comparatively small quantities of
cocaine, cannabis and heroin. 'There was nothing amiss with
the planning,' wrote the loyal man from the *Daily Mail*.[14]

One method the police have of covering their blushes,
according to Jane Goodsir of *Release*, is to hype up the value

of each raid in court so that a common user becomes a supplier and a supplier becomes an international trafficker. As a result more severe penalties are handed out and the police's figures look better. For a force suffering poor clear-up rates, such upgrading becomes a near political necessity.

Substance Round-Up

Alcohol

At the time of writing a new Licensing Bill was about to become law under which the traditional afternoon pause in pub opening (from 3 p.m. to 5.30 p.m.) would be eliminated. This means Monday to Saturday opening from 11 a.m. straight through to 11 p.m., although on Sundays, Christmas Day and Good Friday the break survives and opening hours would be 12 noon to 2 p.m., then 7 p.m. to 10.30 p.m. Proposed backbench amendments might have forced even longer opening.

Is it a good thing? Certainly the old arrangements looked somewhat straitlaced against the regimes in Europe and the US. And given that their original function was to remove temptation from 'idle' factory workers, there are now too many sources of alcohol for that rationale to be sustained. (And too few factories.)

The argument in favour of the old restrictive system is that longer pub hours mean more boozing which in turn means more damage to the individual and his/her family circle – damage that ends up costing the rest of us in terms of health and social security bills. The government itself recognised the strength of this argument when, in its 1981 policy statement, 'Drinking Sensibly', it declared, 'available evidence suggests that licensing restrictions may have a broad influence on both the level of average consumption per head of alcohol and the influence of alcohol-related harm.' It has since U-turned by claiming that the experience in Scotland, where licensing hours have been relaxed since 1977, points to no significant overall increase in consumption. But a proper inspection of the figures reveals the opposite, according to a consortium of voluntary bodies known as Keep Alcohol Safeguards. Women's drinking, they say, has risen by 35 per cent, retired men's drinking by 56 per cent and employed men's by 9 per cent. Only a fall in consumption of 28 per cent by the unemployed forestalled a massive overall increase. As it is, the across-the-board jump was 13 per cent, which, it is claimed, has already translated into an increase of one third in the death rate from cirrhosis of the liver.

Undistracted by the new pub laws, Alcohol Concern has detailed a 12 year strategy aimed at halving the number of people drinking above the recommended levels of 21 units a week for men and 14 for women (for an explanation of a unit or 'standard measure' see page 54). It calls its programme the Drinking Revolution and believes it is already underway (south of the border) inasmuch as the number of individuals declaring themselves teetotal has risen, as has the sale of non-alcoholic drinks and mineral water: a reflection of the '80s health ethic.

The most intractable problem is that of teenage drinking, generally a bingeing activity which, apart from being associated with reckless driving, young homelessness and suicides, is increasingly identified as the trigger for late night mob violence, often directed at police. Even in the sleepy caucasian villages of the Home Counties, large scale bust-ups have occurred, often where a licensed club or disco spills out into an all night fast food joint. A chief inspector with the Thames Valley force told me that in the last eight months of 1987, a total of 1000 youths had been involved in pitched battles with police on dozens of different occasions. The scale of the phenomenon can also be judged by calculations from BBC TV's *Panorama* that the country's 15 to 18 year olds now spend around £277 million a year on alcohol, while a fifth of 13 year olds and half of 15 year olds drink in pubs.

'The government must tackle the blatant advertising campaigns aimed at the young,' said Alcohol Concern. 'During the 1987 Christmas period the breweries spent 10 times as much on promoting their brands (£50 million) as the government spends in the whole year warning people of the dangers of too much drinking.' AC also wants more funding for alcohol services since it claims 'as few as one in 20 problem drinkers receive the help they need.'

Amphetamine

After years of disinterest, the amphetamine scene has been rediscovered by government and media. There have been more raids, more possession and supply arrests as well as hints of a public don't-do-it advertising campaign. One informed suggestion is that the authorities – notably the police – have an agenda for getting amphetamines upgraded from Class B to a Class A substance under the Misuse of Drugs Act. Lots of court and media action would be of assistance. Meanwhile, the price and purity of street supplies have undergone some curious gyrations. Release report grammes on offer at £3 or £4, but at purity levels of perhaps 7 per cent. Such low prices, as well as reflecting a production malfunction, would also be aimed at preventing cocaine, a rival stimulant of foreign extraction, taking root. So far amphetamine's hegemony continues.

Barbiturates

The new factor is the appearance of this drug as an almost routine adulterant of heroin. Dealers feel they can pass it off because it has similar soporific effects. It is, however, far dirtier, problematic to inject and liable to precipitate, when taken in high doses, chaotic, violent behaviour. Over-dosing is especially easy when consumed with alcohol.

Cannabis

There is still no evidence to suggest that moderate use by adults produces any serious health risk although Release report more calls from people 'terribly worried' about their regular smoking.

While some of these callers are indeed leaning on the weed too heavily much of the panic, the agency believes, is prompted by the prevailing anti-drugs mood: the suggestion that all drug use, except for tobacco, caffeine and alcohol, is profoundly hazardous.

Meanwhile, the quest for the long-lived 'cannabis psychosis' continues. This is a condition, according to one UK researcher,[15] characterised by 'confusion, delusions, hallucinations and emotional lability (instability)'. His prescription? Lots more publicly funded research to add to the truck-loads already produced. For front line drug workers the willingness of psychiatrists to diagnose cases of CP is a worrying one since this could lead to individuals being sectioned – initially for 48 hours – under the Mental Health Act. Invariably, those put away are black youths, about whose culture and modes of expression the average middle class white psychiatrist knows next to nothing. Once 'binned' in the system, and contained by licit drugs, it can be difficult to break loose.

Cocaine

It is, of course, the putative crack invasion that has made the news since I wrote my chapter on derivatives of Erythroxylum coca. Aided by a massive free ad campaign in the editorial pages of the tabloid press, crack dealers have nonetheless been unable to find a receptive market. Easy availability of the far cheaper and longer-acting amphetamine was part of the reason. Then again, as Colin Hewitt, co-ordinator of the UK's National Drugs Intelligence Unit, remarked in March 1987,[16] 'it has been forgotten by the pessimists that the trail from the coca fields to the cocaine dealers here is a long and difficult one and the return journey for the profits is equally hazardous.' Hewitt posited that the drug has remained a minority indulgence among the affluent of the big cities, as had cocaine itself. But while the predicted deluge hadn't arrived, there were signs of hydrochloride (ordinary coke), if not crack, spreading beyond the elite into poorer white and black areas – the latter traditionally having eschewed all controlled drugs except herbal cannabis. Cocaine paste or pasta is also reportedly finding a market there. In fact the spectre of blacks and cocaine, which first surfaced 80 years ago in the US, is likely to become a chief panic factor in the next few years. Already there is some excitement about 'Yardies' – the suggestion being that here is an organisation equivalent to the disciplined transnational networks operated by the Chinese and Italians. The evidence points to a variety of ad hoc West Indian groups – ruthless but disconnected.

What also needs to be put in perspective is the reported 261 per cent increase in Customs seizures of cocaine in 1987 over the previous year. Not only did a single seizure account for 60 per cent of the haul, but it is not known how much of the total was simply passing through the UK to another market. The 60 per cent seizure itself was destined for Holland – even though Customs suggests a 'substantial part' could have been re-exported to Britain.

Pharmacologically speaking, crack is another form of free-base (see pages 150–1) only less complicated and dangerous to produce. Instead of a four or five step process employing volatile solvents, ordinary cocaine is mixed with water and baking soda or ammonia and then heated. The end product comes as small white rocks or nuggets. The processing, while removing sugar cuts, will not excise other common adulter-ants such as the synthetic local anaesthetics procaine and lidocaine. It will also probably preserve a residue of sodium bicarbonate which, when smoked, makes the crackling sound that gives the product its name. Being non-soluble in water, and therefore unsnortable, crack is smoked – generally from a pipe. This pipe might be something grand or composed from a flattened beer can.

Like everything else about crack, the danger it poses to health and sanity has been over-hyped. Death is not an automatic consequence of use, even repeated use. Nor is addiction. But it is a powerful, short-lived drug (a five to ten minute high) and thus the ensuing rebound or crash will entice some users into damagingly repetitious use. Being of uncer-tain purity, it can also cause potentially fatal toxic reactions: the heart and respiratory system would suffer. The heat of the smoke and/or the impurity of the product also lead some users to 'complain of sore throats, chest pains and black or bloody sputum'.[17] According to a report in the *Journal of Pediatrics*[18] 'cocaine abuse in humans significantly reduces weight of the fetus, increases the stillbirth rate related to abrupto placentae (hemorrhage during pregnancy) and is associated with a higher malformation rate.'

The last few years have shown, above all, that cocaine and its more robust offspring continue to generate vast profits. This is true of Colombia where the 'drug barons' have set up an alternative economic and paramilitary structure powerful enough to neutralise the central government. But it is also true of North America where, in the delicate phrasing of a couple of well versed academics,[19] 'cocaine abuse treatment has been become big business, with numerous programmes of questionable ongoing efficacy.'

Hallucinogens

The average LSD dose now seems to be considerably weaker as the trend towards casual, almost daily use grows. Conversely, high potency 'tabs' are still around and can cause distress in users who are anticipating something weaker. The drug is now particularly favoured as an accompaniment to alcohol.

Heroin

The main changes on the heroin front relate to questions of HIV infection and the efficacy of supplying clean needles and maintenance doses of methadone. These are dealt with above. There has been another interesting, although entirely predictable, development: the discovery of other substances for weaning users off opiates – products that are supposedly superior to methadone. Followers of clinical fashion will be familiar with many such false dawns. Morphine was supposed to have been a safe pain killing substitute for opium yet resulted in hundreds of thousands of addiction cases. Heroin was supposed to have been a dependable alternative to the problems of morphine dependence. And now methadone, which users report is even more difficult to withdraw from than heroin, is the state's 'cure' for opiate addiction. One of the new miracle products is clonidine (brand names Catapres, Dixarit) which was originally used to treat raised blood pressure and migraine. Naturally enough blood pressure problems result from its prescription to addicts, while other adverse effects include constipation, drowsiness, impotence, swelling of the throat and face, nausea and dizziness.[20]

A second methadone alternative is Naltrexone, an opiate antagonist – that is to say a product which is able to block the effects of opiates and can actually provoke withdrawal symptoms in someone who already has opiates inside them. Hence its use in overdose cases or as a guide to whether a patient undergoing treatment is as cleaned-up as they may have professed.

Both clonidine and Naltrexone – which are sometimes used in concert – are claimed to be non-addictive, even though American trials have shown former opiate addicts are selecting to continue Naltrexone use 'on a long term basis'.[21]

Amyl and Butyl Nitrite

There have been further calls to control these drugs under the Misuse of Drugs Act or to outlaw them altogether. Notably, an Old Bailey judge in May 1987 urged the Home Secretary to act after hearing the case of a 19-year-old Bromley youth who, having apparently pepped himself up on amyl nitrite, attempted to have unlawful sex with a 14-year-old girl and then murdered her. He then tried to slash his own wrists. Seven months later the issue was put in the hands of the Advisory Council on the Misuse of Drugs which had already rejected the idea of control in 1984. Even as they were pondering the question a second time, social services minister, Tony Newton, reported in the House of Commons that while the inhalation of nitrites can cause 'a fall in blood pressure leading to fainting, nausea and vomiting, palpitations, deeper, faster breathing, sensations of numbness and tingling, the effects are transitory and it is not thought that the abuse of these substances would lead to any lasting ill effects in the majority of cases.' Elsewhere it has been found that swallowing rather than sniffing the liquid can be hazardous, sometimes fatal, which is why in Australia the product is not available in open mouthed bottles that could cause spillage down the throat.

Solvents

The picture since the middle of the decade has been one of waning public interest coupled with a steady increase in the number of fatalities 'associated' with the sniffing of glues and other volatile solvents. In 1981, total deaths were 46. By 1985 this had jumped to 116. While there was a drop the following year, the upward trend looked like resuming in 1988. A bigger proportion were due to the direct consequences of sniffing rather than to accidents or suffocation, prompted by inhalation of vomit or plastic bags placed over the head. A note of caution is worth sounding over the term 'death associated with solvent abuse'. In some cases,[22] it won't be clear what role, if any, solvents played in causing the fatality. In others solvents will be just one of several contributory factors.

The significant enforcement development was the enactment, from August 1985, of the Intoxicating Substances (Supply) Act. Among the first to sample its remedial powers was a Southwark newsagent, convicted of supplying four or five bottles of Tipp-Ex thinner to a local 14 year old. The boy died after sniffing with his friends in a local park. The newsagent received three months' imprisonment. It remains to be seen whether the act will be effective against purveyors of bulk lots of butane gas, hair spray, etc. to teenagers; and whether, in fact, young sniffers will turn increasingly to these more lethal products because of curbs on glues and thinners.

Tobacco

The issue of passive smoking (i.e. the involuntary ingestion by non-smokers of stray fumes) has come to dominate. The argument as to whether it is possible to get damaged in this way hung in the balance at the time of my first draft. Now the question seems to be settled given the results of the fourth report of the Independent Scientific Committee on Smoking and Health. The committee concludes that passive smoking increases the chances of non-smokers contracting lung cancer by between 10 and 30 per cent. This translates into several hundred deaths a year out of the UK total of 40,000. The committee's prescription is for more smoke-free areas and, where smoking is permitted in enclosed places, for the smokers rather than the abstainers to be treated as the aberrant strain, and segregated. Generally the reverse is the case. The committee, knowing the colour of the government's thinking, stopped short of recommending legislation. Instead it expected local environmental health departments to take up the issue. Several of those departments soon replied that they were too pressed with other matters.

There were, nonetheless, a number of smoke-free initiatives in the wake of the report, notably on some of British Airways' routes.

The poor news for the anti-smoking lobby was that after a decade of steep decline in the total number of smokers aged over 16, the drop has slowed considerably. In fact during the third quarter of 1987, as compared with the previous year, spending on tobacco in real terms increased by £3 million. The no-smoking message seems to be heeded least by girls and women, most by men and boys. Not only is the female abstinence rate lower but the number of cigarettes consumed by each smoker has increased. Speculation arose that an AIDS type anti-smoking ad campaign was in the works, to be aimed principally at teenagers.

Certainly there was a peculiar imbalance in government effort directed at 'drug abuse' compared with the money targeted at smoking and drinking. Total annual deaths from all illegal drugs, heroin included, amount to less than 240.[23] Alcohol, by contrast, kills 6,500 and smoking 100,000 every year. According to the British Medical Association the total expenditure aimed at combating controlled drugs is £411 million (this includes Customs, police and crop substitution programmes). The combined total for booze and cigarettes is a little over £6 million.

Tranquillisers

The news on benzodiazepine tranquillisers, particularly the short-acting temazepam type, gets worse. Reports from as far afield as Plymouth and Glasgow suggest street use of the drug is producing problems familiar from the barbiturate phase of the late '70s.[24] Injecting has become commonplace and, as with barbs, heavily dosed individuals are exhibiting both violence and severe withdrawal symptoms, sometimes including convulsions. While the drug is frequently used as an accompaniment to alcohol, for many it is now a drug of first choice. A Plymouth psychiatrist said temazepam was the most frequently injected substance in his locality.

Supplies have not been difficult to come by. Even though, since April 1986, all benzodiazepines have been controlled under the Misuse of Drugs Act – a development that was supposed to have prompted a cut-back by GPs and drug company sales reps – the message has still not sunk home. Prescription totals for daytime anxiety-relieving products have fallen, but those for the short-acting type used to promote sleep continue to rise. This last category includes the new street favourite temazepam (brand names Euhypnos and Normison).

Another of the benzodiazepines to be specifically fingered is lorazepam (Ativan), a daytime sedative of shortish duration. The problems it provokes, according to psycho-pharmacologist, Heather Ashton,[25] are numerous. Already inherently potent, manufacturers supply it in powerful tablet strengths. These features are compounded by the quickness of its action: between doses blood concentrations fall appreciably triggering a craving for the next hit. Its relative potency and quickness of action additionally complicate withdrawal effects.

Professor Malcolm Lader of South London's Institute of Psychiatry, the man who did much to force his colleagues to acknowledge the addictive nature of benzodiazepines, was another who saw lorazepam as a special case. The drug, he said, should no longer be prescribed because it caused dependency at normal dosage levels. And weaning patients off the drug was twice as hard as with other types of benzodiazepines.[26]

Whatever the particular demerits of lorazepam and temazepam, the last couple of years have uncovered the existence of between one and 2½ million individuals dependent on any one or more of the whole noxious range of benzodiazepines. More than a thousand of these victims joined with lawyers to claim compensation and suitable treatment for their addiction. Some 150 firms of solicitors were initially involved, many acting together in the preparation of joint suits. Among the courses being considered was a case to prove doctors and drug companies had been negligent in failing to accept the 'fact of addiction'; that the physicians caused 'withdrawal hardships' by recklessly pulling their patients off the drugs instead of lowering them gently, and that they failed to warn patients of the drugs' addiction potential and its side effects.

Beyond these questions lay the issue of treatment for those currently attempting to quit the drug. Unlike the costly, elaborate manoeuvres associated with heroin withdrawal, tranquilliser addicts tend to make do with simple self-help groups since nothing else has been available; projects whose success rate is, nonetheless, impressive. Their funding, over the three years to 1988, was one fortieth the sum targeted chiefly at opiate addicts (£500,000 versus £20 million), even though some 20 times more people are afflicted.

More insupportable was the arrival – right-on cue – of a new generation of anti-anxiety product, promoted, as always, as *the* safe, non-addictive pacifier for which the medical/drugs trade has always striven. Safe, non-addictive is what was said about benzodiazepines' chain of discredited predecessors: about ethyl alcohol, chloral hydrate, paraldehyde, bromides, barbiturates and methaqualone (brand names Quaalude and Mandrax). The damage these drugs caused was known years before their distribution was controlled or banned, but such measures were always delayed until the drug firms had a wonderfully profitable new cure in the works.

The new one is buspirone – known, by its action, as an azaspirodecanedione and originally developed as a treatment for schizophrenia. Its anti-anxiety or anxiolytic properties were discovered in the early '70s when it was forced on laboratory monkeys. It has no cross-tolerance with benzodiazepines, which means it cannot be used to relieve the withdrawal symptoms of benzos, and is said to produce no 'rebound' effects when use is stopped, or problems of dependency.

The data sheet made available in Britain lists various side effects, including dizziness, nausea, headaches, nervousness, insomnia, light headedness and excitement. These symptoms have affected between 12 and 33 per cent of those participating in clinical trials. However, the US data sheet lists several reactions missing from the British list. Among them are claustrophobia, stupor, slurred speech, photosensitivity, pressure on the eye and psychosis. The US sheet also warns that 'its central nervous system effects on any individual patient may not be predictable.' Manufacturers Bristol-Myers baulked at the suggestion that they were being economical with their data. The decision about what goes on the British sheet, they said, is that of the Committee on the Safety of Medicines. Nonetheless at the March 1988 British launch, Charles Medawar, director of the drugs industry watchdog, Social Audit, asked the obvious question: 'How can we be sure this is not going to become another scandal like Opren or involuntary tranquilliser addiction?'[27]

But, incredibly, among Medawar's antagonists was Malcolm Lader, the benzodiazepine campaigner, who has apparently learnt very little about empty drug company promises and has decided to lend his support to Bristol-Myers and buspirone (or Buspar as it is branded).

'This drug will certainly expand the options available to practitioners in the treatment of anxiety,' he said at the launch. Trials for dependency, he noted, had been satisfactory and patients taken off the drug had shown no 'rebound anxiety'. 'If we are making a mistake, we are making a new mistake.'[28] No, Dr Lader. It will be the same old 'mistake' wearing a different hat.

Xanthines

Research proceeds to discover links between caffeine intake and a range of often fatal ailments, such as coronary thrombosis, fibrocystic breast disease, fetal abnormalities and cancers of the pancreas and urinary tract. A recent review of these matters gave not so much an all-clear but a 'no clear evidence' of any link. Pregnant women were nonetheless advised to limit their consumption.

Notes

1 Dr Roy Robertson, Aidan Bucknall, Dr James Strachan, 'Use of Psychiatric Drug Treatment Services by Heroin Users from General Practice', *British Medical Journal*, 12 April 1986, vol. 292, p. 997
2 A. Glanz, C. Taylor, 'Findings of a National Survey of the Role of General Practitioners in the Treatment of Opiate Misuse: Extent of Contact with Opiate Misusers, *British Medical Journal*, 16 August 1986, vol. 293 (6544)
3 *Doctor*, 9.1.1988
4 Russell Newcombe, 'High Time for Harm Reduction', *Druglink*, Institute for the Study of Drug Dependence, London, January/February, 1987
5 Annual Report of the Home Office Drugs Inspectorate for 1986, Home Office, 1987
6 Dr Brian Johnston, in letter to *Druglink*, London, January/February 1988
7 Allan Parry, *Druglink*, January/February 1987
8 John Marks, *Druglink*, July/August 1987
9 Raj Rathod, 'Substitution is not a Solution', *Druglink*, November/December 1987
10 'AIDS and Drug Misuse, Part 1', Report by the Advisory Council on the Misuse of Drugs, Department of Health and Social Security, HMSO, London, 1988
11 Paula Hendry, *Druglink*, September/October 1987
12 Annual Report of the Home Office Drugs Inspectorate for 1986, HMSO, London, 1987

13 H. Parker, R. Newcombe, K. Bakx, 'Heroin and Crime: The Impact of Heroin Use on the Rate of Acquisitive Crime and the Offending Behaviour of Young Drug Users', University of Liverpool 1986, available from Misuse of Drugs Project, University of Liverpool

14 Peter Burden, *Daily Mail*, 18.11.1987

15 A. Hamid Ghodse, 'Cannabis Psychosis', *British Journal of Addiction*, 1986, vol. 81, p. 473–478

16 *The Guardian*, 19.3.1987

17 Michael Gossop, *British Medical Journal*, vol. 295, 17.10.1987

18 N. Bingol, M. Fuchs, V. Diaz, et al., 'Teratogenicity of Cocaine in Humans', *Journal of Pediatrics*, 1987, vol. 110(1), p. 93–96

19 J. Grabowski, S. I. Dworkin, 'Cocaine: An Overview of Current Issues', *International Journal of Addiction*, vol. 20 (6–7), pp. 1065–1088

20 Peter Parish, *Medicines*, Penguin, London, 1980

21 Hans Agren, 'Clonidine Treatment of the Opiate Withdrawal Syndrome: A Review of Clinical Trials of a Theory', *Acta Psychiat. Scand.* 1986, vol. 73 (supp. 327)

22 *Druglink*, January/February 1987

23 'Comparative Mortality from Drugs of Addiction', Action on Alcohol Abuse and British Medical Association, 1986

24 *Druglink*, November/December 1987

25 *Druglink*, March/April 1988

26 *Pharmaceutical Journal*, 24.10.1987

27 *The Observer*, 27.3.1988

28 *The Observer*, 20.3.1988

2 ALCOHOL

Intro

FOR ANYONE caught in possession of a joint or, for that matter, a wrap of heroin, the special, almost exalted place alcohol occupies in society will be a perpetual irritant. What other drug that can floor a full-grown man within half an hour is so freely available, so freely advertised and dressed up not as a drug – with all the concomitant health implications – but as a happy social lubricant?

The case of alcohol is exceptional in regard to the hundreds of thousands of 'problem drinkers' – a good proportion of whom die early – and the thousands more who get mangled on the roads in drink-related accidents. Yet it is not easy to dismiss a drug that has been a good companion to people all over the world for thousands of years, calming nerves, lifting spirits and conjoining groups in merry insobriety.

When we speak of 'alcohol' we are referring to beverages that are for the most part concoctions of flavoured water, with the alcohol content of that water amounting to no more than 40 per cent in whisky and as little as 3 per cent in beer. Consumed in this way, alcohol inevitably gets rated by most people as less awesome a substance than it really is. This feeling is reinforced by the fact that neither ale nor spirits lend themselves to comfortable injection; the pure undiluted stuff never has been tried intravenously on a grand scale by even the most ardent users.

Alcohol gets its special place in society because of its particular intoxicant effect. In unshackling normal social restraints of behaviour it causes an initial lift in spirits. But, fundamentally, it is a dulling, stupefying drug. It provokes no contemplation or dreaming experiences as do LSD and certain magic mushrooms, and while there are other drugs that are equally unastounding and thus safe in their perceived effects, these either came along after Western society had drawn up its 'approved' drugs list, or in early times they were too closely identified with the diabolical pagans of the New World to be accepted.

Only the Moslems have decided to shun booze completely. Prohibition works – at some considerable cost – in the Islamic world, but elsewhere temperance and prohibition movements have only modified the drug's pattern of use. Accepting this fact, other societies create a fabric of rules and rituals that make mass use of the drug more manageable. To further this process they also put the shutters up on other strong intoxicants, except when used in a medical context. The justification for such action comes via an elaborate mythology that says alcohol is less dangerous than it is, and other drugs much more so. It probably doesn't need to be stated again that alcohol is potentially as physically damaging, as addictive and as hazardous to withdraw from as practically any other intoxicant substance.

Because a whole range of drugs have seeped out from the surgeries or from Third World growers on to the streets, it is becoming more and more difficult to sustain the lie that alcohol is the one mass recreational drug in use, and that the new ones – illicit or not – on the market are merely a temporary aberration. This is like pretending the motor car isn't really a major form of transport – that we're all still living in the horse age. For good or for bad, alcohol is now only one part of the story.

What Is It?

Alcohol is a hydrocarbon compound derived from fermented sugar. The chemical polite people drink is *ethyl alcohol*, composed of the elements carbon, hydrogen and oxygen. More dispirited types resort to *methyl alcohol* whose legitimate uses are as a solvent in paint stripper and as an anti-freeze. The attraction of methylated spirits (a combination of methyl and ethyl alcohol) is that you can get drunk cheaper. One drawback is that the intoxicant rating is actually lower than regular drinking alcohol. The methane in methyl alcohol (commonly called methanol) also upsets vision – sometimes in a total and permanent way. A third option for alcohol fanciers is *iso-propyl alcohol*, found in after-shave preparations and toilet waters. These are sometimes drunk down straight like a shot of scotch, though this is considered less sophisticated than splashing it on the face.

So it is ethyl alcohol (otherwise called ethanol) that is the intoxicant factor in the beers, wines and spirits, liqueurs, etc. that we consume so abundantly.

Beer

There are three main types of beer – the traditional English ale, the heartier stouts and the light, bright lagers that are the premier choice in most other parts of the world, and increasingly so in Britain. The major raw material in all these is malted barley, made by a process of germination during which stored compounds are converted into fermentable materials. The germination is arrested by kilning or drying, and the malt then extracted with a hot liquor to produce a sweet wort. This wort is now boiled with hops to produce typical bitter compounds and to precipitate unwanted protein. The hopped wort is next cooled and pitched with yeast. Fermentation is allowed to proceed and this produces a green beer which awaits conditioning. 'Real' ales are those that are left to condition in the cask and are still alive when reaching the pub. The sanitised version is pasteurised, filtered and chilled to death in the breweries where it will be packaged in kegs, cans and bottles. Lager is a variation on the ale theme, calling for a different type of yeast and a longer, colder storage and conditioning period. Stout is either made from a more deeply coloured malt or from barley that is not malted at all, but roasted. Guinness is an example of the latter.

Cider and Wine

Cider is made from fermented apple juice. Wines are fermented grape or other plant juice. Sparkling sorts, such as champagne, undergo a secondary fermentation during which the by-product carbon dioxide is retained in the bottle under pressure.

Fortified wines like sherry, port, Madeira and vermouth combine wines with either brandy or neutral spirits, as well as flavourings.

Spirits

The potency of spirits, as any adult from planet earth must know, is considerably greater than either wine (which is about 10 to 12 per cent alcohol) or beer (which runs from 2½ to 8 per cent).

Spirits range from 35 per cent of total volume to 75 per cent in the case of certain highly inebriating rums. They are made by the literal 'spiriting' away of alcohol from the flavoured base in which it sits. Alcohol boils at a lower temperature than water, so if an already fermented liquid such as a grape wine is heated in a vat, the alcoholic spirit will be released before the solution which contains it can evaporate. This spirit is then trapped and cooled. Its character will depend on the style in which it is boiled off. If done quickly in a continuous process a neutral, featureless spirit will result, such as gin or vodka. Various flavourings can then be added to pep up the taste (juniper berries in gin) or it can be sold straight, as per vodka.

If the distiller wishes to preseve the special quality of the original fermented material (grape base for brandy, barley and corn for scotch) then the boiling-up is done more slowly, and the result is a 'noble' spirit. After distillation, the noble ones must be aged in wooden casks for several years. Malt whisky is at its best only after ten years, and the best cognacs need fifty to peak. But since such a fiddlesome method cannot produce a beverage within the price range of the world's masses the distillers will eke out the precious noble nectar by mixing it with cheaper, mass-produced 'neutrals'.[1] French grape brandy, for instance, is made by mixing noble cognac with industrial alcohol distilled from the EEC's wine lake, while blended scotch, like most Irish whiskies, takes the classier route of mixing pot-stilled malt with grain whiskey that has been 'continuously' produced.[2] Also falling between the noble and neutral traditions is bourbon whiskey, popular in the States, which is continuously distilled from legally specified grain and then aged in casks. Rum can be a straight neutral, though this too is sometimes aged in wood.

Liqueurs

Liqueurs are spirits buoyed up with various and usually secret combinations of herbs. In some cases the process starts with the fermentation of herbs in sugary water – a mixture which is then distilled. Sometimes the herbs are added to the spirit after it has been extracted. Their origins lie in herbal medicines concocted in the Middle Ages.

Congeners

Congeners are chemicals vital in determining the taste, smell and appearance of an alcoholic beverage. Present in tiny quantities in virtually all drinks, they are a natural part of the fermentation process. Among the most omnipresent are tannic acid, fusel-oil, ethyl acetate, various sugars, salts, minerals and B group vitamins. While they play no part in getting you drunk they probably contribute to many of the typical hangover symptoms – headache, wobbly stomach, drowsiness. The amount of congeners in a given drink depends on its base material as well as the manufacturing process. The drink with the lowest rating is the neutral spirit vodka. Also low in the congener ratings are gin and beer. Vastly more congener-loaded is bourbon, while wine falls somewhere in the middle range. But contrary to the notion that red wines hurt more in the morning than whites, it is the latter which contain the bigger quantity of an especially noxious congener called acetaldehyde.

Potency

There are two popular methods of indicating the potency of drinks. The simplest is to specify a percentage of alcohol by volume. The one that is guaranteed to bamboozle is the proof system. This dates back to the days when spirits were graded against gunpowder. Water and gunpowder will not ignite, but alcohol and gunpowder will. When mixtures of alcohol and water are soaked in gunpowder there is a point at which enough alcohol has been added to the solution to enable it to blow up. When it reaches this point the solution has 'proved' itself and is known as 100 degrees proof (100°). This has been found to be at 57.15 per cent alcohol. However it is possible to produce spirit drinks in excess of 100° proof as well as below it. Typical British whisky is 70° proof, which means the alcohol content is about 40 per cent of total volume. To complicate matters, the American proof system rates differently from the British. It has nothing to do with gunpowder; every two degrees of proof equals one per cent alcohol.

Standard Measures

If working that out gives you a headache, the British Health Education Council has devised a simpler method of rating drink power. This establishes rough equivalents between different types of beverage, so allowing people to determine how much alcohol they are actually consuming. The comparisons are crude, but they work out as follows: one half-pint of ordinary beer or lager equals a single measure of spirits, which is the same as a medium glass of wine or a small glass of sherry, vermouth or aperitif. The term used for any of these is One Standard Drink.

Sensations

Aldous Huxley had a high-minded angle on what drunkenness was all about when he wrote, 'Sobriety diminishes, discriminates and says No. Drunkenness expands, unites and says Yes. It is in fact the great exciter of the Yes function in man . . . The drunken consciousness is one bit of the mystic consciousness and our total opinion of it must find its place in our opinion of the larger whole.'

Too true, although it helps to be sober when approaching that particular passage. It is also a fact that while alcohol might excite the Yes function it also releases the No function, the Maybe function and the Get-the hell-out-of-my-way-or-I'll-stick-you-in-the-eye function. Inhibitions that normally curdle in the belly jump out when drunk. It is because of this releasing action that alcohol is often called a stimulant when, physiologically, its effect is to depress the central nervous system. Disinhibition comes at low doses and most social drinking doesn't go beyond this point. In most cases the atmosphere will be all the happier for having dispensed with the leg-irons of etiquette, but in certain settings an inebriated group can perform the kind of mercilessly cruel acts that wouldn't be countenanced when sober. Its members become attracted to a certain course of action and little impressed by possible sanctions. Football gangs are a case in point.

From the very first drink there will be a deterioration of mental and physical performance and, as the dose is increased, these functions are progressively dulled. Death from respiratory collapse would ultimately result. On the way, memory, body coordination, the senses, concentration and judgement will all go.

Occasionally drivers or machine operators insist that their performance is actually enhanced by a tipple, but such claims are a product of their ailing judgement which ails all the more as they continue drinking. The biggest boasts often come from s/he who is most hammered.

Some people exhibit more obviously drunken symptoms than others. A lot depends on social setting and the way the individual chooses to steer the experience. Someone sitting alone in a rented room is unlikely to get garrulous, witty and amorous. Similarly, a heavy drinker at work will do his/her best to conceal any signs of excess consumption. Saturday night down the pub is something else. There we are more likely to see the traditional excitement, emotion and perhaps a little kick-fighting if the stimulation – real or imagined – is present. Men who terrorise their wives after drinking do in some respects have a pharmacologically-based 'excuse' (disinhibition, lack of judgement, etc.) but in reality the violence wasn't put there by the alcohol, it was simply let out.

Capacity

A person's level of drunkenness depends on the concentration of alcohol in the body. Sobriety is recovered when the alcohol is discharged. It follows therefore that people will get more drunk if they take in high levels quickly. It also follows that they will sooner be able to walk the white line again if they can hurry the alcohol out of their body. In terms of alcohol absorption we don't all start out equal. Women absorb it faster than men, as do lean individuals against the obese or muscular. There are other factors that affect the rate: food slows it down, especially carbohydrates like bread and potatoes. Milk does, too. But while getting drunk can be slowed or quickened, sobering up works at a steady, unvarying rate. Generally speaking, the average-sized male takes approximately one hour to recover from One Standard Drink. This time scale relates to the work rate of the liver, the organ which metabolises 90 per cent of alcohol. The balance is peed out unchanged or excreted through the breath and in sweat. In emergency cases hospitals have been known to inject fructose – a simple fruit sugar – to speed up the metabolising, but this is risky unless done by trained personnel. Coffee has some merit in stunning people awake, but it won't improve coordination or judgement, so driving is still hazardous.

Health Effects

It need hardly be stated that the majority of people handle their drink well enough, causing no injury to themselves or to others. This illustrates the comparatively mature attitude we have towards this drug. But when things go wrong, then the implications for health are serious.

Hangovers

There is some debate about the part congeners play in laying on the traditional head-thumping symptoms. Some believe congeners are most of the problem, but it seems clear enough that dehydration also plays a large part. Alcohol is a powerful diuretic, prompting water to vacate the body cells and accumulate in the blood. As to hangover cure, the best one is to avoid further irritating the stomach with more drink or explosive foods. A cup of hot water (already boiled) some-times helps. Otherwise, relax and in five to ten hours you'll be on the up.

Alcoholic with Other Drugs

Doctors warn against taking alcohol in conjunction with most of the other central nervous system depressants such as barbiturates, tranquillisers and the opiates, since the action of one is accentuated by the other. Alcohol taken with heroin is *especially* dangerous: there is a possibility of vomiting while in a coma. Alcohol also reacts adversely with the MAOI drugs (see pages 84–5), and with anti-histamines.

Pregnancy

Babies, being a product of their parents and everything they consume, run a risk of damage when one or both of those parents indulges in heavy drinking.

So far, practically all measurements and research have been done on women, but if the child can have its father's nose it can also bear the genetic scars of its father's alcohol habit. The most carefully examined consequence of heavy parental drinking is what is known as Fetal Alcohol Syn-drome. The term was coined in the 1970s, although the condition has been recognised for centuries. Generally, the baby when delivered will be small and light, and a year later will still be under par. Facial features are also distinctive: including a broad, flat midface, low nasal bridge, short, upturned nose, and 'mongolian' folds at the inner corners of the eyes. Mental impairment is the most serious outcome of the full syndrome. Although the link with alcohol appears proven, the risk is believed to be small.

Drinking and Driving

A word of warning to drivers about the creeping-up syndrome. The legally permitted amount of alcohol a driver can have in his/her bloodstream is 80 mg per 100 ml. This will be accumulated from about five Standard Drinks for a man, three for a woman; fairly smartly consumed. If such an amount is taken at lunchtime a residue will still be present in the blood at going-home time. If, before getting behind the wheel, the driver should take a top-up it could send him/her over the legal limit. More importantly, it could get an innocent person killed. Blood alcohol levels can be worked out by looking at amounts consumed at a given time, set against the work rate of the liver. (Bear in mind that it is possible to be registered drunk while driving to work the morning after a heavy session.)

Body Heat

Alcohol causes the blood vessels near the surface of the body to widen, leading to heat loss. For someone falling down drunk out of doors on a cold night this can prove fatal. The elderly who drink are also more prone to hypothermia.

Long-Term Heavy Drinking

In regard to longer-term effects, alcohol intrudes into numerous illnesses either as the actual cause or as a complicating factor.

The DHSS notes[3] that up to 30 per cent of men currently admitted to hospitals are either 'problem drinkers' or physically dependent on alcohol. Among the dependent ones the death rate on a comparative age basis is twice as high as the rest of the population. Nutritional and digestive troubles may be the first signs of illness arising from prolonged heavy drinking, for although alcoholic drinks do contain small amounts of iron and magnesium and some of the B vitamins, their principal food value is as a sugar, i.e. empty calories. Consumed on top of normal eating, drink will deliver excess flab. Taken *instead* of food – which is the style with many serious drinkers – malnutrition will follow. This can be aggravated by further loss of appetite as a result of inflammation of the stomach lining (gastritis) together with sub-normal absorption from the gut caused by irritation of the bowels. Vomiting, nausea, loss of appetite and diarrhea are common warning signs of damage.

The best known consequence of heavy, long-term drinking is cirrhosis of the liver. It usually takes from 10 to 15 years to develop and presently kills about 2,500 people each year in the UK. Although this is a low rate compared to, say, France, since 1970 the number has been climbing fast. Cirrhosis is a progressive and potentially lethal condition in which changes in the fat content of the liver damages its cells, which are then replaced by scar tissue. The problem with the scarring is that it cuts off the blood supply to those areas responsible for producing and storing nutrients. Alcohol is not the sole cause of liver cirrhosis. Indeed, some researchers prefer to blame it on malnutrition, pointing to a high incidence among prisoners of war. Nonetheless, as with smoking and lung cancer, while the relationship isn't exclusive, it's a close one.

Other parts of the body suffer from prolonged heavy drinking. Bronchitis, pneumonia, tuberculosis and diseases of the heart may all occur more frequently.

More research is also being done into alcohol's effect on the brain. It is now understood that the great organ shrinks from imprudent drinking, causing intellectual impairment. Evidence for an increased risk of certain cancers is also turning up. The parts most vulnerable are the tongue, mouth, throat, voice box and liver.

The other major physical ailment resulting from heavy use is called peripheral neuritis. This is the condition that has alcoholics missing their step and crashing to the ground. Basically it's about nerve fibres being starved of vitamins and, as a result, failing to perform properly. The condition mainly affects the toes, feet, fingers and hands. It starts with tingling and progresses to numbness. Treatment is by rest and vitamin B therapy.

Apart from this catalogue of physical hazards, alcoholism also inspires a range of maladies that affects the emotional life of the user and those closest to him/her. Typically, there can be anxiety, depression, guilt, paranoia, memory blackouts, agitation and, quite often, violence visited upon the spouse. It is not an exaggeration to say that the impact on the home life of a heavy drinker is the heaviest of all.

Alcoholism

Alcohol is much like any other potent mind-altering drug in that a proportion of those who use it will return to it too often and with too much relish so that a tolerance to the desired effects develops. If this attachment isn't controlled the tendency is to keep on increasing the dose, which strengthens the bond and weakens the mind and body. A point is reached where to be without the drug is to suffer deprivation. This syndrome can be called dependence or addiction, but in the case of alcohol it has more usually been called alcoholism. An equivalent term would be heroinism or benzodiazepinism. Since the 1960s alcoholism has been thought of and treated as a disease – one that could be defined in medical terms.

The disease idea was a reaction against older notions that said heavy drinkers were bad or weak people, but the notion is now falling from fashion. 'Disease', it is being argued, is a rigid concept that promotes rigid systems for dealing with it. It suggests some alien factor eating away at the passive victim, whereas 'alcoholism' allows for a host of psychological and physical moving parts that vary from person to person and over which the 'victim' can and does have control. More contentiously, it is now being stressed that total abstinence may not be advisable for some chronic drinkers, unless they have extensive liver damage; it would be better to get the dose down and steady. This coincides with the intellectual drift among workers dealing with other drug problems. With it goes the demystifying of the medical apparatus: the 'treatment' centres, the detox units, perhaps even the rehabilitation houses. And as those balloons are pricked the hope is that all kinds of people in society will understand more fully the causes of dependence, and how it can be handled. A Government-commissioned report in 1979 was following just this line when it stated: 'Treatment is not an answer to alcohol problems. Services cannot cope now and are never likely to be able to. And not all those offered treatment will benefit. Help can be given to alcoholics by people in a wide range of different capacities and not just by those in the medical profession . . . The main task is to develop services so that awareness of alcohol problems amongst those coming into contact with alcoholics is enhanced, and the spectrum of facilities is brought to bear on those who may benefit from them as early as possible.

Platitudes? The translation into something tangible depends on how serious 'society' intends to be. If the existing treatment modules are rubbished to the extent that the government has an excuse to pull out the fiscal plug then we could be left with nothing but platitudes to offer the problem drinker.

Sudden Deaths

As with other central nervous system depressant drugs, an extremely high dose of alcohol quickly consumed can kill. Again there is no amount you can point a finger at and say: this much is lethal. It depends on constitution and how much tolerance has been built up. However, anything in excess of one bottle of spirits in one bout and death is a possibility. Alcohol has other ways of despatching people in a hurry. It is often a factor behind murders, suicides and accidental deaths. Drownings and alcohol are a common duo, as are drink and road casualties. One-fifth of all road deaths is related to excessive drinking, and the young male, above all, is frequently disposed of in this way. Alcohol plays a part in about half of the road accidents involving males aged 15 to 24.

Withdrawal

Once a person becomes physically dependent on alcohol the problems incurred by suddenly withdrawing supply are as severe as from any other drug. They are almost identical to the results of barbiturate withdrawal, including the risk of convulsion, hallucination, and delirium. The first symptoms can occur a few hours after the last drink, typically with the morning shakes. A drink will steady these. If one is not forthcoming the alcohol dependent will get increasingly jumpy and agitated, unable to hold a cup or tie a lace. While in the throes of the shakes something like a quarter[4] will suffer accompanying hallucinations. They'll probably be short-lived and take the form of distorted shapes, moving shadows, snatches of music or shouted remarks. In this state, note Kessel and Walton in their classic little volume *Alcoholism*[5], the sufferer will be prone to reading threats into the most casual glance or remark from innocent bystanders. More awesome still is the condition known as *delirium tremens*. This, they say, 'is one of the most dramatic conditions in the whole calendar of medicine.' Kessel and Walton's own description cannot be bettered.

'The symptoms are florid. There is great restlessness and agitation. In the hospital ward the patient, weak as he is, may have to be restrained by two or more people before he can be got into bed. He is never still, tossing and turning restlessly, constantly engaged in conversation, switching from person to person, from subject to subject at the smallest stimulus and frequently shouting salutations and warnings to distant passers-by. His hands, grossly tremulous, clutch at the bedclothes; continuously he tries to pluck from them imaginary objects, shining silver coins, burning cigarettes, playing cards or bed bugs. He is prey to ever-changing visual hallucinations and may shield his face from menacing or attacking objects, animal or man. He is completely disorientated. He may not know where he is, the time of day, the date or the month.

'No words can do justice to the picture of fully developed *delirium tremens* during the hours or days before the patient falls exhausted into a deep sleep. He generally emerges from this little worse and with his memory for the recent events mercifully blunted.'

Left to run their course, the DTs generally take three to four days, but drugs can ease the suffering. The main dangers arise from other illnesses that might be present at the same time, and from possible convulsions. They can prove fatal if unattended. Also, a frequently registered cause of death is the inhalation of vomit.

Earliest Use

To trace the history of alcohol consumption is to trace the origins of the human race itself. There is reasonable evidence to show beer and berry wine being drunk as far back as 6,500 BC (some say to 9,000 BC)[6] while the first historical account of alcohol production is in an Egyptian papyrus dated 3,500 BC. The distillation of spirit is thought to be a mere 1,000 years old, although it wasn't until the late 1880s, with the introduction of improved transportation and mass production of bottles, that the first internationally famous brand names emerged – Martell, Hennessey, Haig and Johnny Walker. The common folk of Britain have supped on nut-brown ale for centuries; it was as much a staple as red meat and was said to be the difference between the imperial Briton and the insipid continental. Between 1720 and 1750 the gin epidemic took hold, during which establishments vied to produce the cheapest and most explosive beverage, and supplied premises where the recipient could lie puffing and steaming until the faculties returned. The worst excesses were checked by an Act of Parliament in 1751 which put a high tax on the drink and curbed its retail sale. But even after this move, up to an eighth of all London adult deaths were said to have been caused by excessive spirit drinking.[7]

The introduction of coffee and tea helped to sober the population, but a great liquor resurgence came about during the industrial revolution. For the toiling, uprooted masses of the expanding cities, drink seemed the logical recourse. In the latter part of the nineteenth century the national binge inspired temperance movements with doctors, clergy and other moral upholders imploring the public to acquire better habits. Closure of public houses between midnight on Saturday and noon on Sunday came in 1848 for England and Wales, and by 1872 there was a ban on weekday drinking between the hours, roughly, of midnight and 6 a.m.

The modern system of licensing and opening hours developed through the Defence of the Realm Act(s) of the 1914–18 War. In 1921 they were consolidated under the 1921 Licensing Act which handed over powers to local magistrates. From this emerged the basic pattern of nine hours' drinking per day divided into two sessions – one from about 11 a.m. to 2 p.m., the other from 5.30 p.m. to 10.30 or 11 p.m. More modifications came in 1961 and 1964. Then in 1976 came the hotly debated Scottish reform which relaxed the whole system of opening times north of the border. Under the new measures, individual premises can apply to open earlier, close later and trade all afternoon, Sundays included. In other words, virtually round-the-clock drinking in some cases. The idea had been to appease tourists and lure families in to upbeat establishments.

The effect at ground level has been altogether different. According to *New Society* magazine[8] some 99 per cent of all regular extensions in the Strathclyde region (which includes Glasgow) were granted to ordinary bars that did not admit children and the first establishment to get an all-day licence was not in Tourist-ville, but opposite the Govan docks. The impact on death and crime of the relaxed hours is almost impossible to calculate, though it is reported that fewer drunks are to be seen on the streets. This could merely indicate that they are holed up longer in the pubs, then wobbling home when most folk are in their beds. Convictions for drunken driving rose by nearly a third between 1971 and 1981, but they also rose in England. Convictions for drunkenness fell, but again they fell too in England. Actual consumption of liquor seems not to have risen, but this can be credited to the recession. A similar pattern exists for England. A possibly clearer consequence of the new hours has been the rise in deaths from the drinkers' disease, cirrhosis of the liver. Between 1976 (the year before the reform) and 1981, fatalities increased by 40 per cent against a 17 per cent rise for England and Wales.

Cirrhosis generally takes 15 years of heavy drinking to develop, but given that there is a constant pool of individuals with the disease, a sudden increase in consumption, caused for instance by longer drinking hours, could work through into the death figures quite quickly. But consumption figures are stable! Yes, but even though they are stable, there are indications that more is being drunk by committed drinkers. The moderates are cutting down, but the hardcore are taking up their slack.

The relevance of the Scottish reforms is that they are now being wished upon the whole of the United Kingdom by those parties with an interest in tourism – notably the Department of Trade and Industry. The medical profession ranges against the idea. The Home Office, whose final decision it is, was saying (at the time of writing) it intended tapping the Scottish public for its views and then mulling the whole question over.

Patterns of Use

The pattern of drinking in the south of the UK is allegedly more genteel, with an even spread of what's consumed among the masses. The traditional watering hole has been the pub. However, this institution has been forced to rehabilitate or die. Young drinkers want more than padded plastic chairs and sick-stained carpets. Many pubs have resorted to flash video games or flash food to supplement the primary recreational pursuit of boozing. Others have gone for the complete facelift and now pose as continental bar-cafés or American nightclubs with checkered tablecloths and extremely tall, expensive novelty drinks. Discos in the '80s are taking more young people's liquor money, but the brewers are wise to that one and are buying into them; of course, they already own or control most of the pubs.

Pubs have also been losing trade to supermarkets and off licences. Twenty years ago the country's 76,000 public houses represented 60 per cent of all licensed premises. Today there are about the same number, but they account for only 44 per cent of all retail drink outlets. They still do well from beer (about 87 per cent of total sales) but less so from other drinks.

Still, the pub remains irreplaceable for that great proportion of Britons who don't merely wish to consume, but also partake of an atmosphere. Whether it feels like the Battle of the Somme or is the sort where you get croutons in your soup, there are still few other 'leisure' options to beat the pub's drawing power. For young people, especially males, entry into the pub is one of the traditional ways of celebrating the transition from childhood to manhood: you smoke your fag, buy your round, yap loudly with the mates and you're made. Surveys indicate about one-fifth of all 13–16-year-olds have – or claim to have – drunk alcohol in licensed premises. (An even bigger total drink on a regular basis, buying from other outlets.) This rite of passage is likely to become more, not less important as the recession continues biting into school leavers' job prospects. Getting a job is another 'adult' event. Deprive young people of it and they will start looking for other ways of imposing themselves on an uninterested world.

Not only is the pub a grown-up place to be, the young customer now has more time to inhabit it. The same, of course, goes for individuals of any age when thrown onto the dole. Take a town like Corby in Northamptonshire. In September 1982 Corby registered one of the highest unemployment rates in the country following the closure of its steelworks. It was also estimated that one in five of the town's adult unemployed was an alcoholic: the UK's highest rate.

'It normally takes between five and fifteen years to become an alcoholic,' David Young, director of Northants Council for Alcoholism told *New Society*,[9] 'but when a man is made redundant with a sizeable payment, he has the time, the money and the frustration to drink. He is depressed, perhaps unused to regular heavy drinking and therefore vulnerable.' A former worker at Corby's steelworks was a case in point.

He used to be a two-pints-on-a-Saturday-night man. Within two years of his redundancy he was on two bottles of spirits a day.

The women of Corby are less likely to be found down the local hostelries. They have traditionally found such places inhospitable, even threatening. Instead, women have been lured on to pills or have been obliged to turn their pain inwards. But lately there has been a jump in female consumption. Admissions to hospital for alcoholism are also sharply up (about 35 per cent between 1965 and 1979) as are deaths from alcoholism (600 per cent in the same period) and cirrhosis (about 40 per cent). Welcome to the club, women of Britain.

Policy

While drinking is a major habit in the UK, national consumption still falls some way below countries like France, Hungary, Italy and Spain. Each individual in those countries is on average consuming the equivalent of 20 pints of 100 per cent alcohol every year. For Britons the total is a little over 12 pints. The pattern within the UK shows a continuous rise in per capita consumption from 1950 up until 1979, by which time the intake had nearly doubled. Then, in most categories, it dipped and levelled out. Spirits have peaked in this way, beer too. Wine, however, was still moving upward at the time of writing. More interesting, perhaps, is the condition of the manufacturers' profits. No matter the foibles of the market-place, profits were still rising sharply in 1984, and that's after adjusting for inflation.

The physical and social cost of Britain's drinking is proving increasingly embarrassing to the authorities as the health lobby gets more and more exercised. One especially unnerving report was prepared in 1979 by the Central Policy Review Staff (the Prime Minister's Think Tank). Commissioned by the Labour Government, it was shelved by the incoming Thatcher administration who also abolished the Think Tank itself. Four years later her ministers were still refusing to publish the report, thus obliging journalists and other interested parties to root around the continent for copies.

Drinking in the UK, it said, was a story of two halves – rising profits and rising damage. Some 700,000 people were directly employed in an industry which drew in at least £7,500 million a year and benefited the Exchequer by thousands of millions; the 1983 figure for Customs and VAT income was about £5,000 million. As to the damage that accrued from this massive activity, for every person the industry employed, another one was 'suffering in some way' due to the consumption of alcohol. Deaths from liver cirrhosis rose 50 per cent in 20 years. Hospital admissions for alcoholism or related problems doubled for men and more than doubled for women in the preceding decade. Alcohol was playing an enormous part in driving accidents, as well as acts of violence, and the costs to industry through lost time could be as much as £500 million. Another £51 million was going in health care and a further £648 million on policing and punishing offenders. These were the visible costs. As to a counter-assault, Britain, said the report, was seriously lagging behind other Western countries in mounting a coherent programme to control excess drinking. Specifically, it recommended: increases in the cost of drinks by means of increased duties. (Prices had fallen in real terms since the 1939–45 war.) No relaxation in the granting of licences and no lowering of the minimum drinking age, as had been suggested by a Government committee. The adoption of 'model policies' for work places, with the lead being taken by the Health and Safety Executive. The use of random breath testing. More publicity about the dangers of drunken driving with simultaneous research into the effects of both advertising and sponsorship schemes by alcohol companies. Most of these recommendations were still awaiting action in 1985 and some, such as the increase in drinks prices, were speedily rejected. 'Any social, legal or fiscal measures to contain or reduce consumption could have an adverse effect on the output, employment and investment of the drinks industries,' explained the Department of Health (sic).[10]

The Industry

Booze, fags and food look increasingly like one giant mega-industry with a handful of key corporations dominant in all three sectors. A typically diversified giant is the Imperial group which has about 9 per cent of the UK beer market through Courage, runs a chain of American hotels (Howard Johnson's), operates Ross and Young's frozen foods, as well as a tobacco division incorporating John Player Special and Embassy.

The major spirits company in the UK is Distillers Company Ltd (DCL) whose 1984 turnover was £1,134 billion. Brand names include Dewar, Johnny Walker and White Horse Scotches, Cossack Vodka, Gordons and Booths Gin, Hine Cognac, and Pimms. DCL is also staked out in frozen foods and yeast and carbon monoxide additives.

While it leaves little room for other gin makers, the UK scotch market is big enough to allow in several other organisations. About 23 per cent of the total is taken by the independent company Arthur Bell and Sons with its Bells Extra Special. Allied Lyons take about 26 per cent through Teachers, and the rest is mopped up by the beer brewers and by the Lonrho mining group (Whyte & Mackay).

The major brewers number six. Guinness makes seven, but unlike the rest, Guinness owns no pubs. The company had been declining steadily for a decade until 1983 when it halted the slide through a celebrated advertising campaign based on the 'Guinnless' theme. Though the project cost £7 million, taxable profits were up by the end of that year by 24 per cent, to £58.8 million.

The pub-owning Big Six are as follows:

Bass – operates thirteen breweries and owns 7,500 tied houses. Brand names include Carling Black Label, Bass, Tennant's, Charrington IPA and Worthington Best Bitter. Accounts for about 21 per cent of the UK beer market. The Bass group also controls Hedges and Butler wines and spirits company, Canada Dry and Rawlings soft drinks, Pontins and

Holiday Club International holidays, and the Bass Leisure squash clubs and amusement arcades.

Allied Breweries – operate six breweries and an estate of 7,250 managed and tenanted houses. Brand names include Double Diamond and Long Life. Accounts for about 16 per cent of UK beer sales. Part of a larger group whose interests include J. Lyons Foods, Grants wine shippers and Harveys sherries.

Watney, Mann & Truman (subsidiary of Grand Metropolitan) – operates nine breweries and owns an estimated 6,800 pubs. Brand names include Webster's, Coombe, Truman's, Mann's and Phoenix. Market share estimated at about 14 per cent. Grand Met's other interests include Berni Inns, Schooner Inns, Gilbey Vintners and Mecca.

Whitbread – operates eight breweries and owns 6,000 tied pubs. Brand names include Trophy, Tankard, Mackeson, Stella Artois and Heineken (the last two traded under licence). Market share about 12 per cent. Other interests include the wine merchants Stowells of Chelsea, the off-licence chain Thresher & Co., as well as Beefeater's Steak Houses, the Roast Inns and a joint share with Pepsico in Pizza Inns.

Scottish & Newcastle – operates four breweries and 1,400 managed and tenanted houses. Brand names include Younger's, McEwan's and Newcastle. Market share about 10 per cent. Other interests include Thistle Hotels, the Waverley wines and spirits group and two distilleries. Best known whisky: McKinlay's.

Courage (a subsidiary of the Imperial Group) – operates three breweries and owns 5,000 tied houses. Brand names include John Smith's Best Bitter and John Courage. Market share about 9 per cent. Imperial's interests include John Player cigarettes, Ross and Young's frozen foods and the Howard Johnson Hotel Group in the US.

Promotion and Trends

While beer and lager ads constantly beseech the TV viewer, the spirit makers divert more of their promotional muscle into road hoardings and the print media. 'There is almost an agreement between them to stay off the TV,' a well-placed advertising executive tells me, 'so that they won't cut each other's throats.' TV is in any case a difficult medium on which to advertise strong liquors because the rules of engagement are more ruthlessly applied: there must be no extravagant claims about increased sexuality or physical prowess; there must be no buying of rounds, no suggestion of anyone being drunk and, most stringently, no actor under the age of 25 taking part in the commercials. Young, 'witty' drinks like Bacardi and lager can overcome these problems by putting on an entertainment. The sober-minded whisky makers, however, seem to be getting more and more lost in self-consuming close-ups of bottles and steaming ice cubes. Getting reliable figures on total expenditure is difficult, but according to the research company, Media Expenditure Analysis, the tally for all media in 1984 was £147.1 million.

The factor that has probably done more to push up consumption and the problems that flow from it has been the growth of supermarket and off-licence sales. What could be easier than to pop a vodka bottle and couple of tonics into the wire trolley? Or better yet, one of those sweet, creamy new beverages that are not like booze at all and which the distillers are aiming directly at women. Bailey's Irish Cream is one lip-licking example. The growth of novelty drinks is a consequence of the distillers finding themselves with what they call a 'maturing market'. By this it is meant that there is now more than enough whisky, gin, vodka, brandy and rum sloshing around the UK to meet demand. But while the novelties are there to tempt certain groups who might not have a taste for the strong stuff, the great mass of spirit drinkers will need to be shown a vision of paradise before they shift from their entrenched habits.

Whisky is overwhelmingly the most popular spirit – accounting for 50 per cent of all sales. Gin, vodka and then

rum split most of the balance between them. And it's whisky
that draws back the customers after they've had their fling
with the mixable neutrals. Whisky, not to put too fine a point
on it, is for the older drinker. Lager ads are remorselessly
witty because its makers wish to push the drink as young and
fresh. This has paid off. While the bedrock of pub sales is still
the pint of bitter, lager sales continue creeping up and are
soon expected to reach 40 per cent of the total beer market.

Help

Bad drinking habits derive from a dangerous spiral. They
could have their roots in social ritual that got out of hand, or in
pain. Good drinking habits derive from understanding –
understanding what alcohol is and its potential for good and
for harm. Good habits also derive from self-awareness and
the determination to confront problems and overcome them
in a healthy way.

There is a range of statutory services to help in this regard,
financed by central as well as local government. There is also
an important voluntary sector that – as in the non-alcoholic
drug field – constantly walks the fiscal tightrope. The main
plank of the government's response are the Alcoholic Treatment Units (ATUs) which are usually sited in the psychiatric
departments of major hospitals. They normally include a
detoxification unit, and although the tradition has been to
hospitalise patients, many are developing out-patients services in an effort to 'go into the community'. ATUs have
never succeeded in serving the whole of their designated
catchment areas and so other hospitals sometimes take it
upon themselves to service the problem drinker either in the
psychiatric or general wards. GPs also lay on a service of sorts
but, like social workers, they tend to be less able to recognise
drink-related problems and/or unwilling to get involved when
they are spotted. Probation officers are more sharp-sighted
and the probation service does get involved in the running of
special hostels. But it is through the voluntary sector – that
part which is neither securely funded nor responsible under

statute – that the major facilities are laid on. There are, for instance, about forty local Councils On Alcoholism which provide information, advice and counselling as well as referral to special care facilities. A person may simply show up with or without a doctor's letter. Then there are several residential 'dry' houses where problem drinkers can live-in for six months to a year and grapple with their problems.` Some, like Turning Point and Aquarius, run units in different parts of the country. Alcoholics Anonymous is a mutual help group that is entirely self-funded and organises small local gatherings which meet all over the country, usually weekly but sometimes more often. It works on the Twelve Steps to Recovery principle – employing an amount of spiritual deep-thinking and the unshakeable belief that alcoholism is a 'disease' rather than a simple indulgence. AA's kith and kin are Al-Anon – for the families of problem drinkers, and Al-Ateen – another mutual support fellowship for teenage drinkers.

The other important services are the handful of detoxification units used by the single homeless to dry out in, and by the autorities as an alternative to prison. There are just three in the whole country.

Notes

1 Nicholas Faith, 'Gentlemen's War: A survey of the world's trade in distilled spirits', *The Economist*, 22.12.1984
2 Ibid
3 *Drinking Sensibly*, Dept of Health of Social Security, HMSO, London, 1981, p. 12
4 N. Kessel & H. Walton, *Alcoholism*, Penguin, 1965, p. 34
5 Ibid
6 *High Times Encyclopedia of Recreational Drugs*, Stonehill Press, New York, 1978, p. 91
7 Kessel & Walton, *op. cit.*, p. 54
8 Jeremy Laurance, *New Society*, 16.8.1984
9 Andrea Waind, *New Society*, 2.9.1982
10 *Drinking Sensibly*, *op. cit.*, p. 57

3 AMPHETAMINE

Intro

AMPHETAMINE IS a booster, hence the street name, speed. It boosts energy levels, confidence levels and the powers of concentration by stimulating the central nervous system (CNS). And yet above any other drug it epitomises the maxim that there is no such thing as a free lunch: the additional zest is not conferred by the drug but is borrowed from the system's finite stocks. Thus the inevitable aftermath of a 'speed' trip is exhaustion and depression.

This price might be considered worth paying. For instance, a truck driver hauling a load from Penzance to Aberdeen might find an extra burst of energy useful; similarly the writer struggling to meet a deadline, or the young night-clubber who doesn't want sleep to interrupt the beat. If these individuals can repair their bodies with a long sleep or perhaps ghostwalk through some undemanding tasks over the next day or two then they might estimate they got a good deal from their drug.

Certainly the pharmaceutical industry was at one time extreme in its advocacy of amphetamine products. A 1946 report[1] was able to list 39 different disorders for which Benzedrine – one of the three main kinds of amphetamine – was *the* recommended treatment. These included night blindness, seasickness, migraine and impotence. Even battle campaigns have to some extent relied on amphetamines. During the Spanish Civil War they were dispensed to overworked troops to provide verve and ferocity. Some 72 million tablets were issued to British forces during World War II,[2] during which conflagration German and Japanese forces were also being supplied. Hitler himself is said to have been unable to function without his daily injections of methylamphetamine (up to 5 a day, plus tablets)[3] which would account for at least some of his paranoid ravings. The pattern continued with the Americans in Korea and Vietnam, by which time there had been two absolutely typical developments: first, after years of wanton mass production and mass prescription the pharmaceutical/medical industry 'discovered' that amphetamine was excessively dangerous and suitable for only the most limited dispensing; and second, it had become an undislodgeable street favourite.

What Is It?

Amphetamine is a chemical compound that acts as a central nervous system stimulant. Structurally it closely resembles the body's own chemical transmitter norepinephrine (NE) which plays an important role in the fight/flight response to stress and emotion. Amphetamine (and also cocaine) appears to mimic or potentiate the action of NE in the brain and thus is able to charge up the central nervous system. It divides into three main pharmaceutical classes (their chief trade names are in brackets): laevo- or 'l-' amphetamine (Benzedrine), dexamphetamine (Dexedrine) and methylamphetamine (Methedrine). The three vary greatly in their absolute potency with the strongest, weight for weight, being methylamphetamine. This delivers about twice the kick of dexamphetamine which in turn has double the force of laevo-amphetamine.

In addition to the original amphetamine compounds numerous derivatives have been developed, some of which have been mixed with vitamins, others with CNS depressants, to deliver a smoother ride. One of those in the up/down class was the '60s princeling Drinamyl (*Purple Heart*) which became an enormous street favourite. In the '70s its place was taken by Durophet-M, which too has been withdrawn.

By far the most common street speed these days is amphetamine sulphate, containing equal amounts of laevo-amphetamine and dexamphetamine and recognisable as a whitish crystalline powder. It is not a particularly difficult product to make. Someone with a good knowledge of chemistry can synthesise it in a domestic bathtub from raw materials available without licence from various warehouses supplying the pharmaceutical and cosmetics industries. However, while no licence is required, the Home Office encourages wholesalers to keep an eye out for and report on unusually large purchases, as well as gauche or seedy-looking customers. The sulphate being discussed is rarely pure. On the other hand it is unlikely to contain really foul additives – strychnine, ground glass – used as 'cuts' (economy measures) by dealers in the States. The traditional UK cut is glucose powder.

Other Amphetamine-like Stimulants

The main speed-related substances found on the streets of the UK today are listed below:

Methylphenidate (trade name: Ritalin)

Closely related structurally to amphetamine, Ritalin is a less potent stimulator of the CNS – a quality that made it a drug preferred by doctors for the treatment of hyperactive children. Though production has now ceased, there are still relatively plentiful stocks in existence, some of which find their way on to the streets. In adults methylphenidate was prescribed for listless, senile behaviour, mild depression and narcolepsy. In virtually every respect the drug produces the same adverse and positive effects as amphetamine, though of a slightly lesser magnitude dose for dose. Street users often describe Ritalin as a 'cleaner high' and it is especially fashionable among the hardcore 'polydrug' users who'll inject it as a companion to a downer. Comes as a white 10 mg tablet marked A/B on one side and CIBA on the other. Intravenous users dissolve them in water and attempt to filter out the chalk through cotton wool.

Diethylpropion

Similar to Ritalin in that it is a moderately less potent version of amphetamine. Once prescribed as a safe diet pill, it is now recommended for short-term use only in severely obese patients. Main trade names are:

Tenuate – a 25 mg tablet marketed by Merrell. It was deleted in 1981, but is apparently still around.

Tenuate Dospan – known as *tombstone* and comes as a white, oblong, sustained-release 75 mg tablet.

Apisate – a 75 mg two-tone yellow sustained-release tablet with added B vitamins (thiamine and riboflavin).

Pemoline

Another slightly less potent amphetamine variant. Like methylphenidate it is used widely for hyperactive children, and less often to lift the sleepiness of people being treated with morphine or other opiates for severe pain. Claimed by street users to stimulate the memory and the loins. It goes under the trade names:

Kethamed – 20 mg small white tablet (deleted in 1981).

Ronyl – 20 mg white tablet.

Volatil – 20 mg white tablet.

Filon

Trade name for a combination of phenbutrazate hydro-chloride and phenmetrazine. The first is a mild stimulant. The second has the potency of amphetamine. Prescribed as a slimming aid and taken less formally for a mildish high. Comes as a plain yellow sugar-coated tablet.

Durophet

The drug trade's licit speed tablet, containing laevo-amphetamine and dexamphetamine in equal parts. Comes in white 7.5 mg, black and white 12.5 mg and black 20 mg capsules.

Durophet-M

Officially deleted but illegal stocks are still around. It is the latter-day equivalent of the '60s *Purple Hearts* except whereas *Hearts* contained amphetamine and barbiturate, Durophet-M mixes amphetamine with methaqualone, an extremely potent hypnotic. Comes as 12.5 mg green/brown and 20 mg red/brown capsules.

Sensations

A standard 5 mg dexamphetamine tablet will yield results within 15–30 minutes, which is fast for an oral drug. The lift from snorted amphetamine sulphate occurs quicker still. By either method the effects usually last for around six hours and produce similar sensations. It starts with a tickle in the gut and the feeling that energy is being pressed up through the body – clearing the mind and making it more powerful. The teeth start grinding. The jaws clench. There is a sense of elation, confidence and a desire to communicate fine new insights and witticisms. Libido might be raised, but the erogenous zones could be less responsive than usual. Appetite is suppressed. There might be frequent weeing. If no more of the drug is administered there is unlikely to be more than a manageable level of fatigue and depression when the effects wear off. The temptation on an open-ended weekend, however, or for someone without constant demands upon their time, is to sniff/swallow more as the comedown begins. This makes the rebound more severe when it does occur.

Regular Use

There are various patterns of amphetamine use, many of them fundamentally harmless. But not all who come into contact with it are able to keep it in check. Someone drawn to the drug initially because it overcomes feelings of powerlessness or social ineptitude may keep returning to it for a lasting 'solution'. Because amphetamine can't possibly deliver long-term euphoria, a ragged cycle of use is set up causing emotional and physical sensations that alternate between soaring and crashing. One victim of the up/down syndrome in amphetamine use is a rock music journalist we can call 'Richard'.

'I am quite lazy by inclination and have had confidence problems at various stages of my life. Amphetamine seemed to solve both these problems. I didn't get tired and I didn't get self-conscious. In fact, I felt witty, energetic, powerful, amusing. For six months I thought I was God. I wrote masses, lost a lot of weight, which was bothering me at the time, and didn't have to miss out on anything through the mundane need to sleep. The use gradually escalated until I was only sleeping about three nights a week. I would start out taking speed on a Friday and generally write or party most of the weekend, keep going through Monday, generally stay up all night Monday, go to the printers Tuesday to help get the paper out, then gradually come down – sleeping or staggering through from Tuesday night until Friday morning – when I would start going up again.

Between me and the person I was living with one £10 gram a week was consumed, which made it an incredibly cheap drug compared to coke. It has to be said, though, that coke is a much subtler, less disgusting experience than snorting sulphate, which is like sniffing powdered razor blades off the toilet floor. It stung and put this horrible pissy smell right inside your nose.'

After six months' use, Richard lost his feelings of magnificence and started becoming 'mildly psychotic'. His gums began bleeding, he had constant colds, spots, eczema, his hair was like straw and he developed a 'really violent temper' that luckily was directed at objects rather than his companion. That speed offers nothing for free was illustrated perfectly by his struggle to recover. The depression and fatigue it involved is explained later.

Taking It

Sniffing

The snorting method involves chopping up the crystalline powder so that it is fine enough not to scrape the nose. Chopping is done on a mirror or hard board with a razor blade. A thin 'line' two or three inches long is formed and this is drawn up through the nose either via a rolled-up banknote, a ballpoint casing or – for those who don't care for ceremony – without any accoutrement.

The Needle

The needle never appealed to Richard, and doesn't to most sulphate sniffers, even those who use heavily. Those who do take to injecting will probably find themselves locked into an even more chaotic pattern of use. Though crude sulphate can be injected by dissolving it in water and filtering it through cotton wool to remove the chalk, it is the more potent and difficult to obtain methylamphetamine (Methedrine) that is prized among the cognoscente. This is principally because of the exhilarating 'rush' the drug affords at the moment of injection. Adepts claim the hit is like no other and comparable to an entire body orgasm – an electric spasm. It occurs immediately the liquid is injected and is gone within half a minute. But then such superlative claims are made on behalf of several other substances or combinations. In the US, Methedrine has developed something of a cult following, but since the epidemic year of 1967–68, illegal stocks have been virtually impossible to obtain in the UK.

Also vanishing from UK recreational circles is methyl-phenidate (Ritalin), which has been withdrawn by its manufacturers. It is often mixed with the synthetic opiate methadone. Methadone plus Ritalin is the up/down combination that is supposed to issue a strong but not too jarring experience – and being 'pharmaceutical', will be less polluted than underground stock. The combination is modelled on the original *speedball* – heroin plus cocaine.

Injectors are known to use a whole variety of substances in order to achieve an up, down or 'out' condition. In Glasgow I heard accounts of kids injecting themselves with talcum powder, and with crushed-up travel sickness pills – sometimes between their toes. In Bradford young 'freakies' are apparently shooting up whisky, Tuinal, methylated spirits, indeed whatever substance can be put into a syringe. But users of needles are comparatively rare so far, and among that fraternity it is rarer still for a person to be an amphetamine purist.

There are health risks common to injectors of any substance. It can contain insoluble particles which lodge in the small blood vessels at the periphery of the lungs and brain. Abscesses are common, as is inflammation of the walls of the vein, and infections in or around the site of injection. Any of these problems can be caused by inept injection techniques, by the use of unsterile needles or by repeated attacks on the same spot. Long-term injectors will run out of suitable entry points. Heavy users have low resistance to disease, and when unsterilised needles are shared the problems are passed around. One almost indigenous problem is viral hepatitis. This is a debilitating ailment that incubates for as long as six months and then takes several weeks of rest and good diet to recover from. Some cases of cirrhosis of the liver may have started with hepatitis.

Runs

The phenomenon of the speed 'run' is well known in drug circles. It lasts for several days and is an attempt, by repeated injections, to hang on to the initial feelings of exhilaration and mastery. By the second day there is no more rush and the high feelings are replaced by agitation in body and spirit. These sensations intensify over the next three to five days, during which time the user won't eat or sleep and will usually inject more speed more often. The run ends when the supply or the user is spent. Sleep will follow – for 48 hours or more. Upon awakening there will be a ferocious hunger and depression.

Amphetamine Psychosis

Some individuals can trip into what the professionals call an 'amphetamine psychosis', so named because in most respects it is comparable to the symptoms expressed by schizophrenics. In both cases there are vivid auditory hallucinations as well as paranoid delusions. The major difference between the two conditions is that the drug user's symptoms will vanish once the body is free of the substances – usually within a few days, rarely more than a week. Also, in amphetamine psychosis consciousness and memory stay clear and there is an accurate appreciation of time, place and self-identity. Such elementals can become fudged in the true schizophrenic.

The onset of amphetamine psychosis is frequently related to heavy, long-term use. However, those in the novice class, but with a predisposition, are also vulnerable. A more serious problem is that amphetamine use could trigger an authentic schizophrenia in such persons who are latently inclined.[4]

Long-Term Effects

Amphetamine psychosis aside, most of the problems associated with the drug have more to do with the pattern of living and thinking it encourages rather than the toxic effects. In fact amphetamine has a remarkably low toxicity and is rarely the chief substance in poison/overdose deaths. Unlike CNS depressants such as barbiturates or the opiates it rarely causes vital body functions to close down. And an advantage it has over cocaine – another short-acting stimulant – is that, lacking coke's anaesthetic properties, high doses are less likely to cause respiratory depressions and convulsions.

Where overdose deaths do occur they are usually attributed to the collapse of blood vessels in the brain, to a sudden, extreme rise in blood pressure, to heart failure or to fever.

Until 1979, only 79 such cases had been recorded worldwide,[5] and these also included 'secondary complications related to the route of administration.'

None of this is to say amphetamine is a drug without hazards. Long-term regular users experience chronic sleeping problems, bursts of ill temper, persistent anxiety, malnourishment due to suppressed appetite, skin rashes, speeded-up and erratic heartbeat, plus numerous other complaints associated with poor eating and sleep.

Doctors warn about taking amphetamine when certain medical conditions are present – in particular, severe hypertension (high blood pressure), hyperthyroidism (over-activity in the thyroid gland), urinary retention, glaucoma (eye disease), arterio-sclerosis (hardening of the arteries) liver and kidney disorders and diseases of the heart.

Tolerance

Amphetamine is a drug against whose effects the body quickly builds up a tolerance. This will necessitate an increasingly higher dose to get stoned, but as with many other drugs the tolerance fades during gaps between use. Thus, someone who has worked up to a 1,000 mg daily dose would be unable to manage that quantity after a lay-off. Curiously, it has been found that children given amphetamine for hyperkinetic syndrome (hyperactivity), and in those administered it for the sleeping disease narcolepsy, tolerance does not develop, i.e. a rising dose is *not* required to keep them normalised. This could be due to the different rates at which the psyche and the body become tolerant. Yet overweight amphetamine users looking to suppress their appetite will find they can't keep a lid on their hunger unless they up the dose.

Dependence/Addiction

Just as the lure of heroin for those who dabble in it has been over-dramatised, so the pulling power of amphetamine has been understated. As with heroin, the attraction is a combination of the physical and psychological, with the user – if s/he is not wary – becoming dependent on the release of energy and confidence while feeling more and more uncomfortable with the correspondingly low periods between use. This, as explained earlier, can produce an escalating pattern of 'abuse'. When withdrawal is undertaken the result will be precisely the reverse of what the drug was offering: instead of euphoria and the curbing of the need to sleep or eat, there will be depression, excessive hunger and fatigue. While of a different nature from heroin withdrawal, there is no doubt that it is equally distressing.

In Association with Other Drugs

The interaction of one drug with another in the body is still little understood, but there are certain agents with which it is known amphetamine and its ilk react poorly. These include substances prescribed for high blood pressure and certain diuretics whose effectiveness is decreased when taken at the same time as speed.

Even more serious problems can arise from the simultaneous use of amphetamine with drugs classified as MAOIs (monoamine oxidase inhibitors). This is a fairly complex though important phenomenon to outline: the body produces an enzyme called monoamine oxidase (MAO) naturally in the digestive juices. It is responsible for destroying potentially harmful fatty acids (amines) that occur in many common foods such as aged cheese, wine, pickled herrings, broad bean pods, beer, beef extracts, avocado pears, bananas and drinks containing caffeine-like alkaloids. If MAO didn't combat them, the toxic amines these foods contain would build up in the body, causing blood pressure to soar to a potentially fatal level.

Some drugs interfere with the MAO function and so allow the amines to accumulate. Such drugs include certain non-stimulant anti-depressants, some obscure hallucinogens such as yohimbine, the harmaline alkaloids and various tryptamines and blood pressure drugs. Patients being prescribed any of these should be (but aren't always) clearly warned about which foods to leave alone. However, apart from reacting badly with numerous foodstuffs, the MAOIs also fail to get along with many other drugs. They either distort the effects or cause them to hang around in the body for long periods. Amphetamine is one drug which is affected like this and the outcome can possibly be fatal. Other drugs to be avoided in the company of the MAOI's are barbiturates, tranquillisers, sedatives, hypnotics, anti-histamines, insulin, narcotic analgesics and more.

In Association with Medical Conditions

Amphetamine can be hazardous for people suffering from heart diseases, hypertension, hyperthyroidism and glaucoma. Doctors are also cautious about issuing to patients with anorexia where kidney function might be impaired.

History

Amphetamine is structurally related to the naturally occurring stimulant ephedrine (from plants of the Ephedra genus) and adrenalin (a bodily hormone). It was first synthesised in 1887, but it was in 1927 that its therapeutic potential was realised when it was discovered that the drug raises blood pressure, constricts blood vessels and dilates the small bronchial sacs. This last characteristic prompted the pharmacautical manufacturing company Smith, Kline and French to go into the bronchial dilator business with their Benzedrine Inhaler[6] – an item of widespread abuse. Not only did asthmatic sufferers turn to the 'B-Bombs' for relief, it was soon learnt the contraption could be invaded and the amphetamine-saturated wadding soaked in water, coffee or alcohol for a mighty beverage. The Inhaler was but one of an ever-growing range of products using amphetamine during the '30s and early '40s. These were the decades of Depression and then global war, and it was little wonder that amphetamine looked to be the perfect pharmaceutical accompaniment to such dismal times. As early as 1935 it was being used to tackle narcolepsy, whereby the sufferer lapses into sudden, unpredictable sleeping bouts. Amphetamines could keep them awake. By 1937 researchers had discovered the drug's paradoxical quality of being able to 'tame' hyperactive children. A decade later it was being prescribed for depression and to suppress the appetite of the obese. Chemists were also working on refining the original crude amphetamine mix. Laevo- and dex-amphetamine had already been separated out; now the search was on for a central nervous system stimulant that didn't also increase heart rate and blood pressure.

As the '40s ended and memories of the war receded, industry and government became progressively less rapturous about the drug. From 1939 onwards it was increasingly obvious that amphetamine was capable of causing hypertension, dependence, psychosis and suicidal depression, but it wasn't until 1956 that the UK government ordered that amphetamine drugs be available on prescription only.[7] The one exception was the street-celebrated Benzedrine Inhaler[8] – a curious exclusion since its wadding contained several hundred times the dose of amphetamine sulphate found in the average tablet. It continued to be available not just in chemists but in general purpose corner stores. The result was a surge of recreational usage followed by a call from the Pharmaceutical Society for manufacturers to either withdraw their products, alter the formulation or include indigestible additives. The trade complied.

The very first great speed epidemic occurred in Japan when a hoard of amphetamine, often in injectable form, and no longer needed to fuel the war effort, was dumped on the open market.[9] In Britain the first 'speed freaks' were exhausted, isolated housewives. Or they were marathon performers such as truck drivers and politicians like Prime Minister Anthony Eden who reported that he was 'living on Benzedrine' during the Suez Crisis of 1952.[10] Other notable users were the frenetic US comedian and narcoleptic Lenny Bruce,[11] as well as that zesty statesman, John F. Kennedy, who is believed to have made regular use of injectable methylamphetamine.[12] It would be interesting to know what drug-induced decisions are made in our own momentous times by the world's political leaders.

The 'pep pill' fad among '60s R & B mods centred on a pill called Drinamyl. This was not actually a straight amphetamine, but an exotic mixture of amphetamine and barbiturate. On the street the pills were called *Purple Hearts* due to their colour (blue) and their shape (triangular). The use of *Purple Hearts* by thousands of ordinarily wholesome youths of every class amounted to the country's first underground drugs craze of the modern era – and it scared the elders. Notwithstanding the previous widespread use via legitimate channels the authorities now expressed great alarm. There were questions in Parliament and the introduction in 1964 of a new piece of legislation called the Drugs (Prevention of Misuse) Act. This made unlicensed possession and importation of amphetamine an offence, but placed no restriction on the drug's manufacture, storage or prescription. These constraints would have to come voluntarily from the trade itself and from GPs. The manufacturers responded by altering the shape of their product. (Young users simply switched its street name to Blues or French Blues.) Prescriptions began falling – from 4 million in 1966 to 2.5 million in 1967. But, like every drug that's pumped into the culture and then withdrawn, alternative sources developed. One was forgery of prescriptions, another was pharmacy thefts. Thirty theft cases were reported in Nottingham alone in 1968, while in Lancashire one young gang are said to have broken into 20 chemists in six weeks, netting some 30,000 tabs.[13]

By the mid '60s London was seeing its first wave of needle-fixated cocaine and opiate users. Many used both drugs simultaneously to achieve a stronger initial rush and for a smoother subsequent ride. Their source – prior to the advent of Chinese black market heroin and South American street coke – was pharmaceutical stock, most of it prescribed by a handful of grasping or badly informed private practitioners. By the later part of the decade more doctors began issuing prescriptions for ampoules of injectable methylamphetamine. Some did so in the belief that it was a safer accompaniment to heroin, others because they appreciated the consultancy fee. The epidemic year, according to a Government report,[14] was 1967–68 when the habit began spreading from London and the Home Counties to other large towns. Numerous cases of 'amphetamine psychosis' began showing up in hospitals, and in Brixton prison during 1968, 400 intravenous *meths* (methylamphetamine) users were logged.[15]

The youth underground movement of the day borrowed a phrase from San Francisco and warned, 'Speed Kills'. The trade itself reacted by withdrawing general supplies of injectable methylamphetamine and confining the product to hospitals only. The fad was efficiently curtailed. At Brixton prison in 1969, not a single intravenous *meths* user was registered.

Yet, as we keep seeing, once the taste for an intoxicant has been whipped up, no amount of curtailment or penalising will remove it. To replace those pill stocks previously derived from GPs and the ampoules of *meths* available from the small coterie of mainly London practitioners, a thriving underground market in amphetamine sulphate developed. Today it is the undisputed market leader in the high speed stakes.

Current Use

Amphetamine has been discredited as a palliative in all but two major areas of medication – narcolepsy and for hyperactive children. While there is little argument among medics as to its use for the first syndrome, its use for (or 'against') hyper-active children is coming increasingly under attack, particularly in the US where some 600,000 children are under treatment for Hyperkinetic Syndrome (HKS). A number of researchers are claiming that HKS doesn't actually exist and that the use of drugs on children who prove 'excessively disruptive' in school and on the streets amounts to a medical form of social control. These children are also said to run an increased risk of suffering stunted physical growth.

Away from the consulting rooms, speed's unpretentious efficiency made it a big favourite with washed-out flower children in the early and mid '70s, providing them with a physical and mental lift. From about 1975 it became popular with the dance-crazy Northern Soul crowd, and by the first and subsequent waves of punks who found they could pogo, spit and shout more fiercely on it and, of course, would no more be seen snorting that overpriced, bourgois stimulant cocaine than wear a Paul Smith suit. Amphetamine's staying power has also made it a winner in the smart London dance and record clubs. Meaty bikers appreciate it because it tells them they are Thor or Odin. Lads of the Heavy Metal ranks go for it for related reasons, although their traditional brew has been alcohol and/or barbiturates. It is an appealing drug for exam crammers and is also an acceptable 'hit' for those individuals who consider themselves neither young, deviant, in need of therapy nor part of the 'drug culture'. Such people needn't go to weird places for their purchase. It can be obtained from their local pub.

Sources

While there have been occasional batches of speed pills available, virtually all the amphetamine used since the early '70s up to the time of writing has been crude amphetamine sulphate. Much is manufactured in the London and Essex areas from raw materials bought or stolen from wholesalers. Certain biker bands are known to derive much of their income from this practice and will defend their business with bloody vigour. From Wiltshire, for instance, come reports of local bike gangs battling to keep heroin out of their area because, unlike speed, this is a drug they have no hope of commanding from source to street-level sale. Ugly scenes are anticipated since some of the gangs – to quote my local contact – are composed 'of the kind of "nail-your-head-to-the-floor" merchants from Monty Python. Unbelievably vicious and disgusting.'

· Establishing how much amphetamine sulphate is actually in circulation is an especially difficult task since most stocks are derived from 'precursor' chemicals obtained in this country. Where they are domestic in origin Customs has no chance of an interception. Nor can the pharmaceutical trade easily monitor how much is around since the purchase of a precursor from a supply house (which can be done across the counter without a licence) does not necessarily indicate that it will be converted into speed. Items such as perfumes and antibiotics call upon the same materials. The authorities' figures on seizures and raids therefore offer more of a clue to the authorities' diligence rather than how much speed is around – and by most anecdotal accounts the quantity is formidable. In a report to the UN Commission on Narcotics the government revealed it had detected 11 clandestine amphetamine laboratories during 1983. During that same year the police report they seized 22.6 kg, while Customs intercepted a further 12.3 kg. Provisional Customs figures for 1984 show their figure had topped 20 kg.

Tip-Off Signs

You can recognise an amphetamine user by the odd hours s/he keeps – up and bouncing for long periods and then marathon sessions of sleep from which s/he'll wake ravenously hungry and dispirited. Depending on how much is being used there will be unaccountable mood spasms: joyful and confident; anxious and irrational with outbreaks of temper. Heavy, long-term users, or those who are susceptible even at low doses, will express fears of being persecuted: *what's that noise? why is that person following me?* Then the panic will pass and you'll probably see another elevation of mood.

Coming Off

Most moderate users of amphetamine, whether snorters or tab takers, will face no great hardship if they decide to quit. In most cases their sleeping cycle is jarred and they'll have some depression accompanied by a sense of deprivation which soon passes. But those who have remodelled their lives to suit the pharmacological ups and downs of the drug can expect severe disruption. In the early stages there'll be a depression that has been known to lead to suicide. There could be such fatigue that much of the day will be taken up by sleep. Richard, referred to earlier, had a half-gram-a-week snorting habit that caused him to reprogramme each week into sleep and no-sleep portions. His habit developed over 18 months and it took exactly that time to recover.

'I woke up one day and decided I couldn't stand it any more. The person I was living with was also a speed freak and she got hit a lot harder by the psychological factors than I did. We decided to sort of quit together, which was extremely messy. Apart from informal advice from people I knew, I went to see my GP, who said he didn't know anything about it but gave me notes to stay off work, and prescribed a lot of vitamins. When we first stopped, the day consisted of getting up at five in the afternoon, just in time to go out and buy some groceries. I'd suddenly re-discovered this appetite for food. Then we'd stay up watching TV, listening to records and smoking dope until about one o'clock, and then fall over again. There was this complete lassitude and depression in the first couple of days. I don't think I've felt quite so low in my life. The way it was explained to me was that there was so much ampheta-mine in my body that it had almost packed up producing [structurally related] adrenalin, because it wasn't required. It had to adjust itself to naturally producing adrenalin again. The period was completely uncreative. I could hardly write. I could do virtually nothing, but what I would do was get up as early as possible, which effectively meant that after week two I was getting up at four instead of five, and a week or two after that, at noon. When I actually got to the point where eight hours' sleep was enough and I could get up at 9 a.m. I went back to work. This took about two months, but it was 18 months before I felt I was restored to the kind of human being I'd been before taking the speed.'

He admits to backsliding a couple of times, tempted by the demands of work, but he got through and is now ampheta-mine free. His new drugs of choice are hash, alcohol ('I drink more than I like') and the occasional nose of cocaine – though he 'wouldn't dream of buying or seeking it out.'

Help

Heavy users going through abrupt withdrawal should first settle their minds about what lies ahead; do their calculations as to whether they truly want to be rid of the drug and then guard against succumbing to the depression that will follow. They could do with help from a friend who understands what is happening. The problems of relapse and depression were emphasised in a key document produced in the 1970s by the government's Advisory Committee on Drug Dependence.[16] It warned doctors: 'The onset of depression [during withdrawal] may bring the risk of suicide. Attention must be given to the social and psychological factors which have led to the drug abuse. Follow-up of patients is essential as relapse is the rule rather than the exception if and when supplies of amphetamine become available. Some 6 to 12 months aftercare may be required, and it seems likely that some cases will require continuous psychiatric supervision and treatment.'

The Advisory Council's warning is legitimate although exaggerated as well as brutally mechanistic in language. It assumes practised speed users will be for the most part defeated and can only draw succour from the authorities. In fact, the best long-term 'cure' for amphetamine addiction is for the user to set about developing an improved opinion of him/herself. Friends and family can help generate this confidence by encouraging whatever piecemeal progress is achieved and by offering constructive assistance rather than keeping a morbid watching brief. Ultimately, the process is about seeing and believing in an amphetamine-free future.

Notes

1 T. Duquesne & J. Reeves, *A Handbook of Psychoactive Medicines*, Quartet, London, 1982, p. 217

2 M. Gossop, *Living With Drugs*, Temple Smith, London, 1982, p. 162
3 Ibid, p. 163
4 'The Amphetamines and LSD', Report by the Advisory Committee on Drug Dependence, London, 1970, p. 6
5 Cox *et al.*, *Drugs and Drug Abuse*, Addiction Research Foundation, Toronto, Canada, 1983, p. 161
6 *High Times Encyclopedia of Recreational Drugs*, Stonehill Press, New York, 1978, p. 237
7 'The Amphetamines and LSD' *op. cit.*, p. 8
8 Ibid
9 *High Times Encyclopedia of Recreational Drugs, op. cit.*
10 *Living With Drugs, op. cit.*, p. 164
11 *A Handbook of Psychoactive Medicines, op. cit.*, p. 218
12 Ibid, p. 277
13 'The Amphetamines and LSD', *op. cit.*, p. 15
14 Ibid
15 Ibid, p. 14
16 Ibid, p. 6

4 BARBITURATES

Intro

DRUG AGENCY workers are notoriously bashful about ranking recreational drugs in what might be called the League Table of Harm. They would argue that so much depends on the user's expectations, the environment in which they are used, plus a host of other factors ranging from personal body chemistry to the laws of chance. But when pressed a little, most of these workers will expose a deep abhorrence for the barbiturates. If ever there was a class of drug that in actual use has refuted much of what was claimed for it by the pharmaceutical industry, it is the barbiturates. Conceived as sedatives, they are capable of rousing furious and chaotic behaviour; as an aid to sleep, they might bring on slumber for the first two or three weeks, but then begin to suppress the normal sleep function, including dream sleep. Barbiturates are a favourite drug of suicides; they are practically the most lethal of all injected substances, and one of the most dangerous to withdraw from. Given the confused state of the UK's drug laws it will come as no surprise to learn that until January 1985 barbiturates were not considered dangerous enough to control under the Misuse of Drugs Act 1971, unlike virtually every other substance examined in this book. Now that they have been brought within the MDA's ambit, they have been placed in a class drawing moderate penalties for the punter and lax regulations for the professionals who prescribe and dispense them.

What Is It?

'Barbiturate' designates a substance derived from barbituric acid, which was discovered in 1864 following the unlikely marrying of urea, a principal component of urine, and malonic acid, a by-product of apples. Barbituric acid itself does not sedate, but many of its literally thousands of derivatives do. They are divided into three main groups according to the time they take to get absorbed by, work upon, and pass through the body. The first are called ultrashort-acting. They get their name because, being extremely soluble in fat, they quickly penetrate the fat-laden barrier to the brain where the sedation work takes place. They also quickly evacuate the brain, after which they are redistributed to other parts of the body. It is this talent for rapid brain entry and exit that makes this category attractive for quick surgical procedures or as 'softeners' for more substantial anaesthetics. The patient goes out and comes round within a few minutes of an injection. The traditional after-surgery grogginess is caused by the drug continuing to haunt the body in concentrations too low to induce sleep, but high enough to make the limbs feel leaden. Eventually it is metabolised by the liver and excreted unchanged through the kidneys. Because of their fast, incursive nature the rapid-acting type are rarely picked up by the recreational user.

At the other pole are the long-acting barbiturates. These circulate in the blood primarily in water soluble form and thus take longer to penetrate the brain's fatty defence. Because they are not easily picked up by muscle and body fats they carry on circulating through the blood in concentrations sufficient to keep the individual sedated or sluggish for 12–24 hours – and it can be many days after that before the drug is finally excreted. The slow, unexciting nature of the long-range type again makes them unappetising to pleasure seekers. They are prescribed chiefly to control epileptic seizures.

The barbiturate group that street users find irresistible are those in the short-to-intermediate range. These fall midway between the other two groups both in terms of speed of brain penetration and the duration of bodily hangover. Their 'effective duration' is said to be 6–8 hours and, depending on dosage, doctors issue them as sleepers (in 50 mg to 300 mg doses) and, now rarely, as daytime sedatives (at about 15 mg to 50 mg).

All barbiturates achieve their hypnosedative effects by depressing the central nervous system (CNS). But unlike the opiates, which also depress the CNS, they are not effective against pain. They might make the user sufficiently drowsy not to care, but they don't appear to lock on to the pain receptor sites deep inside the brain as do morphine and heroin (see page 205). Nonetheless, many heroin users consider them a valuable piece of weaponry to supplement their arsenals when supplies of the real thing run short.

Identifying the Products

Barbiturates come in a multiplicity of plain and coloured tablets, capsules and dry ampoules. The four leaders, as far as street users are concerned, are listed below.

Tuinal: This combines two barbituric acid derivatives, amylobarbitone sodium and quinalbarbitone sodium, in equal portions. It is made by Eli Lilly and comes in a red/blue capsule that is coded F65 (100 mg strength). Known informally as *Tueys, traffick lights*.

Tuinal was singled out for a special mention by the Committee on the Review of Medicines in its 1979 report,[1] saying it can lead to 'increased dependency and addiction potential' and a 'particularly high risk of abuse'. Tuinals are, indeed, the top-ranked street corner barb.

Nembutal: Made from pentobarbitone sodium by Abbott. Comes as a 100 mg yellow capsule which is marked with the maker's name and symbol. Known as *Nembies* or *yellows*.

Seconal: Another Lilly product, featuring quinalbarbitone sodium. Produced as an orange capsule in 50 mg (coded F42) and 100 mg (F40) doses. Known as *reds*, *sekkies*.

Amytal: Also from Lilly, made from amylobarbitone in five strengths. All are white tablets. T40 is 15 mg, T56 is 30 mg, T37 is 50 mg, T32 is 100 mg and U13 is 200 mg. There is also a Lilly amylobarbitone sodium compound at 200 mg, (coded U15) which comes as a white tab.

Other Hypnosedatives

The pharmaceutical industry will not rest until it has found a safe, non-addictive soporific. Consequently it has searched diligently for a barbiturate replacement since the 1950s. The most discredited – because of its massive appeal to the young – is methaqualone. This drug was first synthesised in India in 1951 as an anti-malarial agent. It was discovered that rats got sleepy on the stuff, and so it was swiftly introduced to the market as a hypnosedative. It reached Britain in 1965 where it was loudly advertised as a reliable cure for insomnia; a product that would cause no dependence and few of the toxic hazards associated with barbs. One product soon came to dominate – Mandrax. Mandrax juiced up the basic methaqualone formula with a sedative antihistamine known as diphenhydramine. By 1968 it was the most widely prescribed hypnotic in the UK, and just as big a hit on the streets where its quirky euphoriant high was much appreciated.

   The effects of methaqualone are close to those of barbiturate, but users claim that it is less inclined to dowse the spirits, more likely to lead to laughter and lovemaking. In New York City in the early '70s it was branded the *Love Drug*. The British pet name for Mandrax, apart from *Mandies*, was *Wallbangers*, a reference to their tendency to make the user oblivious to bumps acquired by walking into solid objects. (An acquaintance in Bristol tells me that he and his girlfriend used to play a game of seeing how many stairs they could jump down in a single bound. Neither of them ever felt pain – until the drug wore off.) In 1970 the authorities took fright at methaqualone's cult following and controlled it under the Drugs (Prevention of Misuse) Act, making possession and dealing without prescription an offence. A year later, when this statute was updated by the Misuse of Drugs Act, metha-qualone was listed in the least serious Class C category. In January 1985, however, it was upgraded to Class B in the MDA, alongside the newly-controlled barbiturates. Metha-qualone is today recognised as matching the destructive force of barbiturates on most levels, but it is perhaps marginally less hazardous to suddenly withdraw from, and its ability to depress respiration is not as great. But, like the barbs, it is a favourite drug to commit suicide with, and there is the same danger of plunging into the pit of increasing dosage combined with deepening melancholia. It is also hazardous for sufferers of epilepsy.

Though methaqualone is also a controlled drug in the US, it seems to be easily and massively available over there. The brand leader is Quaalude, and *Luding-out* is now a stock rock'n'roll phrase. Availability in the UK is at a low level and the new upgrading to Class B of the MDA is likely to choke off the already diminishing 'licit' channels. They some-times arrive from Europe as 250 mg or 275 mg tablets marked RL and MX, or as two-tone blue capsules similarly marked.

In addition to legal supplies there is an enormous traffic in underground methaqualone. Colombia is believed to be the world's leading manufacturer, using base materials originat-ing in Hungary and China. As a measure of the US's ap-petite, some 100 tonnes of the drug are believed to have illegally entered the country in 1980,[2] enough to make some 200 billion doses.

Sensations

Given that only the short-to-medium acting barbs are widely used in recreational circles these are the ones discussed below. Brands include Tuinal, Seconal, Amytal, and Nem-butal, which sell from 20p to 50p each. At small doses (usually one tab) they direct themselves at mental tension, producing tranquillity without too much drowsiness. When the dose is increased, the depressant effect spreads to all parts of the central nervous system and the inclination is to sleep. If this is resisted, the results are remarkably similar to a high intake of alcohol. In fact, loading up on barbs is just another way of getting drunk. Inhibitions are released, thinking and speech become clumsy, the limbs go numb, emotions soar and dive and there is a tendency to bounce into walls, fall off chairs, etc. While there can be spasms of sexual hunger, the body will be less likely to perk up as desired. Quarrelsomeness and spates of violence are common, so much so that of all drug cases that fall into hospital casualty departments, the barb user is the one most feared by staff. One-fifth, according to a mid-1970s survey,[3] behaved aggressively. The usual duration of the barb experience is three to six hours, which is followed by sleep and a thudding, alcohol-type hangover. But the experience can be terminal if enough is consumed, for as the dose goes up, the recipient will lurch into coma and death. All the sensations so far described increase markedly when alcohol is taken at the same time. And it is not just a question of calculating one plus the other. The net results are greater than the sum of the parts.

Health

The greatest danger from barb use is the relatively minor difference between the therapeutic and the lethal dose. Whereas a doctor might prescribe a 200 mg tablet for sleep, roughly ten times that amount can kill the patient – or at least send him/her to a dangerous overdose. There is an inbuilt enticement to reach a lethal level, for while tolerance to the intoxicant effects builds up quite quickly, a comparable resistance does not develop for the drug's depressant effects on the central nervous system. This means that as the user takes more of the stuff in an effort to retrieve an ever more elusive stoned feeling, the drug is banging down his/her respiration to, ultimately, a lethal level. The dose that finally breaks the user's back could be just one more 100 mg tab than was taken last time.

Injection

Injecting barbiturates brings all the familiar risks of septi-
caemia, collapsed veins, viral infections, AIDS, etc. However,
there is also a range of problems peculiar to barbs which rank
them among the most dangerous of all commonly injected
drugs. The main hazard comes when the needle user has spent
his/her easy-to-aim-at veins and turns to the femoral vein in
the groin. Since this corresponds closely to the femoral artery,
it is easy to hit the latter by mistake. Should this happen, the
barb will send it into spasm, causing a drastic loss of blood
supply to the leg below. 'Quite a few people', a doctor who
until recently was attached to a drugs agency tells me, 'have
had legs amputated as a result.' A similar outcome can derive
from hitting an artery in an arm.

Babies

Since barbiturates cross the placental wall, it is possible for a
child to be born dependent if the mother is using. The risk
to children is believed by some researchers to extend back to
the moment of conception (all drugs which affect anxiety
have been incriminated as possibly leading to malformed
offspring).[4] This could implicate either male or female
parent.

With Other Drugs

Doctors generally advise that barbiturates should not be
consumed together with alcohol or any other drug which
depresses the central nervous system. Each drug multiplies
the effects of the other. Barbs should also be avoided, they
say, with 'major' (otherwise known as neuroleptic) tranquillisers, certain anticoagulants, corticosteroids such as Corti-
sone, contraceptive pills and the anti-inflammatory drug
phenylbutazone.

With Other Conditions

Barbiturates are not recommended for people suffering
from severe liver disorders or respiratory problems, kidney

disease, prostate enlargement, hyperthyroidism, diabetes, severe anaemia, heart disease and raised pressure within the eye of the sort caused by glaucoma. They are also a problem to the elderly, increasing the risk of falls through grogginess, and hypothermia.

Overdose

When an overdose does come it will be signalled by a weak, rapid pulse, sweaty skin and breathing that is either very slow or rapid and shallow. In contrast to opiate poisoning there is no straight antidote to a barbiturate OD, but with quick treatment hospitals have enough in their kitbags to bring about a recovery.

Long-Term Health Problems

Problems of long-term use include pneumonia, because the cough reflex is suppressed, and hypothermia, because the normal responses to cold are blocked. There is also believed to be severe repression of dream or REM sleep. The consequences of this are not well understood, but it does appear that if the full quota isn't had, some psychological impairment can occur. This manifests itself during the day in symptoms ranging from vague restlessness to full-blown psychotic episodes. Some researchers believe that if REM sleep is cut down for other than short periods a phenomenon known as 'REM rebound' occurs. REM rebound is said to equal 'intense, often horrifying nightmares.'

Addiction

There are real physical and psychological incentives to continue dosing on barbiturates, and if the supply is abruptly withdrawn, both physical and mental trauma sets in. The time it takes to get barb-dependent varies according to the constitution of the user. However, it seems very few are resilient beyond an 800 mg daily dose taken for a couple of months.

The physical incentives to reach towards such levels are the sort that spring from the use of most other mind-altering drugs whose effects not only diminish as the body builds up a tolerance, but cause real discomfort unless there is an increase in dosage. The momentum towards higher doses that comes from psychological factors is also considerable. Barbiturates are usually acquired, whether from doctor or dealer, to provide an emotional lift. While they might do this in the short term, on a medium to long-term basis they will heighten anxiety and depression. The tendency then is to take more, which sends the user deeper into the trough from which the apparent escape is more drugs: after all, curing the blues is their stated function. In this way not a few individuals have been caught in a downward spiral which has ended either in accidental overdose or suicide.

Earliest Use

The development of barbituric acid derivatives since the 1920s is an example of science's search for the safe, non-addictive agent to calm the human spirit. At the time there was room for a promising new item. Opium, in the form of laudanum, had been discredited as an all-purpose tranquilliser, and ethyl alcohol, chloral hydrate and paraldehyde were also proving problematic after initial great expectations.

Yet to be unfrocked were the bromides, which, since the 1850s, had been sold in the form of inorganic salts. Like barbiturates, they were also prescribed for sleep and daytime sedation, but their prime function was in the management of epilepsy. It was believed then that the root cause of certain forms of epilepsy was masturbation. Since it appeared that potassium bromide reduced the sexual drive, and thus the need to manhandle the private organs, it followed that the drug would help alleviate the seizures. And this it did, but not, we have to assume, because it quelled sexual fervour, rather for its ability to depress general CNS functioning. Bromides were still considered the efficient fix until the 1950s when the phenomenon known as bromism was finally recognised. It was caused by the body's painfully slow action in breaking down and excreting the drug. Symptoms included trembling, delirium and rashes that could cover the entire body.

Just as bromides began dipping in popularity, the barbiturates were lifting off as the hypnosedative of medical choice. By the '60s there were literally hundreds of them in an array of sizzling shapes, colours and sizes. By 1971 English doctors were handing out an annual 12.9 million prescriptions, even though the United Nations in that same year proposed that barbs, along with certain other psychotropic (mind-altering) drugs, should be more strictly controlled.

Policy

The UN proposals were embodied in what was called the Convention on Psychotropic Substances, which required the consent of forty member countries before it took on legitimacy.[5] These were forthcoming in 1976, and the countries concerned then set about implementing the new measures through their own domestic legislation. Along with most other developed nations, Britain held back from signing – a reluctance that still survives, even though in January 1985 she took most of the necessary measures for controlling barbiturate use that would allow her to sign. Why the continued standoffishness? The British case is one of financial logic. To agree to the 1976 Convention proposals would mean the elimination of unnecessary and unhealthy prescribing, and while barb prescription totals have sunk to such levels that would permit ratification, there is now the problem of a voluminous traffic ('licit') in tranquillisers. The UN is just beginning to get interested in the enormous worldwide business in these psychotropics, and has set in motion the first of a series of (so far) mild controls. For Britain to ratify now could subsequently mean having to beat down 'trank' traffic to levels the pharmaceutical trade would never countenance.

The reluctance of Britain and other Western nations to conform to the guidelines of the Psychotropic Convention can be contrasted with their relative enthusiasm for internationally agreed controls on the 'narcotic drugs' (opium, cannabis, cocaine) that are mainly produced by Third World countries. The message here is that substances made by the West are 'medicines', whose free flow through 'licit' channels are tampered with at the peril of the 'patient'. Those substances emanating from the Third World are 'dangerous drugs', with no redeeming value.

With barbiturate-linked deaths in the UK rising to 2,000 per annum by the early '70s, even doctors were disposed to rethink. In 1975 the Campaign on The Use and Restriction of Barbiturates (CURB) was undertaken by a group of eminently well-placed specialists who barracked members of their own profession for wanton prescribing of 'these outdated drugs . . . which are now killing far more people than heroin.' By then they accounted for more than half of all fatal poisonings – something like 27,000 lives between 1959 and 1974.[6] At the same time as CURB was going to the loudhailer, the Committee on the Review of Medicines (CRM) was also casting its eye over the barbiturates. In 1979 came their assessment.[7] Under normal circumstances barbiturates (they then named all those being issued at the time as sleepers, anti-anxiety agents and sedatives) should not be used in any medical treatment of the following groups: children and young adults; the elderly and debilitated; women who are pregnant or breastfeeding; patients with a history of alcohol or drug abuse. In the end the only use the Committee could find for the drugs was in the treatment of 'intractable insomnia'. It also warned about the 'potentially fatal' withdrawal symptoms which could occur on abrupt cessation in all ages, and was scathing about the 134 combination drugs in which barbiturates were but one constituent, declaring that it might revoke licences for such preparations. Most manufacturers now seem to have found alternative formulae.

Prescription totals were already tumbling by the time of the CRM report – down to 9.5 million in 1974, to 5.1 million in 1978, and even lower to 2.5 million during 1980. (Government statisticians no longer give separate barb figures.) Doctors were switching to the new benzodiazepines (Valium, Librium, etc.) and since these new agents were far more expensive than barbiturates the drug companies were not exactly itching to keep the outmoded barb deployed any longer than was embarrassingly necessary. They didn't even baulk at proposals to control them under the Misuse of Drugs Act. The biggest whine came from chemists who feared they'd have to lock up these low-yield drugs in expensive safe storage to prevent their robbery.

Patterns of Use

Barbs landed on the streets in a big way during the mid '60s when they were combined with amphetamine in a famous combination called *Purple Hearts* (Drinamyl). The *Purple Heart* rage was essentially the beginning of the mass street drugs scene (discounting alcohol and tobacco). It was the first elephantine kick for youth, the first piece of intensive tutoring about what drugs are and how their effects call for mastery and respect. Some learnt. Some didn't. The authorities tried to come to grips with the fad, but their angle of attack was at the racy amphetamine, as though the barbiturate part of *Hearts* was of no consequence. In fact the barb element was considered essential by consumers to avoid jagging out on a diet of pure speed.

New controls quite soon put a stop to the wide availability of Drinamyl, but not to the taste. Within a few years a 'licit' pill with almost identical effects was on the market called Durophet-M (see page 78). Although this too was deleted in 1981, there are now countless other ways of acquiring the up/down fix; the combination has become a permanent feature of the drugs culture.

Barbiturates are popular on the Manchester club scene, into whose virtually free all-night joints recession kids pour several nights a week charged up with snorted amphetamine sulphate (known locally as *gear*). It helps them get on with their furious jazz dancing. On the way home, still charged up, they'll swallow a barb such as Tuinal, which allows them to present themselves back home in a credibly worn condition. They might even get some sleep in what remains of the night. This is a comparatively softcore use of the drug.

Up a couple of notches, barbiturates also appeal to classic speed freaks – that is to say, to those whose preferred fix is an armful of amphetamine sulphate. If speed is injected, it usually follows that the barbiturate will also be injected. This might be done simultaneously or when the individual is in need of 'cooling out'. Conversely, there are 'barb freaks' who use speed to bring them up from a drowsy low. But soon it is difficult to tell the cart from the horse; a barb addict using speed or a speed addict using barb? Since there are often a variety of other drugs being thrown down, such as alcohol, cannabis, tranquillisers, the only statement that can be made with certainty is that on such a terrain there are few substance purists. Instead, there are varying states of physical and mental disrepair which the user attempts to redress by what-ever apparently appropriate remedy comes to hand.

Historically, however, speed is an older street drug than the barbiturates. The latter came along as its companion or its remedy. Indeed there is a fairly well-trodden path from speed, not simply through to barbs, but from there on to heroin. It works like this: after a spell of injecting barbiturates to counteract the violence of the amphetamine experience, the user starts suffering from the chemical characteristics of the downer drug. Painful abscesses develop where the needle misses a vein, killing the pleasure the barbs are supposed to offer. So the speed user starts looking elsewhere to relieve him/herself. S/he alights upon a downer drug that is poten-tially less 'filthy', but in any case brings with it (short-term) painkilling properties. Such a drug is heroin.

The speed-to-junk-via-barbs route is most easily spotted when looking at the punk fallout of the late '70s/early '80s. British punks got po-going in 1976, selecting no-nonsense speed as their Number One drug because it gave them the chemical zest to stay the hard, sharp course. But as punk withered and its exponents either cleaned up or got more frenetic, barbs came more into their own. The peak of the uptake occurred from 1981 to mid 1982 when such drugs were *the* sought-after item on the London Piccadilly scene. One support agency worker told me that six of his teenaged clients died from barbs during this period, five of them girls, one of whom walked sleepily into a bus.

To meet the demands of the barb epidemic a special centre was set up in North London called City Roads. Though not exclusively for barbiturate consumers, some 85 per cent of their early traffic were registering this drug as their main problem. Today, in keeping with the line we are plotting, it is heroin that gets the most 'mentions'. One young man who ran the speed-to-barbs-to-junk course is a fellow I met at City Roads early in 1983 called Eric. Eric's drug career began five years earlier following a family trauma he didn't care to talk about. Conflict developed at home, and after being kicked out, he moved into a squat with some older 'hippy types' who helped him score hash and amphetamine sulphate.

It was not long before he'd moved on to barbiturates and started overdosing regularly. Then it was on to fixing heroin and Diconal. The gap between himself and the hippies widened to the point where he had to move into another squat with an equally dismantled friend. They set about establishing a network of easy-going GPs from whom to coax drugs, and partly supported themselves with burglaries. By degrees things got uglier. A friend was stabbed to death by a couple of teds and, 'before it was too late,' Eric called upon City Roads. Of that first time he says 'the counselling wasn't a lot of help, but they were all nice here. I could see they were trying to help me. I suppose I went out a bit more open-minded. But then I got in with me mates and, you know, I've been coming in and out ever since. This is my twelfth call here in less than a year.' But this time, he swore, he was now that much more determined to stop; for his new girlfriend. The last reports I got were promising.

At the same time that barbs were hitting the West End of London, they were also appearing in towns such as Bradford where in addition to punk fallout there is a particularly severe recessionary frost. Bradford's social erosion goes back nearly 30 years to when many local industries began collapsing. Prior to late 1980, £1 used to buy three or four barbs in a pub. Then suddenly there was a rash of chemist break-ins and they were going for £1 for 100. In a letter to the music paper, *New Musical Express*, a young local poet, Joolz Denby, reported 'children of 14, 15, 16 hurtling headlong to death by their pathetic ignorant use of barbiturates, especially Tuinal. In the last 18 months we have had many in hospital with colossal overdoses, three in intensive care. They seem to regard this as some kind of a test of street credibility, of how cool they can be. A hospital overdose bracelet is the latest fashion. They flirt with death as if it was nothing.' When I checked back in late 1983, Bradford's young were still doing barbiturates, but now it was more common to inject rather than to swallow them, and since that time heroin has reached town.

Though we have been examining the speed-through-barbs-to-heroin syndrome, this is only one of an incalculable number of patterns. Once a person starts loading up heavily on any sort of drug there is little incentive to remain a purist. Thus, while some people mount and dismount barbiturates on their way to a 'superior' kick, others reserve a central place for them. Equally, people latch on to heroin without ever having tried another drug, and once the heroin habit is acquired they might then turn 'backwards' to barbiturates for relief during heroin shortages. A particularly large number of people use barbs together with alcohol for an extremely ribald high. It is due primarily to the unappealing spectacle of drunken barbheads that the drug has achieved its gutter reputation among the great mass of conventional drug users. For drug moderates, barbiturates are for the headbanging lunatic fringe. They are about falling off chairs and squaring up to innocents. No doubt, because of such a reputation, barbs will continue to be cherished by those who feel themselves cut off from more wholesome options.

Controls

The new laws against possession of barbiturates are a logical consequence of increasing worries about their wide availability. But apart from criminalising another drug group, the penalties are unlikely to have any lasting impact on usage. A likely effect is that some foul and extremely noxious compounds and pseudo varieties will quickly blossom in home labs to compensate for the reduction in official supplies.

Some twenty barbituric acid derivatives find themselves with a class B ranking under the Misuse of Drugs Act, along with cannabis, codeine, Preludin, Ritalin and amphetamines. Although barbiturate penalties are medium tough, the constraints placed upon chemists are outrageously slack. Instead of being required to lock them away in safe, locked storage boxes, they are being permitted to stash them in a place of their own choosing. It was argued that to include them in safe storage would involve enlarging the special cabinets, and for a drug that retailed so cheaply, it just wasn't worth it. Given that most barbiturates, prior to criminalisation, were finding their way on to the black market via chemist thefts, the new policy seems bereft of logic.

The requirements placed upon doctors are tougher. A prescription has to be in the physician's own handwriting, and for clarity's sake words as well as figures must be used when stating quantities. But the handwriting requirements are relaxed on long-acting phenobarbitone since this is a drug used heavily by thousands of epilepsy sufferers, and not one generally of interest to pleasure seekers. If a person can demonstrate to a pharmacist that s/he suffers from the condition, s/he can still get the drug without a prescription. Other measures control imports and exports. There is also moderate tightening-up for hospitals. But the gap that remains unplugged – in addition to the slack lock-up rules for chemists – is in the supply of the base material that goes to make up the drug. There are chemical suppliers that will still sell an individual all that is required without asking to see a licence or authority. While these suppliers are encouraged to closely 'liaise' with the Home Office, a person with the right credentials, say an employee in the drugs industry, is quite capable of making a safe purchase.

Coming Off

Physical withdrawal symptoms can be eased considerably by special treatment (details of which can be had from a doctor or local drugs advisory agency). Without it, sudden cessation of the drug will produce a range of symptoms that, again, depend on how much has been used, for how long, and general bodily repair. Typically, they start within 12–24 hours of the last dose and involve shakiness, anxiety and inability to sleep. At a more profound level there might be fluctuations in blood pressure, fever, seizures and *delirium tremens* (DTs). The most dangerous time is between one and three days after the cut-off point. During this time it is possible for death to occur, although it is rare, and usually only happens when vomit is inhaled during a seizure. Once over this peak, all physical symptoms should gradually clear. Then there comes the more lingering business of patching those parts that are in psychological/emotional disrepair.

It is worth restating that barbiturates are one of the most dangerous of all recreational drugs to inject. They also cause particularly savage problems when a dependent person's supply is abruptly withdrawn. This is not an advertisement to ensure plentiful stocks, but a recommendation that special help be sought from a doctor if withdrawal – voluntary or compulsory – starts up. It is also worth being very cautious about any unknown substance passing itself off as a barbiturate. Now that they have been controlled under the Misuse of Drugs Act, encouraging a drop in prescription rates, the chance of disgusting concoctions reaching the streets is greatly increased.

Notes

1 'Recommendations on Barbiturate Preparations', Committee on the Review of Medicines, *British Medical Journal*, 22.9.1979, vol. 2, pp. 719–720

2 A. McNicoll, *Drug Trafficking: A North-South Perspective*, North/South Institute, Ottawa, Canada, 1983

3 A. H. Ghodse, 'Drug Dependent Individuals Dealt With by London Casualty Departments'. *British Journal of Psychiatry*, 1971, vol. 131, pp. 273–280

4 'Barbiturates in Obstetrics and Gynaecology', Campaign on the Use and Restriction of Barbiturates (CURB), April 1980

5 'Barbiturates – from Valuable Medicine to Dangerous Drug', *Druglink*, Institute for the Study of Drug Dependence, Spring 1979

6 Ibid

7 'Recommendations on Barbiturate Preparations', *op. cit.*

5 CANNABIS

Intro

CANNABIS IS by far the most dangerous of all the recreational drugs in its effects upon the authorities. By continuing to penalise it as a dangerous substance, despite a lack of supporting evidence, they are left politically without a stitch. There is no substantial medical case against moderate use by adults any more – not even from the World Health Organisation. And neither does the general public succumb to the old dark invocations about brain damage, deformed births or the rocky road to heroin addiction. Cannabis is just as likely to lead to a pinstriped job in the City as to subterranean junkiedom.

An indication of just how rapidly the dope phenomenon has grown can be learned from the 1969 edition of Peter Laurie's very readable *Drugs*.[1] He notes that cannabis is 'now probably the most widespread illicit drug in the United Kingdom, with 30,000 regular users.'

The up-to-date, regular-user figure is now put at around 2½ million. The drug agency, Release, believe the number of individuals actually involved in various levels of street dealing to be around 40,000.

Even if these figures take the truth and double it, the authorities are still left with an extremely damaging situation. A law that is ignored by so many millions may be called a bad law. At the heart of the lawlessness there is organised trafficking involving the transport of perhaps 600 tonnes of material annually worth £1 billion or more. These levels provide the ready elements of large-scale corruption of officialdom. We can see what has happened to Bolivia and Colombia as a result of a vast underground cocaine trade. Sections of the public are complicit; cocaine has made such a hole in their economies, the coke barons can literally make and unmake governments.

This is clearly not the scale or even the flavour of the UK cannabis market, but neither is it safe to assume that because there are no overt signs officials are not being baited and bribed. This is all some way from the 'evangelical' epoch of the late '60s and early '70s when hippies would meander over to North Africa or the Indian sub-continent to procure a pound or two of hashish for a few friends. Today the market is judged to be governed by harder, more organised people who have access to sealed juggernauts, large, specially adapted seacraft, and to a pool of willing 'mules' who do the physical hauling and invariably take the legal rap when things go wrong. The men who control them will have links with professional groups in other countries – the Sicilian and Neopolitan Mafias, the Corsican gangs of France – and will probably be shifting heroin too. The difference between heroin and cannabis, however, is that whereas the first is a drug at which the majority scowl, the case against cannabis is less clear.

And so what options do the authorities have? They can slacken up on criminal penalties, which has already happened in many countries in Europe, and even contemplate some kind of licensed distribution, which could reap millions in extra tax. Or they can seek to justify the existing penalties by ever more closely scrutinising the medical surveys for helpful glimmers.

Both options have their problems. To back off might, it is feared, signal that the UK is soft on drugs – which no government of whichever complexion wants to contemplate. However, to press on with the argument that cannabis is a dangerous narcotic loses the authorities more credibility with those millions who believe they've got the drug's measure. It also makes a hash of the law. For with so many millions at odds with it, the law cannot be applied systematically, only selectively – which in practice has meant against suspect groups like the young unemployed and young black males, for many of whom 'herb' smoking is practically sacramental.

What Is It?

Cannabis is the name the international regulatory agencies give to the group of intoxicating products derived from *Cannabis sativa*, a green and bushy plant with saw-toothed leaves, fluted stalks, ranging in height from 3–20 feet. It is the male that produces the tough fibres from which hemp rope is made, the female which generates the sticky aromatic resins. Most of the resin is exuded from the flowering tops, but some is also found in the leaves. Botanists have argued that there are two more distinct cannabis species other than *sativa* – one they call *Cannabis indica* and the other *Cannabis ruderalis*. The first is the finely formed and extremely potent plant originating in India. The second is the tough, stocky type that has traditionally grown wild by the roadside in central Asia, whose seeds are capable of surviving icy Russian winters. As far as the US Federal Bureau of Narcotics is concerned, there is just one cannabis species, *sativa*, and its seeds, wherever in the world they might be planted, will eventually acclimatise and assume the characteristics of the local variety.

The cannabis product most often found in the UK is the caked resin of North African plants that comes in slabs, chunks, sticky balls or powdery flakes and is called *hashish*. Here it is smoked, but in its home regions it is often eaten in a spiced, fruity confection called *majoon*. In India hash is known by its Hindu word – *charas*. The other domestically consumed cannabis product is made up of the dried and chopped leafy parts of the plant. It is home-grown or imported from as far afield as the West Indies and Africa. Many are its names: *ghanja* , *ganga*, *marijuana*, *draw*, *blow*, *weed*, *grass*, *dope*, *bush* . . . Most people know it as an unpredictable mix of sticks, seeds, leaves and flowering tops, but some fine distinctions are made. For instance, *ghanja* and marijuana are apparently not the same thing at all. Marijuana should be devoid of seeds and twigs, whereas *ghanja* can have everything thrown in.

There are several more cannabis variables, but these are rarely found on the streets of the UK. There is, for instance, *bhang*, which is the leaves of the plant pounded into a fine powder, spiced and brewed into a beverage like tea. *Bhang* also refers to a smoking mixture of leaves plus stems and twigs – complicated?

Five times more concentrated than the resin is *hash oil*, also known as *honey oil*. This is made by boiling finely powdered hash in a solvent such as alcohol and straining out the cellulose solids. The solvent then evaporates, leaving behind a sticky greeny/brown oil. This can be further refined down to colourless, tasteless tetrahydrocannabinol (THC) which is the plant's main psychotropic ingredient.

First isolated in the 1940s, it was not until 1966 that THC was first reproduced synthetically. Since then it has yielded up somewhere between 35 and 80 derivatives (accounts differ). Several are being used experimentally for the treatment of drug withdrawal, depression, anxiety and convulsions.

It is not generally realised that until 1973 one of the most potent products of the plant was available on general prescription in the UK, chiefly for 'exploring psychiatric states.'[2] Known – like the plant species – as *Cannabis indica*, it came as a green tincture or as a green extract. Both comprised the flowering tops of the best Indian cannabis, pounded, sifted and treated with alcohol. One London man tells me his doctor prescribed it for him 'to relieve the paranoia that overcame me at the thought of being busted for possession of illegal dope.' In fact the prescription of medical cannabis goes back to the mid-nineteenth century, when it was considered the standard treatment for migraine.

Source Countries

The Lebanon

The Lebanon has been an important source of hash from earliest times. Civil war in that country has failed to disrupt production, indeed it has jumped from a 200 tonne annual output prior to the hostilities, to something in excess of 2,000 tonnes.[3] Egypt gets the choice resins, with much of the remainder being directed at Europe. Lebanese resin now outsells any other in the UK.

Production is concentrated in the Bekaa valley in the north of the country. Plots vary from a backyard acre to vast expanses run by those such as the 6,000-strong Jaffra family. Some 80 per cent of the dry and dusty upper Bekaa and the hills of Hermil are planted with *C. sativa*, providing a livelihood for perhaps two-thirds of the region's 100,000 inhabitants.[4] A good deal of what reaches Europe is believed to exit via the Syrian capital of Damascus, and is then moved through Budapest, Rome or Amsterdam. Various professional organisations employ a variety of modes such as air freight, sealed trucks, yachts and container ships. Since the murder of the Christian Phalangist leader Bashir Gamayel (believed to have been the major trafficker in the area) the aforementioned Jaffra family seem to have risen to prominence. Magazine writer Michael Kienitz describes[5] a visit to their estate and factory off the main highway out of Ba'labakk. He saw a lush fortress bristling with microwaves and Sony Trinitrons, plus an anti-aircraft gun mounted in the living room. A family elder told Kienitz of deals done with Soviet and American secret service agents and that the key to the family's success was the way they have standardised production. Every half-kilo slab is stamped with the family's seal – one year a star of David, the next the logo from the American Express card. Quality is guaranteed, and thus they have stopped the family's front parlour from being crowded out with gangsters from all parts of the world, haggling over whether they'd been fairly treated.

Morocco

Morocco is the second biggest supplier of resin to the UK, supplying some 30 per cent of the market. Cultivation is centred in the Rif Mountains on mainly small plots. As many as 150,000 people derive all or part of their income from the trade.[6] The country's total production per annum is put at between 50 and 65 tonnes. Native middlemen strike a deal on the grower's own property and then sell off to foreign tourists or, increasingly, to professionals.

Pakistan and Afghanistan

Afghanistan is famed for producing both quality grass as well as a black, sticky hashish that is prized above most others in the UK. Neighbouring Pakistan is another source of the once ubiquitous black: its street price has risen from £12 to £100 an ounce since 1969. Both countries have been supplanted in Europe by The Lebanon, but the professionals have found a lucrative alternative with heroin.

India

No longer an important UK supply point for hash. Along with Thailand, India supplies Asia and the Far East.

Colombia

During the '70s, this nation reputedly became the world's leader in marijuana production, benefiting in the most spectacular way after the US got the Mexican government to spray its own land with paraquat where marijuana was thought to be growing. Until that time Mexico had been America's main supplier. In recent years, however, Colombia has also suffered a financial penalty due to the massive growth of American home growing. This home-grow phenomenon has a limit. Experts believe the US will never be able to produce much more than 10 per cent of her own needs without attracting domestic paraquat spraying (pilot schemes are already under way).

Jamaica

In 1974 the US took a personal hand in trying to demolish the Jamaican *ghanja* trade with a 'search-and-destroy' programme called Operation Buccaneer. It included the use of American helicopters, and the erection of pillars along the sides of the main roads on the north coast which were intended to bust the wings of *ghanja* planes trying to use the highways as landing strips.

Cannabis cultivation is big in Jamaica. According to a

report by the North/South Institute[7] it is the country's main cash crop and possibly the most important source of foreign currency. From an export volume of about 800 tonnes in 1978, production is believed to have risen to 4,800 tonnes in 1981. The UK, together with the US, takes the greatest share, which helps to support some 8,000 farmers who depend on the crop for their livelihood. Most of these growers operate small plots in the valleys of the Blue Mountain area. This land once bore small banana, coffee and cocoa plantations, but the local farmers report they can no longer compete with the large estates. Making the cannabis connection with foreign customers works at both the tourist and the professional level.

South of the Sahara

The considerable returns from cannabis against cash crops such as coffee or bananas have drawn several newcomers into the dope market. Among those nations south of the Sahara tipping their hat are Kenya, Lesotho, Nigeria, Swaziland and South Africa.[8]

Home-Grown

There are no reports of commercial hash production in the UK, but the domestic industry is developing steadily as ordinary consumers learn how relatively easy it is to husband quality weed. It can be done under lights indoors, in window boxes, on farmland, and even on high, stony ground where few ever venture. Virtually any type of seed can be used since the progeny will quickly adapt to local conditions, but starting with seeds from a quality batch is an advantage.

Exotica

Aside from the above-listed standard fare for UK consumption, there is a whole range of cannabis products which rarely turn up commercially in this country, or having once visited briefly, have since flown. In the latter category are *Tibetan Temple Balls* – dark, soft nuggets from the Chinese-occupied realm of the Dalai Lama. A more lingering item is the *Thai Stick* – an extremely potent herbal cannabis tied by hemp fibres to a stick. The 'stick' formula is now used for other grasses to kid the consumer s/he is purchasing a quality product.

Another rare grass is the seedless *sinsemilla* made from the unpollinated flowers of the female plant. It resembles *Thai*, but without the stick, and is said to be extremely elevating. Rarer still are the high-powered Colombian grasses, *Chiba* and *Gold*; and *Oaxacan Red* from Mexico (rated Number One in the *High Times* Top 40). Then there are the famous blasts from Hawaii – *Maui*, *Oahu* and *Maui Wowee*, *Surfboards* from Afghanistan, *Moon Discs* from Kanhairi, *Finger Clusters* from the Himalayas and *Pellet Rubbings* from Nepal. There is no end to the varieties in which this most uncommon weed materialises.

Buying It

The amateur trafficker will probably deal in no more than one-kilo blocks of grass or half-kilo blocks of hashish at a time. S/he'll likely be purchasing – whether direct from source country or from a bigger UK trafficker – on behalf of a cooperative venture. The professional might import literally tons at a time if, say, a yacht or a sealed truck is available. On the street, hash is bought 'blind' in clingfilm-wrapped £5 or £10 deals. Purchasers of bigger quantities will generally be able to examine the material to check its quality. At the time of writing the price of one ounce of 'black' was hovering around the psychologically testing £100 mark. Grass is also bought blind and generally comes wrapped in newspaper. One ounce costs £60–£70, home-grown usually cheaper.

Methods of Ingestion

Every conceivable route has been used for getting cannabis into the body. It can be eaten in a sweet or savoury concoction, or drunk in tea or other beverages, but smoking is the method employed by those wanting to partake of the intoxicants most efficiently. In the UK this usually involves rolling a *joint* or *spliff* from several cigarette papers stuck together. It will contain tobacco sprinkled with heat-softened resin or a quantity of grass. The ratio of grass to tobacco is usually two to one in favour of the tobacco. For a hash joint, a pellet the size of a barley grain will suffice. Joints are often completed with a half-inch-long rolled cardboard filter.

Both hash and grass are also smoked in pipes. The types include clay *chillums*, brass *grill tops* and the venerable *hookah* which cools and softens the smoke by passing it through a channel of water. Blobs of hash can also be balanced on the hot end of a cigarette and the snake of smoke inhaled straight through the mouth or via a ballpoint casing. These pellets can also be heated on a sheet of foil and the smoke sucked up, or they can be clamped between hot knives, the smoke trapped in a milk bottle and sucked up in an enormous gust.

Unlike cigarette fumes, cannabis smoke is not carelessly blown around the room. It is inhaled deeply into the lungs and held there for several seconds. This often causes the novice to erupt in a violent cough, but the lungs eventually learn how to cope with the experience and veteran smokers are even able to talk, though in a faintly silly voice, while holding the fumes deep inside them.

Sensations

The specifics of the cannabis experience can't easily be set down. This is not simply because of the great range of resins or because of each person's varied response, but because, almost above any other drug, cannabis is supremely responsive to the flickering of human emotions, more so even than the Big Gun hallucinogens such as LSD and Liberty Cap. Mood and environment are rarely discussed in regard to cannabis, because it is rated a 'soft drug'. Yet, while it does not create LSD's big psycho bang, it does create alterations in feelings and perceptions that can be profound. In fact so soft is the drug's reputation it is inadmissible in certain 'experienced' circles to show any outward sign of being affected.

Smoking

Smoking a couple of grains of medium-quality hash mixed with tobacco will less forcefully enter the brain than gulping a lungful of same via the hot knives method. But however it is inhaled, no smoker will have to wait more than about ten minutes if the resin or grass has anything to offer. The initial feelings depend on the quality of the cannabis. Hash is often more immobilising, although there are certain grasses that are capable of pinning the user to the floor after just a couple of 'tokes'. More usually there will be feelings of uninhibitedness, dreaminess, heightened awareness of sound, colour, textures. Music will probably sound more magnificent than usual. Hidden layers and meanings can be revealed and there'll be an impulse to utter profundities, to giggle, and eat a great deal.

Younger, less repressed smokers can close their eyes and witness, for instance, vivid cartoon hallucinations. The communion between fellow smokers is often powerful. Intimacies, both sexual and mental, might occur. Higher doses and/or heavier blends lead to paralysis of the imagination and reluctance to move a single limb.

Eating

While smoking provides almost instantaneous effects, eating hash or grass can take ninety minutes to become noticeable. The results come on stealthily, sometimes deepening beyond what the user desires. A hash smoker who has had too much simply stops toking. A hash eater might already have eaten too much without knowing it and yet continues to fill up. The edible high is often described as more of a 'body experience'. There will more likely be sub-LSD type hallucinations, with objects swelling and shrinking.

But the idea that leaves and sticks can be steeped in water and the resulting solution washed down for the kind of effects described above is unequivocally put down by the cannabis gourmand Adam Gottlieb in his pocket book, *Cooking With Cannabis*.[9] 'If the plant is good quality,' says Gottlieb, 'strenuous boiling might encourage some resin to float off into the water, but this is wildly inefficient.' Gottlieb goes on to claim: 'THC, the active substance in grass and hash, is not soluble in water, but in oils, fats and alcohol. Thus, before combining it with whatever other ingredients are to be used, it should first be either soaked or boiled in alcohol; sautéed or boiled in butter; or combined heated or unheated with an oil/water emulsion such as milk.'

Paranoia

This crops up regularly among dope smokers and is often caused by an inability to relax. It might also be an acquired problem since many long-term users – whatever their disposition – find themselves going into the state from the first inhalation. Bad adulterants are also thought to cause paranoia. It is believed that camel dung is sometimes mixed in with Moroccan resin, while South African grass has been known to contain *datura* – a less marketable psychoactive plant that is renowned as a stupefying agent and poison. *Datura* is one likely cause of what drug professionals call Cannabis Psychosis (CP).

No Effects

In a percentage of resistant individuals cannabis has no psychoactive effects at all. For some it produces nausea. One young woman reports that it did nothing at all for her except it 'made me lose control of my bladder so that I weed myself.'

Regular Use

A large proportion of cannabis users consume it on a regular, even daily, basis, and as a consequence tend to live in a fog. In especially heavy users the fog becomes so thick as to cut off a sharp appreciation of 'reality'. For such users, nights are dreamless, or can be dreamless. It is as though the daytime use of the drug is depleting their finite dream stocks. When the drug is cut off there will usually follow a 'dream rebound' – a bombardment of all the fantastical and perhaps scary dream imagery which the nights had for so long been starved of.

Impact on Health/The WHO Report

In the past fifteen years there have been numerous substantive reviews of cannabis and its general impact on human health. As consequential as anything yet issued was the report[10] that arose out of a meeting in Toronto during the winter of 1981. Chaired by the Canadian Addiction Research Foundation and the World Health Organisation, the resulting document doesn't exactly clear up all the loose ends (the *realpolitik* of drugs research requires ambiguity) but it does have something to say on how cannabis is received and conducted through every imaginable part of the body. Its main findings are as follows:

General Toxicity

Intermittent use of low-potency material doesn't generally produce obvious symptoms of toxicity. Daily or more frequent use, especially of the highly potent preparations, can produce a 'chronic intoxication' taking weeks to clear after drug use is discontinued.

Respiratory System

Cannabis smoke appears to be more injurious to the lungs than cigarette smoke, and hashish (resin) smoke is worse than herbal (grass). Possible consequences are bronchitis and, 'after sufficient exposure', lung cancer.

Heart

Little evidence of a toxic effect on the heart muscles, but users with pre-existing heart disease risk compromising that organ further.

Growth and Body Weight

No reliable data.

Gastro-Intestinal

May produce vomiting, diarrhea and 'abdominal distress'. Chronic use could make the intestine more susceptible to infection.

Chromosomal Damage

Studies to date show no cell abnormality or mutagenic effects attributable to cannabis.

Cancer

'Analysis of cannabis smoke, animal studies and one clinical report suggest that cannabis may have significant carcinogenic potential.' Cannabis tar (the dark, sticky substance that forms as the smoke cools and condenses) is considered the chief culprit, and while no evidence of cannabis-induced cancer in humans exists, it could show up in the future.

Immune System

The body's natural defence systems play a major role in defending it against infection and preventing the growth and spread of malignant cells. There is only 'suggestive, but not conclusive' evidence that consumption of cannabis or THC may produce immune dysfunction.

Allergic Potential

It has some, although it appears 'uncommon'.

The Male Reproductive System

Animal tests indicate 'prolonged intake' leads to decreased sperm production and other disruptions of male reproductive capacity. But these effects are apparently reversible, and in any case tests have been confined largely to immature rats. In humans nothing conclusive emerges.

The Female Reproductive System

There was one report of disrupted menstrual cycles among cannabis-smoking women – otherwise the subject is virtually unexplored in human females.

Fertility

No consistent evidence of decreased or increased fertility.

Driving Ability

It can and often does impair driving ability and actual performance – even in small doses – but whether this translates into vehicle accidents and how often hasn't been satisfactorily demonstrated.

Intellectual Function

'A host of studies have demonstrated impaired functioning on a variety of cognitive and performance tasks during marijuana intoxication.' The faculties to suffer include memory, sense of time, reaction time, motor coordination, attention and signal detection. In most laboratory studies 'memory alterations' last just a few hours, but for some there may be 'more lasting problems with transfers of new information into long-term memory storage.' For the most part, cognitive task impairment is 'dose-related', but there are apt to be 'multiple marijuana effects' depending on the exact demands of the task. 'Performance on some cognitive tasks might even improve when low doses are used.'

Amotivational Syndrome

A term used by researchers to encompass apathy, loss of ambition, impaired ability to carry out difficult tasks, neglect of personal appearance, etc. The syndrome cannot be tied plausibly to cannabis use – 'better to discard it and adopt *chronic cannabis intoxication*'.

Psychiatric Effects

The existence of short-lasting panic, and paranoid states arising from cannabis use 'are no longer questioned'. They could be due mainly to the user's lack of experience or 'adverse social conditions'.

Problems of Chronic Use

Most important among them is the cannabis-related psychosis whose symptoms (lasting up to four weeks) include mental confusion and impulsive behaviour. In Western societies the incidence is 'quite low'. It seems to affect mainly very heavy users who already have a disturbed personality. The higher frequency in, for instance, North Africa and India, 'may soon disappear as the validity of this diagnosis is being questioned and the use of this term is being abandoned in that region'. However, the West will likely show a rising incidence as the numbers of heavier users in the population increase.

Tolerance

Tolerance to most of the effects of THC (the main psychoactive ingredient) develops in much the same pattern as that for opiates, nicotine and alcohol. So-called 'reverse tolerance' (the effects of the drug coming on more easily for the practised user instead of needing an increased dose), 'if it occurs at all, is likely to be due to conditioned responses linked to familiar cues'. (Namely, the user responds not pharmacologically, but to the setting and the ritual.)

Dependence

Although scientific opinion is divided, there is now 'substantial evidence' that at least mild degrees of both psychological and physical dependence can occur.

Withdrawal

Some reports note elements of withdrawal similar to those caused by opiates, alcohol and sedatives, with reports of sweating, nausea and muscle spasms. Other studies have found only 'post-drug' irritability.

Vulnerable Groups

Fast-growing adolescents and older people who metabolise drugs more slowly may be more sensitive to the drug's effects, while a variety of conditions in the general population can be exacerbated. These include mental illness, heart disease and epilepsy.

WHO Summarised and Evaluated

The use of moderate doses of cannabis produces intoxication associated with dose-related impairment of driving and machine operating ability. The desired state is euphoria, although in some situations the user experiences short-lived reactions ranging from mild anxiety to an acute psychosis. Daily or more frequent use, especially of potent material, can produce chronic intoxication taking several weeks to clear after use is discontinued. Respiratory toxicity is observed in heavy users and may depend on smoking techniques and the combustion properties of the particular material. Effects on hormonal, reproductive and immunological states of heavy users is unclear. Chronic administration can lead to the development of tolerance to a wide variety of the drug's effects, although opinion is divided on dependence. To a mild degree, at least, physical and psychological dependence is believed to occur.

Certain groups such as the young and old are 'susceptible to the effects of cannabis', but in general a low prevalence of adverse effects has been observed even among heavy users. 'Given that millions of individuals are now using the drug, even relatively infrequent but serious adverse consequences could be of public health significance.'

Many users of cannabis, as well as experienced workers in the drugs and medical field, would consider the ARF/WHO vision of cannabis obsessively strict. The report, and others like it, omits from its brief an analysis of the drug's therapeutic potential which, according to some surveys, is looking strong in the areas of depression, anxiety, asthma, glaucoma, appetite stimulation, relief of pain, possibly as an anticonvulsant and as an antibiotic. It also omits an analysis of the wounding effect its illegal status has on relations between smokers and the authorities. Research into adverse medical consequences nonetheless carries on apace with the focus of concern settling, at the time of writing, on the impact on pregnancy and 'cannabis psychosis'.

Pregnancy

There have been suggestions that marijuana affects the length of pregnancy, the relative difficulty of delivery, the early condition of the newborn and the rate at which the mother recovers. There have not so far been strong suggestions of long-term impairment. The problem when conducting research has been in trying to separate the effects of cannabis from other drugs likely to have been taken by the mother, such as alcohol, tobacco and coffee. The physical fitness of the male in the partnership has also been neglected. One authority in the field who claims to have taken account of most of these variables is P.A. Fried of the Department of Psychology, Carleton University, Canada. His study, which began in 1978, has looked at 420 'predominantly middle-class women'. The results: 'Marijuana was associated with a shorter gestation period and a decreased maternal weight gain. No adverse effects on birth weight, length of labour or difficulties in birth were observed. Consistent with earlier reports, babies born to women who smoked more than five joints per week during pregnancy demonstrated marked tremors, startles and altered visual responsiveness at 2–4 days of age. These symptoms had attenuated by 30 days.'[11]

Cannabis Psychosis

The issue cropped up in some detail during an important Old Bailey trial during the summer of 1984 in which a publisher, Tony Bennett, was charged with trading in a number of obscene titles contrary to the Obscene Publications Act; these were not sexual in content, but drug related.

Among the prominent witnesses called by both sides was Professor James Griffith Edwards, a senior psychiatrist in charge of the Addiction Research Unit in South London. Appearing for the prosecution, Edwards claimed that cannabis could cause a psychosis lasting for several weeks. The prosecution further implied that countless thousands who had been mentally damaged by the drug could be resisting treatment because of possible trouble with law. Edwards dwelt on a survey carried out in South Africa in 1982, known as the Rottenburg Report. Yet when it came to proving the existence of cannabis psychosis the authors themselves were ready to admit that their study fell some way short.

Even as the legal case was being fought, the same argument was occupying the pages of the *British Medical Journal.* A doctor from the Caribbean insisted that treatment of psychosis following cannabis use was 'a normal part of psychiatry in the Caribbean', while two British physicians from Guy's Hospital were complaining that the term 'cannabis psychosis' had 'without justification' insinuated itself into medical literature. The case for cannabis psychosis has still not been proved or disproved.

History

Like the coca shrub and the opium poppy, *Cannabis sativa* has been recognised as a plant of great utility for thousands of years. There is no part of it that has not been coopted, most often for hemp and medicine, but even for the production of fibrous wands used to drive out demons. The wild version is believed to have originated in Central Asia. Further abroad it was carried and planted by nomads. The ancient Chinese are believed to have been especially adept at cultivation, under-standing from the earliest that when sewn close together, tall thick-stemmed plants resulted – ideal for hemp fibres. From these twines came textiles, fishing nets, ropes and mats. The seeds of the plant were extracted to make oil for cooking as well as herbal therapies for fever and menstrual cramps.

Aryan nomads are credited with taking the plant into India[12] during the second millenium BC. Here it was appreci-ated for its therapeutic properties. It also formed the basis of spicy beverages that were consumed by both mortals and gods. Knowledge of the plant is then believed to have spread to the Near East, Africa, Europe and the New World.

The ancient Greeks used juice from the seeds to cure after-dinner flatulence. The Romans took a more utilitarian view, using the fibrous stems to make sailcloth and rope. It was they who brought hemp to Britain, but it was the Anglo Saxons who inspired widespread husbanding.

While there have been no arguments about using the cannabis plant to make rope, there have always been rumb-lings about making use of the plant's psychoactive properties. Any substance that can alter mood and perception is poten-tially injurious to the orthodoxy. We can see this problem as clearly in the 1980s as we can imagine it some one thousand years ago in the Near East.

It was at this time (c. 1090) that a furiously zealous order was founded in the Persian mountain fortress of Alamut by one Hasan ibn-al-Sabbah, leader of an Ismailite sect of the Shi'ite Moslems. The precise ambitions of the order and the part hashish played in them are now impossible to ascertain since all its books and records were destroyed when the fortress was sacked in 1256 by the Mongolian Hulagy. Nonetheless, the ripening myth of Hasan tells us plenty about the deep-rooted suspicion with which hashish is viewed to this day. The very word *hashish* (as well as *assassin*) is claimed to have been derived from Hasan's name.

Lester Grinspoon, in his scholarly *Marihuana Reconsidered*[13] describes Hasan's organisation as a quasi-spiritual dynasty and notes that it was called by its members, 'the new propaganda'. Hasan's personal motives were apparently 'ambition and a desire for vengeance' while the 'agnosticism of the organisation sought to liberate people from the rigidity of the doctrine, enlighen them to the super-fluity of the prophets and encourage them to believe nothing and dare all.' Below the Grand Master (Hasan was the first of seven) came the Grand Priors, each in charge of a district; below them came the common propagandist. On the bottom rung were the thoroughly trained young fanatics known as *fida'is*, who stood primed to undertake whatever the Grand Master required of them. Much of their work was the execu-tion of prominent Moslem targets, and so mysterious and bloody were these deeds that the Islamic world was plunged into terror, while the order's political impact grew throughout Syria and Persia.

The role of hash in these murderous enterprises is usually given thus: in a valley set into the Alamut mountain fortress lay a garden filled with every variety of fruit and tended by faithful servants, with free-flowing wine, honey and milk, and sweet-singing beautiful damsels. It was to this place that the Grand Master had his young fida'is brought after they'd first been delivered into a deep sleep by a 'certain potion'. When they awoke and were left to dally with all that goodness they thought they must be in paradise – the very idea the Grand Master sought to impress upon these simple hill people.

Some accounts record that the young men were by this point softened for their murderous tasks. Others, more plaus-ibly, say the garden served as a reward for services rendered, and that having dallied the devotees would again be knocked unconscious by the potion, brought back to the palace where their account of the paradise-in-waiting – just as Mohammed had described it in the Law – was used to bait new initiates into obedience. While folk history has insisted the 'certain potion' was hashish, it seems more likely that an opiate was used for the knock-out. Equally, there are no plausible accounts that the assassins actually went about their business stoned. A clear head, or perhaps one filled with a stimulant, would in any case seem to be the better equipment. Boccaccio, Dante, Rimbaud and many others have alluded to the work of the fida'is. Such accounts are inevitably enriched with fabrication and gloss, and the whole story of Hasan has long since been woven in with ancient myths that derive from all parts of the East.

A defence of the assassins is put up by the US magazine *High Times* in their *Encyclopedia of Recreational Drugs*:[14]

'The alleged etymological connection between assassins and *hashishiyyun* (hash heads) glosses over the fact that their enemies wished to blame hashish for politically motivated crimes. This would be rather like the establishment officials today calling any young radical a 'dope fiend'.

With the sudden proliferation of sea traffic during the sixteenth century *Cannabis sativa* in all its forms began travelling to those parts of the world where it hadn't yet been seeded – notably South America. The Europeans were chiefly interested in cultivation to make hemp for rigging on the ships, and encouraged their own populations as well as those they colonised to grow it. But with the revival of classical learning there was also a new appreciation of cannabis' medicinal properties. Knowledge of its intoxicant effects was even more widely dispersed as the African slaves of those European plunderers introduced the practice of smoking both to their masters and to the indigenous peoples of the new South American colonies.

Of all the Europeans it was the sybaritic French who took most joyfully to the metaphysical dimensions of cannabis. While Napoleon was cutting a swathe through the hashlands of North Africa the people back home were immersing themselves in all that was Arabian, bowing to the style and the artefacts.

A man who travelled to those new Arab outposts and had witnessed for himself the effects of hashish was the physician Jacques Joseph Moreau de Tours. So convinced was Moreau of the similarity between hash intoxication and mental derangement that he felt certain the study of the first would help the treatment of the second. He turned to his friend, the novelist Theophile Gautier, who was so enthralled by the idea that he helped to establish a club dedicated to thorough immersion in the hash experience. It was called Club Des

Haschischins, a weightier forerunner to Leary's acid-based League For Spiritual Discovery, and had a membership that included Dumas, Balzac, Baudelaire and Flaubert. They gathered in the Hotel Pimodan, Paris, where their hash experiments were observed by Moreau, and gave rise to descriptions such as this from Gautier:

> 'My body seemed to dissolve and I became transparent. Within my breast I perceived the hashish I had eaten in the form of an emerald scintillating with a million points of fire. My eyelashes elongated indefinitely, unrolling themselves like threads of gold on ivory spindles which spun of their own accord with dazzling rapidity. Around me poured streams of gems of every colour, in ever-changing patterns like the play within a kaleidoscope. My comrades appeared to me to be disfigured, part men, part plants, wearing the pensive air of Ibises . . .'

The British tended to be more earthbound in their approach to the plant. Romantic youths such as Coleridge and De Quincey weren't above sampling a pellet of hashish, but mostly it was important as the base for sailcloth and – later – tinctures. Edinburgh was a key centre of research for cannabis' therapeutic properties. Queen Victoria's personal doctor, John Reynolds, a leading advocate of what came to be marketed as *Cannabis indica*, described the drug as 'one of the most valuable therapeutic agents we possess.'

The prime source of the raw material were the cannabis fields of Bengal (also the source region of the opium the British pressed on the Chinese). But at the height of the *indica* rage, Bengal was so stretched that other outposts of the empire had to be employed.

Pharmacologists, meanwhile, worked harder and more hazardously to obtain the best possible extracts from what were often inferior crops. Some died in the attempt – blowing themselves to pieces. Not until 1966 was the key psychoactive alkaloid – THC – able to be reproduced synthetically.

Though the British didn't take to cannabis as an intoxicant in the manner of the smart French, they were responsible for introducing the habit to the Caribbean. It was an indirect introduction; affected by indentured Hindu workers the British were shipping out to the West Indies from about 1840 to work on the sugar plantations. The black people of the Caribbean, who perhaps dimly remembered the plant from their African homeland, welcomed its introduction both as a tonic and to smoke the laborious day away under the British.

But while it's true the descendants of those black slaves did bring *ghanja* with them to the UK, they consumed it very much in a private way. The cannabis rage among young British whites, starting from the early '60s, was learnt from their Caucasian counterparts in the US, from the hipsters, beats and their flower children spin-offs. But where did the American whites learn it?

They learnt it from their black fellow countrymen, who probably got it from Africa.

The American Scene

Like France, America also seems to have experienced cannabis fever in the mid-nineteenth century. There were the usual medicinal therapies made from *C. indica*, but in addition there grew a fashion for chewing quids of ground betel nuts mixed with cannabis's flowering tops. Straight hash smoking through a hookah was also in vogue in the most fashionably dissolute circles.

A sharp downturn in the reputation of cannabis came as a reaction to the political/racial exigencies of the day. There was no serious problem while smart New York ladies were smoking *bhang* in their uptown apartments, but Mexicans and dope, was another matter.

Mexicans had been flowing into the South-West states of the Union from the turn of the twentieth century and were welcomed as a source of cheap farm labour. They brought with them their smoking pleasures, and although there were local statutes outlawing the weed, these were not seriously enforced until the Depression years of the '30s when the migrants and their habit were suddenly surplus to national requirements. The chase for jobs between whites and Mexicans set up grave tensions, and just as cocaine had earlier been blamed for the poor humour of American blacks, marijuana was now identified, half cynically, half in earnest, as the cause of the dispiritedness of the Mexicans; thousands were deported.

Black Americans, particularly young jazzers, were also turning themselves on in the first two decades of the century, as an alternative to the prohibited alcohol. In New York hundreds of 'tea pads' opened up in which cannabis was sold, either for consumption on the spot or for carry-out. The city authorities blinked, but they seemed to tolerate these parlours fairly well, again until the onset of Depression. A new commissioner of the Federal Bureau of Narcotics called Harry K. Anslinger, also influenced a change in attitude. He was a man reefer-obsessed. He saw marijuana-induced crime waves everywhere and he countered them with tempests of anti-dope propaganda. Squalls were coming in from abroad too. Turkey and Egypt had come before the League of Nations to beg assistance in beating the cannabis menace. Then in 1937 the US Federal government passed its decisive Marijuana Tax. From now on licit traders such as doctors, druggists and birdseed sellers would have to register and pay a tax. For the rest, the drug was banned.

Viewed from the UK, America was in a curiously repressed mood by the post-war/'50s period. She seemed fearful of perversions – ideological and sexual – in all places. But then beneath the writhing exterior there was indeed something outlandish taking root. Mescaline and LSD had been discovered. Intrepid beats were penetrating the Upper Amazon to explore native hallucinogenic cults, and figures like the poet Allen Ginsberg and the radical academic Timothy Leary were doing their utmost to cleave a great hole in the body of US society. By the time the '60s arrived, a sizeable proportion of young Americans believed they knew exactly how to articulate their complaints, and to an important degree it involved the use of the medium of drugs. Theirs was a reaction against soulless materialism. American youth dressed up rough and steeped their senses in 'organic' pleasures. The important drugs were LSD and cannabis. But whereas the first was considered a spiritual emetic, cannabis was the dependable companion. It was warm and giggly and, moreover, a badge of affiliation. Smoking 'dope' in '60s America earned instant access to a sub-nation of 'heads'.

The British Scene

Given that the UK has long been infatuated with American youth culture – a compliment that is periodically reciprocated – the US movements of the '40s, '50s and '60s inevitably had their counterparts among British youth. From the '50s there was a semi-flourishing jazz scene in the clubs of Soho where 'pot' was ingested along with cool blues and bebop music. Another strong pro-*ghanja* faction was found among the new young West Indian immigrants – lured into the big UK cities to do the menial jobs that the whites wouldn't do. Just how much *ghanja* was smoked by those Caribbean imports in the early days is difficult to gauge, but there are reports of young black men freely walking the streets of West London's Notting Hill pulling on spliffs. The young smokers would not have found favour among their more proper church-going elders, but local police, in common with the rest of white society, would scarcely have known of the drug's existence.

One of the first serious attempts to provoke a cannabis scare came from the barrister Donald Johnson in his 1952 opus, *Indian Hemp, a Social Menace*. I am indebted to the author Peter Laurie for uncovering this work which included extracts from a series of articles in the *Sunday Graphic*:[15]

> 'After several weeks I have just completed exhaustive enquiries into the most insidious vice Scotland Yard has ever been called on to tackle – dope peddling.
>
> 'Detectives on this assignment are agreed that never have they had experience of a crime so vicious, so ruthless, so unpitying and so well organised. Hemp, marijuana and hashish represent a thoroughly unsavoury trade.
>
> 'One of the detectives told me: "We are dealing with the most evil men who have ever taken to the vice business." The victims are teenage British girls and, to a lesser extent, teenage youths . . .

'The racketeers are 90 per cent coloured men from the West Indies and the West Coast of Africa. How serious the situation is, how great the danger to our social structure, may be gathered from the fact that despite increasing police attention, despite several raids, there are more than a dozen clubs in the West End at which drugs are peddled.

'As a result of my inquiries, I share the fear of detectives now on the job that there is the greatest danger of the reefer craze becoming the greatest social menace this country has known . . .'

He goes on to describe entering a 'tawdry' West End club where he and his contact were among just six white men.

'I counted 28 coloured men and some 30 white girls. None of the girls looked more than their mid-twenties. In a corner five coloured musicians with their brows perspiring played bebop music with extraordinary fervour. Girls and coloured partners danced with an abandon – a savagery almost – which was both fascinating and embarrassing. From a doorway came a coloured man, flinging away the end of a strange cigarette. He danced peculiar convulsions of his own, then bounced on to a table and held out shimmering arms to a girl. My contact indicated photographs on the wall. They were of girls in the flimsiest drapings. I had seen enough of my first bebop club, its coloured peddlars, its half-crazed, uncaring girls.'

Writings such as these, though not particularly plentiful, gnawed away at national policymakers during the '50s, cementing the reputation of cannabis as a dangerous narcotic. Such panics can be seen as echoes of other panics from other parts of the world in different ages: the Spanish encountering the coco-chewing Incas; Napoleon when his troops first discovered the hash-eaters of Egypt (the Emperor tried to ban the drug); the Americans and their black coke sniffers and the English in response to the numerically insignificant Chinese opium smokers of Limehouse who simultaneously were regarded as inert and physically menacing.

No matter the dimensions of the '50s dope scare, cannabis

continued to be confined to a fairly small, outre crowd right through that decade with rarely more than a dozen prosecutions each year under the Dangerous Drugs Act. Aside from hip Jamaicans, there was the odd Nigerian sailor passing through London or Liverpool, and there were the US-influenced white jazzers and shaggy-sweatered beats who perhaps dug CND. Sources were informal – a parcel from Jamaica, a little 'personal' picked up in an African port.

The rapid rise of the drug in the '60s was in one sense part of the sensual awakening of Western youth following the drubbings of the Second World War. It was also linked to what might be called the 'proletarian renaissance'. This was a movement spurred by cheap travel and which saw the hitherto hidebound masses pour into the Mediterranean where they discovered foreigners too have good ideas. They brought back pasta, retsina, mosaics, cuban heels, halva, incense and, a little later, hashish. In the early part of the decade such items signalled cosmopolitan modism. They went with the little skirts, and funny sculpted haircuts. The prime desire then was to be dynamically on the go. Drinamyl became the preferred fillip both through licit channels and on the street where the pills taken were *Purple Hearts*. But by the middle of the decade the mood changed again. Manic fabbism was displaced by something more contemplative. The Commissar was ousted by the Yogi (the Commissar is back once more in the '80s) and as the trails to the Eastern hashlands became more and more comprehensively trod, cannabis started to infiltrate the art schools, the colleges and then sixth forms – places where speed had previously been the essential mode.

The swell had begun in the year 1966. In 1967 the first wave had rolled in, and by 1968 the whole culture was drenched.

Servicing of the new cannabis consumers was still very much an ad hoc business until the early '70s. Hash was being brought back in VW vans from Eastern source countries like Afghanistan and the Lebanon, and divided among friends. A small portion would perhaps be sold on the street to provide for future liquidity. Black dealers could score hash from white dealers, while white youths who wanted a bag of herb could go to certain pubs and clubs where it would be cut up on the back table. (The specialisation of whites in hash and blacks in herb still survives, as does the cross-over effect in times of need.)

Policy

'Straight' society in the late '60s was quick to see the symbolic importance of cannabis smoking and launched many attacks upon it. There was still an idea, lingering from the '20s and '30s, that it was a morally perilous drug, and if masses of British youngsters were going through their weird metamorphosis, challenging every last conceit of society, then the drug which was so vital to them had to be in some large measure culpable. A great disappointment to the Labour government of the day was the 1968 report on cannabis prepared by the Hallucinogenic Sub-committee of the Advisory Committee on Drug Dependency. Chaired by Baroness Wootton, it was the first attempt by any British government to properly investigate the drug since 1894. It came at a time when controls had been in existenc for some 40 years. Home Secretary Jim Callaghan no doubt anticipated a reinforcement of standard policy. Yet Wootton and her panel delivered a political grenade.

There was no evidence, said the report, that the drug, which was widely used by young people of all classes, caused violent crime or aggressive, anti-social behaviour or produced dependence or psychosis requiring medical treatment in people who were otherwise normal. It pointed to a 'body of opinion that criticises the present legislative treatment of cannabis on the grounds that it exaggerates the dangers of the drug and needlessly interferes with civil liberty.' And yet despite the penalties there were no signs the drug's consumption was diminishing. Among the committee's recommendations were that:

1. The association in legislation of cannabis and heroin be ended and a new law to deal specifically and separately with cannabis and its derivatives be quickly introduced.

2. Possession of small amounts should no longer be considered a serious crime to be punished by imprisonment.
3. Preparations of the drug should continue to be available on prescription for research and medical treatment.

The popular press fumed, subjecting Wootton's panel to what the Institute for the Study of Drug Dependence (ISDD) described as the 'most explosive campaign of vilification ever visited upon an official drugs advisory body.' Hundreds of items were generated. George Gale, writing in the *Daily Mirror*, suggested the Committee was part of the 'conspiracy of the drugged.' The 1967 *Times* advert calling for liberalisation and signed by many notables was once more fulminated against.

It was the 'escalation' syndrome – the possibility of cannabis leading to heroin – that worried most people. It worried particularly those who participated in the Commons debate on Wootton during which both government and opposition were at one on the need for holding the line against what Callaghan called 'this so-called permissiveness . . .'

The level of discernment among certain Government ministers can perhaps best be judged from a note in the late Richard Crossman's diary: 'Thursday, August 14, 1968: Barbara Wootton had come to talk to us about the drug problem. She got into trouble with Callaghan for recommending that oh, what's it called, not heroin but one of the other drugs, should be categorised as a harmless drug, although many people regard it as leading to addiction.'

Home Secretary Callaghan rejected most of Wootton's advice, of course, and five years later, in June 1973, the Misuse of Drugs Act came into force, placing cannabis possession, trafficking and manufacture in the Class B category, along with amphetamine, Ritalin and the like. Maximum penalty for possession was now to be five years and/or an unlimited fine. Cannabinol and cannabinol derivatives such as synthetic THC were placed in the more serious Class A category, along with heroin and cocaine. These carried seven years for possession as well as the unlimited fine.

History of Controls

The 'Legalise Cannabis Campaign' traces the origins of Brirish control back to 1912, when an international conference was called to discuss controlling opium traffic. The conference also decided to investigate the cannabis question. There were a lull until 1923 when the South African government proposed to the League of Nations that cannabis be treated as a habit-forming drug and internationally regulated. (The Durban government was apparently concerned that the weed was causing African labourers to slacken off in the mines.)

Britain wanted the matter fully investigated and a decision on international controls to be considered when the League's advisory committee met in 1925. But some couldn't wait. At the second Opium Conference in 1924, Egyptian and Turkish delegates begged and won support for more urgent action. 'The illicit use of hashish,' the Egyptian envoy claimed, 'is the principal cause of insanity in Egypt.' Proposals were drafted which controlled unlicensed consumption, import and export. Britain signed, and in that same year introduced the Dangerous Drugs Act, giving effect to her undertakings. She signed, even though she believed the drafting committee's analysis lacked credibility, and even though Britain herself had produced a more solid analysis of cannabis some twenty years before which argued *against* prohibition. The work was executed by the Indian Hemp Drugs Commission which, in studying the drug's use in India, spent two years interviewing 800 witnesses, reporting in a seven volume work.

In support of its recommendation not to prohibit in India, it noted: 'Moderate use of these drugs is the rule and excessive use is comparatively exceptional. Moderate use produces practically no ill effects. In all but the most exceptional cases the injury from habitual, moderate use is not appreciable. Excessive use may certainly be accepted as very injurious, though it must be admitted that in many excessive consumers the injury is not clearly marked. The injury done by excessive use is, however, confined almost exclusively to the consumer himself.'

Until the Wootton Committee was charged in the '60s with looking at the drug again, the Indian Hemp Commission's report was the only substantial analysis of cannabis in existence anywhere in the world. And yet this did not prevent the League of Nations and its successor the United Nations from further turning the heat up so that signatories became obliged to restrict not just lay consumption and trading, but use in scientific circles too. In Britain for many years the drug was in the same penal category as heroin.

Research Booms

Since the rejection of Wootton, the cannabis investigation market has boomed. There have been something like 15,000 scientific papers as well as cartloads of government-commissioned reports subjecting the drug to the kind of scrutiny that wouldn't pass a broad bean fit. Where a consensus on physical/mental impact does suggest itself, it is that there is no clear and significant damage to be found in adult humans resulting from moderate use of the drug: something the Indian Hemp Commission stated 90 years ago. And where there is a social policy recommendation, it is that locking people up or fining them heavily for simple possession cannot be justified; the drug should be demoted in the penal league table. This suggestion has been made in the US, Australia and in the UK (post-Wootton). In each case it has been rebuffed by a central government too fearful of the political consequences. But informally, at least, there has been elasticity on the part of police and judges who recognise that there would be no room in the jails for anyone else if cannabis smokers were stalked too actively.

The two key UK reports since Wootton were both produced by the Advisory Council on the Misuse of Drugs – the first in 1979 by a technical sub-committee and a follow-up three years later by an 'expert group', saying much the same thing but more elaborately. The 1979 team found 'no compelling evidence that occasional moderate use of cannabis was likely to have detrimental effects' and recommended that magistrates should not imprison for possession. They could either impose a fine or submit the offender to crown court. Since most possession offences are dealt with by magistrates, the proposal would 'reduce cannabis possession to the level of possessing an unlicensed TV – a status that in practice it has already achieved in some parts of the country.'[16] No government action was taken. The 1982 team supported this demotion, and though the format of their report was changed to allow the eight professors, four doctors and one retail pharmacist their independent heads of steam, the gesticulations were familiar '. . . insufficient evidence to enable us to reach any incontestable conclusions . . . research undertaken so far has failed to demonstrate positive and significant effects in man attributable solely to the use of cannabis.'

Regional Penalties

The experts' inability to state, without reservation, that cannabis under all circumstances is harmless to humans gives governments the opportunity to maintain the status quo. Cannabis possession continues to draw a possible three months' imprisonment, plus a £500 fine, even if the on-the-ground reality is often sharply different. In Northumberland and North Wales, cautions are the form for the first and even second stops.

In inner city areas cautions are less likely, but courts are liable, at the time of writing, to confer fines of no more than £25. Even Customs and Excise were experimenting with a scheme in 1984 whereby those caught with a 'small' amount could negotiate an instant cash penalty. But there are also some distinctly illiberal trends. In rural courts, fines for possession are still running at £100+, and the legal advice agency, Release, reports that police will often get on the backs of noticeable 'weirdos', not getting off until the 'addiction' was broken, or those targeted had left town. In the Isle of Man, parts of Lincolnshire and the Scottish Highlands, imprisonment for even first-time offenders is being administered routinely.

Perhaps the most fractious trend of the lot is the part cannabis plays in police relations with young black males.

Official police figures on the numbers stopped and searched throughout the UK disguise the true scope of the stop-and-search operation, since most police interceptions don't get logged. Nor is there any reliable assessment of how many times police are looking for drugs. A London-wide survey commissioned by the police themselves[17] revealed that an unemployed young male is five times more likely to get stopped than the equivalent with a job – even more often if the male is black. And those who are stopped are stopped repeatedly. The research team estimated that of the 1½ million London stop-and-searches in each 12-month period, 90 per cent fail to detect any crime. In 34 per cent of the cases there is no 'proper reason' for making the stop.

The contribution of such harassment to the tensions that led to the 1980 and 1981 riots (and to sporadic outbreaks that have occurred ever since) was noted by Lord Scarman. The specific contribution of cannabis searches is also clear from an analysis of events. The April 1980 riot in the St Paul's district of Bristol followed a drugs raid on the Black & White Café by forty officers, some of them in plain clothes. The cafe was an important meeting place for West Indian youth.

A year later the second and most explosive of three nights of violence in Brixton broke out following a drugs stop of a mini-cab driver; a cannabis stop-and-search campaign was regarded by many in the Notting Hill area of West London as the trigger that set alight that part of town.

The former Chief Constable of Devon and Cornwall, John Alderson, argues that since cannabis has become an unassailable feature of West Indian culture, 'The law for dealing with it should be administered with great discretion and sensitivity . . . It is one way the police fail to understand ethnic communities.' But this was unacceptable to the ears of one Home Office Minister who, following the St Paul's and Brixton riots, told the Commons: 'The legal prohibition may well have been a source of tension between the police and the West Indian community, but chief officers of police are fully aware of the need to enforce the law impartially.'

'It's true that many of the youths here openly flout the law by smoking cannabis on the streets,' the owner of Notting

Hill's Mangrove restaurant, Frank Critchlow, told his local paper in April 1982,[18] 'but that's because they don't see it as a crime . . . The cannabis laws are used as an excuse to stop and search any and every black person in this area.' Critchlow knew of what he spoke. First raided in 1969, his restaurant received forty more incursions during the following five years.

The struggle between black youth and police is not about cannabis any more than the rift in the '30s between Mexican immigrants and the US authorities concerned the drug. But cannabis – which figures in nearly 90 per cent of all British drug offences – does have a clear emblematic value that is recognised by all sides. A young stockbroker may smoke the drug as an alternative to chilled wine and it means nothing politically, but in the hands of a 'dread' or a 'slag' (as the police call them) who attends a summer music festival, it is a noxious insult. Given the widespread dissemination of cannabis throughout the whole of society – at least among the under 45s – this prickliness on the part of the authorities is badly judged. Aside from nourishing a sense of grievance among the target groups it also perverts normally conformist individuals who periodically have to lower themselves into the subworld of cannabis trading in order to 'score'.

Notes

1 P. Laurie, *Drugs*, Pelican, London, 1969, p. 83
2 A. H. Douthwaite, *Hale-White's Materia Medica Pharmacology and Therapeutics*, J. & A. Churchill, London, 1963, p. 178
3 A. McNichol, *Drug Trafficking*, North/South Institute, Ottawa, Canada, 1983
4 Ibid
5 M. Kienitz, *High Times*, May 1983
6 A. McNichol, *op. cit.*
7 Ibid
8 Ibid
9 A. Gottlieb, *Cooking With Cannabis*, Greenham & Gotto, London, 1981

10 'Cannabis Use', World Health Organisation, Addiction Research Foundation, Toronto, 1981
11 P. A. Fried, *Marijuana Use by Pregnant Women and Effects on Offspring: An Update*, Journal of Neurobehavioural Toxicology and Teratology, 1982, vol. 4, pp. 451–454
12 *High Times Encyclopedia of Recreational Drugs*, Stonehill Press, New York, 1978, p. 118
13 Lester Grinspoon, *Marihuana Reconsidered*, Harvard University Press, Cambridge, Mass., 1977, p. 291
14 Ibid, p. 123
15 *Drugs*, *op. cit.*, pp. 88–90
16 'The Cannabis Cover Up', Legalise Cannabis Campaign, London, 1978
17 D. J. Smith & J. Gray, 'Police and People in London' Policy Studies Institute, London, 1983
18 *Kensington Post*, 30.4.1982

6   COCAINE

Intro

COCAINE IS one of the great bogey drugs of the West, periodically rousing episodes of great terror. It derives from the pulped leaf of the South American coca plant and in its unadulterated form is of great utility, particularly for the undernourished Indians who occupy the high Andean plains where the air is thin and the labour hard. Aside from providing mild physical stimulation, a daily dose of two ounces of leaves – the average for 90 per cent of the Indians – is said to yield virtually all the vitamins needed. The greenery is particularly rich in thiamine, riboflavin and vitamin C, and is believed to tone the muscles of the gastro-intestinal tract, aid breathing during physical exertion, act as an aphrodisiac and relieve fatigue of the larynx: hence the popularity of the old coca wines with singers and orators. In fact, the coca plant much resembles the opium poppy which carpets great tracts of South East and South West Asia. Both can offer many blessings, and both are easily abused once the active ingredient is extracted. Equally, they have been subjected to varied prohibitions which have driven the drugs underground, opened up illicit trafficking routes and encouraged the kind of corruption exceeding even that experienced by the US during the great liquor ban of the '20s. The South American cocaine trade has become particularly unsavoury since '70s rock stars made the drug ultra fashionable in North America and Europe. In Bolivia it has attracted veteran and new-wave Nazis, corrupt military and local Mafia-type clans. The 1980 military coup was financed entirely with cocaine money, and when democracy was restored, one of the cocaine barons forcefully threatened to bring down the government unless he was allowed to continue as before.

Among South American expatriates in the US, there is brutal gang warfare as Colombians fight Bolivians fight Cubans for the bigger share of the *Yanqui* market. The authorities there talk in terms of a cocaine epidemic and cite a rash of hospital admissions and numerous deaths. In the UK the drug has always been considered too expensive for the ordinary punter – not so much for its per-gram price, about £65, comparable with heroin – but because its effects are extremely short-lived. Nonetheless, UK Customs report unusually large seizures in the past two years. The figure jumped almost sixfold in 1983, from 12.117 kilos to 71.079. Provisional data for 1984 showed a drop on the 1983 high, but the quantity seized, 34.7 kilos, was well above average for the decade.

So why all the excitement? Does cocaine really warrant the extreme reputation it has garnered both among its adherents and opponents? The short answer is that what applies to cocaine's image applies to every other drug, from yopo snuff to nicotine. That is to say, it is not a question of cocaine's relative potency or toxicity, but the measure of economic, political and social pressures for or against it.

What Is It?

Cocaine is a powerful though short-lasting central nervous system stimulant and local anaesthetic that is not generally physically addictive or particularly toxic. In terms of sustained wallop it pales beside amphetamine, whose effects last six to eight times longer.

The source of much of the West's recreational coke is the plant *Erythroxylum coca*, found in the moist tropical forests on the Eastern slopes of the Andes throughout Peru, Bolivia and Ecuador. A second cocaine-rich species is *E. novogranatense*, which is husbanded in the dry mountainous regions of Colombia along the Caribbean coast and in certain parched areas of Peru.

The coca leaf can be consumed for intoxication in four basic ways:

The Leaf

This is the ancient method employed by some 90 per cent of the Andean Indians. A wad of leaf is moistened with saliva and spiced with a lime-rich material such as crushed sea shell or a cereal. The lime facilitates the separation of the leaf's active alkaloid. The wad is placed between the gum and cheek and gently sucked.

Pasta

All the rage in urban Peru and neighbouring countries where it is mixed together with tobacco or marijuana and smoked. Pasta is the intermediate stage between the leaf and finished hydrochloride cocaine crystal. There seem to be various methods of production. One witnessed by British television producer, Brian Moser, was as follows: The leaves are first salted, sprinkled with sodium carbonate and left to sweat in the sun for three to four hours. They are then poured into a 50 gallon drum where the alkaloid is extracted from the leaves by the introduction of gasoline. The gas is poured off into glass jars inside which the important separation takes place. At the top of the solution is gasoline. In the middle is a muddy alkaloid/petrol mix and at the bottom the sought-after *guarapo*. Further filtering and treatment with hydrochloric acid produces a pasta of variable purity which is sold off for domestic smoking or to the labs for conversion into cocaine hydrochloride.

Cocaine Hydrochloride

This is an odourless white crystalline powder with a bitter numbing taste. Known informally as *charlie*, *snow*, *toot* and, by mid-Atlanticians, as *lady* or *girl* (because of its reputation as a seducer; heroin is known conversely as *boy*).

Snorters chop it up finely with a razor blade, draw it into

two-inch-long lines and sniff it up one nostril at a time using a variety of implements. A plain straw might be used. The conspicuous rich will employ a rolled-up £50 note or specially made jewelled and gold implements obtainable in drug paraphernalia shops.

The hydrochloride is made by subjecting the pasta to further refinement. It is first washed several times in kerosene, then chilled and the kerosene removed so that 'gas crystals' of crude cocaine are left on the bottom of the tank. The next stage, say the authors Philips and Wynne,[1] is to dissolve the crystals in methyl alcohol, recrystallise them and dissolve them once more in sulphuric acid. They go through a further complex procedure of washing, oxidation and separation calling for such materials as potassium permanganate, benzole and sodium carbonate. The result is cocaine at the mid-90 per cent purity level.

Such high-grade material will never reach the street. As it goes through the chain of distribution, getting broken down into smaller and smaller quantities, some traffickers will add a 'cut' to maximise profits. Some of these cuts are inert (glucose, the baby laxative Mannitol), some psychoactive in their own right (amphetamine, the local anaesthetics lidocaine, novocaine), others might provide no 'charge' but when injected prove highly dangerous (cornstarch, talcum powder, flour). Other cuts are just plain pernicious whatever the route of administration (quinine, strychnine, glass). In Britain so far there is no tradition of dangerous cuts. Most often glucose is used to thin out coke.

Freebase

This is a more potent form of cocaine that, because of its indissolubility in water, cannot be satisfactorily injected or sniffed. It is smoked either in a water pipe (to cool it) or from a strip of foil. It's a method said to have been invented by the *Yanqui* traffickers in the early '70s as a means of testing the purity of their South American-purchased hydrochloride. The idea was to divorce the pure hydrochloride salts from the cutting agent by applying a strong solvent. What's left after

the four- or five-step process is supposed to be pure cocaine –
thus the purchaser would know how much dud s/he had
bought. The flaw in the system is that while freebasing
eliminates sugar cuts and Mannitol, it won't expel other salts
such as the synthetic local anaesthetics novocaine and lidocaine. So the fine white powder resulting at the end of the
process could be just as tainted as the original sample.
According to the US drug magazine, *High Times*,[2] the production of freebase is a simple procedure that can 'easily be
brought off in one's kitchen.'

The practice appeals to those confirmed coke snorters
suffering from overworked nasal septums or to injectors who
want the rush without the track marks and the other
hypodermic complaints. Not that freebasing doesn't take its
physical toll – it just happens to conceal the damage (often to
the lungs) for longer.

Reports from the Los Angeles area where freebasing first
took off suggest that it encourages compulsive imbibing. This,
however, could be no more than the expected response of LA
people to a new and exciting fad. 'We hunkered around that
pipe like fucking vultures', says a freebasing 'young magazine
writer' in the *High Times* article. She was speaking of a
three-day smoke party in an extremely expensive tree-house
overlooking San Francisco Bay. 'We were practically grab-
bing it out of our friends' hands. The freebase high is like an
orgasm, but instead of leaving you relaxed and satisfied
you're jumping, with your body screaming for more.' Among
the cultural élite of New York, freebasing has failed to catch
hold. A London publisher who visits the city regularly told me
this had a lot to do with the New Yorker's supercilious
perception of Californians as brainless gluttons, and of
freebasing as an indulgence 'entirely compatible with that
state of being.' Its chances of catching on big in the UK are
more remote – if only because of its extraordinary expense.
Nonetheless it is over here now, and not simply in smarter
areas. Reports are turning up of freebasing in tower-block
country.

Other Routes of Admission

It is possible, though not very usual, to smoke cocaine hydrochloride inside or on the tip of a cigarette. Not usual because of its comparative inefficiency in terms of intoxicant effect per given amount. Other rare ingestion methods are to eat or dissolve the crystal in a drink. Again, these methods are considered inefficient.

The rarely seen pasta is too 'dirty' to inject and impossible to freebase because of its non-solubility. Cocaine hydrochloride, however, is extremely soluble in water, making it possible to inject large amounts for rapid gratification. It is either injected straight or in a *speedball* combination with heroin. Less often a synthetic opiate such as methadone is used in tandem.

A *speedball* is a mixture of heroin and cocaine which is administered through a needle. Known in medical circles as a Brompton Cocktail, it is given orally to 'terminal' patients suffering pain. Said to impart a euphoria greatly surpassing that achieved by each drug taken alone.

Sensations

As usual there is a tremendous subjective element involved here. Most snorters will say of cocaine that it gives them a feeling of exhilaration that comes on within about three minutes and tapers off inside an hour. Like speed, there is the sense of potency – mental, sexual and physical, as well as a suspension of appetite and fatigue. But in comparison with the common amphetamine, it is rated a smoother, more aristocratic ride. Typical users snort repeatedly through a session of fun or work, especially through tasks requiring stamina, concentration and imagination. The problem with the drug, again like speed, is that nerves become jangled the more that is administered in one session, and at high doses, or if the user happens to be susceptible, a 'toxic psychosis' can develop. The effects would include paranoia, confusion, hypersensitivity and the sensation of bugs crawling under the skin.

The cocaine injection 'rush' affects people differently. Some are made nauseous and distressed, while advocates often talk in sexual terms – of 'total body orgasm' or of 'body electrification'. It lasts little longer than it takes to pump in the dissolved hydrochloride.

The higher and longer a person trips on cocaine, the bumpier the landing. But after virtually any dose there are degrees of tiredness, melancholy and hunger.

The subjectiveness of the cocaine experience was demonstrated recently by a team of researchers at the Yale University School of Medicine. In administering doses of various substances to experienced cocaine users they found none 'could distinguish a single dose of cocaine taken intranasally from the same quantity of a synthetic local anaesthetic, lidocaine.'[3] Investigators at the University of Chicago School of Medicine moreover found that their subjects 'could not distinguish the immediate effects of intravenous cocaine from those of amphetamine, although at later times the differences between the drugs were apparent.'[4] Such results, they were satisfied, debunked 'the overwhelming mythology' about cocaine being an exquisitely inimitable experience.

Heath

Toxicity

Cocaine is a drug of low toxicity with deaths from overdose being comparatively rare. The fatal dose is often put at around one gramme, but there are reports that more than 20 grammes of pure coke have been survived.

Yet cocaine, particularly in higher doses, does present a toxicity problem not offered by the stimulant with which it is frequently compared – amphetamine. This is due to coke's local anaesthetic properties and especially its depressant effect on the lower brain centres which control respiration. US drugs expert George Gay[5] notes that while it is primarily the higher centres that are stimulated by low to moderate doses, when more is ingested (or in susceptible people) the low brain centres begin triggering tremors and convulsions. Confusion, dry throat and dizziness may set in, with breathing wildly fluctuating between rapid large gulps and shallow breaths. Erratic heart-beat develops quickly, and the individual could die either from cardiac arrest or respiratory failure. The episode has been called the 'Casey Jones Reaction' – after the puffing locomotive driver. While it is usually set off by injection or freebasing, a sniffer also runs some risk, according to Gay. This, though, would be extremely remote.

Interestingly enough, several researchers have noted that cocaine-related sudden deaths occur considerably more often during the medical application of the drug than among street users.[6] Under medical supervision cocaine is usually given in a large intravenous dose.

The 'Cocaine Run'

A shorter version of the amphetamine run (see pages 81–4) with a correspondingly milder crash at the finale. Again there is the pursuit of the rapidly dissolving euphoria together with the temptation to use more of the drug to counteract the unpleasant feeling of the crash. A coke run suggests the use of a needle but an episode of freebase smoking would qualify, as would a compulsive snorting bout.

Medical Complications

Cocaine presents some risk for people suffering from hypertension (high blood pressure), severe cardiac disease, abnormal activity of the thyroid gland, epilepsy, liver damage, respiratory ailments and muscular diseases.

In Association With other Drugs

Cocaine is one of many drugs and common foods that react badly with the MAO Inhibiting drugs (MAOIs), see pages 84–5. There is also a problem with hypertensive drugs. Cocaine and heroin mixed together in a syringe for a speedball combination can be more than normally hazardous because of the mitigating effect each drug has on the other. The presence of coke can cause an overdose when taken on top of the amount of heroin the user is accustomed to handling. Similarly, the heroin might tend to provoke a dangerous reaction to what in the past has been a manageable amount of cocaine. The greatest proportion of American coke overdose deaths have resulted from this mix.

Long-Term Use

Unlike amphetamine, which demands hours of wakefulness and therefore forces adjustments to daily routine, it is quite usual for cocaine to be sniffed long-term without the dose escalating or the needle/freebasing being taken up. At the same time there is a significant proportion of coke habitués who do develop problems. These would include mood swings, poor sleep patterns, impotence, malnutrition due to suppressed appetite, agitation, bouts of paranoia, confusion, hypersensitivity and the like.

Tolerance

Unlike amphetamine the body does not build up a tolerance to the effects of cocaine, and therefore the 'high' effects can be achieved each time on a stable dose.[7] And yet there is a reverse tolerance syndrome whereby the body builds increased sensitivity to the drug's convulsant and anaesthetic potential.

Dependence

Users do not build a classic physical addiction to the drug whereby they suffer convulsions and other serious bodily traumas when separated from it, but an intense psychological entanglement is possible, particularly because cocaine, for some, spells glamour and success. Abrupt withdrawal from a heavy habit will produce the kind of long-term fatigue and deep depression known to quitters of amphetamine, but the symptoms are likely to be milder.

Earliest Use

Andean Indians have been chewing on coca leaves for 5,000 years or more. During the Inca period the habit was a prerogative of the ruling classes, but in later and current days some 90 per cent of the total population took to it. Known as a *coquero*, a leaf chewer moistens a wad with spit and places it between cheek and gum in much the way quids of tobacco are pulped in the Southern US States. The claimed benefits include increased energy, nourishment, easier breathing while labouring in the thin Andean atmosphere, and improved contact with the spirit world. The invading Spanish *Conquistadors* believed that coca chewing symbolised the Indian people's pact with the devil and that it encouraged unworthy sexual practices such as sodomy and bestiality, representations of which the Moche people of Northern Peru were carving into their sculptures and pottery at least a thousand years before the Spanish landed. Because of these tendencies the Spanish initially prohibited coca use. They later relented when it was found that more gold could be extracted from the Inca mines if the natives were under coca's influence.

European History

Specimens of coca leaves were despatched to Europe soon after Spain's 'discovery' of South America, and yet despite favourable reviews the practice failed to take off. This was perhaps partly a matter of aesthetics, but largely due to the leaves' inability to retain their potency once dried and put on the long boat ride across the Atlantic. Had they travelled as well as tobacco, tea, opium or coffee beans, our view of the drug might have been markedly different. Even when the German chemist Friedrich Gaedcke isolated alkaloid of cocaine in 1855, and fellow German Albert Niemann further refined the process four years later, the drug failed to implant itself into the medical mainstream. Not until the 1880s were cocaine's principal benefits recognised by medical academics.

In 1880 the Russian nobleman and physician Vasili von Anrep noted that there was no pain from a pinprick when cocaine was administered under the skin. In 1883 the physician Theodor Aschenbrant reported on marvellous feats of endurance and energy by cocaine-high Bavarian soldiers. And in the US, physicians were noting the drug's ability to excite the central nervous system, and studying it as a possible antidote to morphine and alcohol addiction.

All these potentialities were pondered by the young Sigmund Freud, at the time a house physician at a Viennese hospital. It is said of Freud that he latched on to cocaine as a means of promoting his name and fortune, and yet his subsequent treatise on the subject – *On Coca* – is scarcely a work of cynicism. Nor was it wholly laudatory in regard to cocaine's effects. He warned that moderate use was reported to cause 'physical and intellectual decadence' together with weakness, emaciation and 'moral depravity'. But to this he added: 'All other observers affirm the view that the use of coca in moderation is more likely to promote health than impair it.'

Specifically, Freud listed the following major therapeutic applications: as a CNS stimulant, for digestive disorders of the stomach, for the wasting disease cachexia, for alcohol and morphine addiction, for asthma, for use as an aphrodisiac and as a local anaesthetic.

It remained for Freud's friend and associate, Carl Koller, to demonstrate the drug's full potential as a local anaesthetic by applying it to the eye during surgery. The medical community was astounded. To this day the drug is used for such procedures.

Freud's attempt to show that cocaine cured morphine addiction didn't work at all. One of his earliest subjects, his friend and colleague Ernst von Fleischl, simply switched from morphine dependence to cocaine dependence and within a year was using up to one gramme a day. Recorded as Europe's first cocaine 'addict', he went into serious psychological decline. Freud also came unstuck in his claim that 'there seemed to be no lethal dose'. One of his own patients died from a quantity of the drug he had himself prescribed. Reports of cocaine 'intoxication' and cocaine 'addiction' began showing up in the medical journals and things reached such a pass that in 1886 Europe's leading addiction specialist, Albrecht Erlenmeyer, accused Freud of unleashing the 'third scourge of mankind' (to go with morphine and alcohol). Erlenmeyer was apparently alarmed at the by now widespread touting of cocaine as a cure for morphine addiction – as if the simple switch of drugs promised a cure.

The touting of one drug as a cure for dependence on another is a recurring theme in pharmacological history. For those hooked on opium, the far stronger morphine was once advanced. For morphine addicts, cocaine, and then heroin, was pushed. For overcoming heroin addiction, Methadone (another potent addictive drug) is currently being dispensed by the State. A similar line can be drawn through the hypnotics/sedatives, starting with bromide on through to the extremely dangerous barbiturates and then to today's new class of tranquillisers: Valium and Librium, whose high dependence potential is at last being recognised.

What is true about all these classes of drugs is that problems rapidly accumulate when the leap is made from the comparatively mild substance found in nature to the synthesised, streamlined product of the laboratory. The problems are further heightened by claims made by manufacturers and by doctors who won't learn the lessons of the past.

American History

Whatever the cocaine backlash of the 1880s, numerous patent remedies containing coca leaf extract proliferated. This was particularly true of the US where the choice was between nose powders, suppositories, throat lozenges and cigarettes. One of the most successful promoters of the drug was the Corsican chemist Angelo Mariani whose tonic wine – bearing his name – became a favourite with the great figures of the day. They include the Czar of Russia, the commanding general of the British army, the Prince of Wales and the kings of Norway and Sweden. Pope Leo XIII called Mariani's wine 'a benefactor of humanity' and presented him with a gold medal. Coca

Cola was among numerous drinks of the late nineteenth/early twentieth century infused with the leaf's psychoactive ingredient. The king of colas was originally sold as a 'valuable brain tonic and cure for all nervous afflictions' when introduced in 1886. But by 1903 the manufacturers were forced by public pressure to abandon the use of the cocaine-rich syrup and instead employ a flavouring derived from the decocainised coca leaves. The same unstimulating leaf extract is still used – the source being a dry valley in North Eastern Peru.

The pressure against Coca Cola was worked up by the American media – the low and high ends of it – in which cocaine was being identified repeatedly with crime-crazy Southern blacks. There were reports of superhuman strength and guile, such as a story of 'black rapists' in the *New York Times* where it was claimed, 'bullets fired into vital parts that would drop a sane man in his tracks failed to check the "fiend".' The same NYT story branded the drug a 'potent incentive in driving the humbler negroes all over the country to abnormal crimes' and indicated that 'most attacks upon white women of the South . . . are the direct result of the coke-crazed negro brain.' There was, of course, a certain political dimension to this panic. As *High Times* puts it, 'the optimism of the Reconstruction era had been replaced by legal segregation and lynchings' and while bullet-proof blacks weren't all that seriously fretted over, there *was* the more worrying prospect of the drug providing the stimulus to a more organised and energetic resistance.

By 1914, 46 states had passed laws restricting the sale and use of cocaine and the federal government was spearheading international moves to curb not just the production and trading of coke, but of a range of opiates too. America, by this time, was experiencing its first great wave of street use of several substances and it aimed to do something about it on a grand scale.

British History

Britain also went through a cocaine tremor. The first jolt occurred in 1901 when two young actresses suffered overdose deaths. A greater shudder came during the 1914–18 war when an ex-convict and a prostitute were convicted of selling cocaine to Canadian troops stationed at Folkestone. That troops charged with the Empire's defence should be using 'heavy drugs' was serious enough. That the likely source was Germany herself – at that time the world's largest pharmacological cocaine producer – gave the episode an even more poisonous odour. There quickly grew the idea, false as it turned out, that an epidemic of cocaine sniffing was raging among British troops. To counter this, and to comply with obligations incumbent upon Britain under the US-led international control initiatives, a new regulation was passed that in effect established the hardline reaction to drugs that exists to this day.

Regulation 40B under the Defence of the Realm Act (DORA) reserved most of its detailed restrictions to cocaine. It made it an offence for anyone except medical persons, pharmacists and vets to possess, sell or give the drug away. In future cocaine could be supplied only on prescription, and these could be dispensed once only.

DORA 40B became defunct after 1918, but it lived on in the apparel of the Dangerous Drugs Act 1920. This was DORA 40B extended to conform to the guidelines set down by the 1912 International Opium Convention.

Though Britain didn't have bullet-proof blacks to contend with it did have the spectre of the degenerate Chinaman living in East London's dock area and peddling drugs and vice to tender young white things. The novels and yellow press of the day were replete with stories enunciating this theme. The Chinese of Limehouse were seen principally to be involved in the opium trade while the roots of the cocaine menace were often attributed to a shadowy Vice Trust centred in London that used female 'drug fiends' as its missionaries. They could be found in certain teashops in all the fashionable areas of the West End, notes Terry Parssinen in his excellent book on the subject,[8] and were apparently recruited to their mischief by wealthy Bohemian types, behind whom was a mysterious Mr Big, often a businessman or aristocrat.

The real-life model for such lurid tales was the case of Billie Carleton, a beautiful young actress who, after attending a 1918 Victory Ball at the Albert Hall, was found dead in her flat, supposedly killed by an overdose of cocaine. The Carleton case combined a delicious cast of characters for the press. At the Coroner's Inquest it was revealed that Billie had begun smoking opium in fashionable West End haunts and had moved onto sniffing cocaine and heroin. There was apparently a Chinese source in Limehouse, while her immediate supplier was a slippery dress designer called Reginald de Veulle with whom Billie was said to be having an illicit affair. The Carleton case triggered off not just a tsunami of newspaper stories, books and films, but created the new 'junkie archetype'. It also made the new laws not only possible but essential.

The reality of recreational cocaine use throughout the early decades of the century is meticulously traced from court records and other sources by the author Parssinen. He finds that while a recreational subculture similar to that existing today was visible in American cities by the 1890s, the British scene didn't really fruit until about 1916, and even then it was comparatively tiny – confined to a few areas of London and centred on cocaine rather than morphine and heroin. But, as in the States, the London street users were typically young working class, or criminal males and prostitutes. The origin of most stock was probably Germany. These, however, were the cases that came before the courts. There was also a certain amount of smart use of the drug by the Bohemian/theatrical set. Billie Carleton made that clear, while Aleister Crowley's *Diary of a Drug Fiend* gives a good indication of use in aristocratic circles. Such smart folk usually had the sophistication and connections to keep a wide berth from the judiciary. They might also have preferred morphine above coke as their habitual indulgence since this could be obtained from private practitioners. Cocaine and heroin were scarcely ever prescribed.

Given the size and fragility of the English cocaine scene in the early decades it was able to be harassed almost to extinction by 1930. Most users decided it was too troublesome a habit, notes Parssinen, and 'while the odd opium smoker popped up and a few elderly morphine addicts lingered on into the next decade, Britain's drug problem was essentially solved by 1930.'

By 'drug problem' Parssinen is no doubt referring to the illicit scene. In terms of the consumption of toxic and habit-forming substances the drugs industry was by now heavily engaged in the marketing of barbiturates, and by the late '30s was pushing amphetamines. This last was the stimulant that in terms of efficiency easily outstripped cocaine. It lasted longer, jerked you higher, was available in pills, powders and injectable form and, though the ride was more ragged, it was at least legal. Yet by the 1950s cocaine began showing up again. It was traded in one or two Soho jazz clubs and used almost exclusively as an accompaniment to heroin – taken through a hypodermic syringe in a 'speedball' combination. The model was the American cool jazz scene. The practitioners here were musicians, a few Nigerians and some early beatsters. Supplies came from hospital pharmacy thefts, so the stock was guaranteed pure. Then some doctors began prescribing and the scene grew moderately, though it rarely strayed beyond the usual haunts in Soho. In the second half of the '60s the circle was suddenly swelled by the arrival of a couple of planeloads of Canadian heroin and cocaine addicts who had been told by a visiting British doctor that both drugs were being lawfully prescribed in the UK. Then in 1967 came another turnaround with the establishment of the government's new drugs policy: special clinics for addicts were opened; ordinary doctors were squeezed out of the picture; security on pharmacy and hospital stocks was tightened and the number of addicts provided with cocaine on prescription reduced down to half a dozen or less. Many switched to Methedrine – there being a glut for a year – but when this source was also stepped on the injectors had to look elsewhere for their stimulation.

Attitudes

The association of cocaine with heroin-injecting 'junkies' had taken the drug down a step in terms of public image. It was equally unfashionable among the new wave of '60s experimental drug users who largely confined themselves to marijuana and LSD. Dealers who traded in those drugs often considered it a matter of principle not to handle cocaine, and for the same reason avoided heroin and injectable methylamphetamine.

Then in the mid-1970s – by which time the '60s 'youth culture' had fractured, and with it the old drug rules and rituals – cocaine re-entered the scene. This time it was as a chic tonic for musicians. It travelled from there into other glossy circles, some of which were entirely unused to drugs other than alcohol and cigarettes. The key to its rehabilitation was the return to a method of ingestion popular in the early decades of the century – snorting. Snorting made the drug seem safer and less sordid (snorting subsequently allowed heroin to get a toehold), and because cocaine still had its dangerous past it could impart glamour to establishment sniffers such as lawyers and City of London brokers, or to the nearly-chic like advertisers and press officers. It said of them, 'I am a rebel. I live (a little) dangerously.' They would have known that taken in moderation, intranasally, the drug not only allowed them to function at their work, it was as safe or more so than many stimulants and depressants available through the health service. Such factors caused cocaine's appeal to widen. It became *de rigueur* wherever smart and successful people worked and played. And because it was now associated with success the lower social ranks began coveting it. (Either that or they came to detest it as a frothy bourgeois thing – particularly true of English punks.) In America, consumption boomed to 'epidemic' levels. By 1983 it was estimated that some 12 million Americans were using the drug, including 16 per cent of all high school seniors. Cocaine-related deaths more than doubled between 1979 and 1983 (the national reporting service is unable to produce a final figure, but indicates something like 500) and hospital emergencies where cocaine is 'mentioned' also doubled in the period to 5,394. The use of terms like *cocaine-related* and *mentioned* is, however, hardly precise. They should not be read as meaning cocaine killed around 500 Americans in 1983, or caused more than 5,000 emergency cases. Somebody dying from gunshot wounds but with cocaine in them could be logged under 'cocaine related'; while inside the bodies of emergency admissions there will often have been other drugs working in tandem with cocaine.

Nonetheless there has clearly been a quantum leap in US consumption of cocaine, and to service it a thorough re-organisation in the South American source countries. So brutally streamlined has production become that the US can no longer absorb the volumes being processed and traffickers are more seriously targeting Europe where they hope to develop a similar proletarian use of the drug.

An important European transit point, due to traditional links with her old colonies, is Spain. Britain too is figuring more prominently. UK Customs report intercepting six times as much of the drug in 1983 as in the previous year – around 71 kilos. How much of this was actually intended for UK distribution isn't known, but there were signs in the first half of 1985 of more and cheaper cocaine in various parts of the country. At summer music festivals, for instance, £10 bags were showing up and even £1 lines, and the quality was reported to be good. From Wiltshire came word of £40 to £50 grammes, representing something like a 15 per cent reduction on what had been the going price. If such figures were to be maintained across the country, cocaine could be on its way to becoming a mass UK drug. Perhaps we would then also see a rise in cocaine deaths. Thus far there has been hardly any disturbance in the official mortality figures between 1968 and 1982. In each of those years there were either no deaths at all, or one death or two, never any more.[9]

The Producers

Colombia

The US frets about the impact of cocaine upon its social infrastructure, but the drug has caused barely a wobble there compared with what has happened inside the countries that actually harvest the coca leaves and process them into either raw paste or snortable cocaine hydrochloride. The major growing regions have traditionally been Peru and Bolivia where around 40 per cent is still grown legitimately for chewing by the Indian populations. Much of the rest, at least until the early '80s, was smuggled north into Colombian laboratories where it was processed for US and European distribution. But riches from the cocaine trade has caused the pattern to splinter, with leaf-producing countries cutting more and more into the lucrative processing and distribution end; with Colombians growing more of their own leaf and other South American countries not traditionally associated with cocaine putting down their own markers. These include Brazil and Paraguay.

The contest for the *Yanqui* dollar has spread to the US itself, particularly to Miami, the chief transit point. Here Colombian, Bolivian and Cuban ex-patriates regularly fire bullets into each other by way of stating their eminence: at present it seems the Colombians are winning. The warfare back home in South America is of grosser magnitude. In Colombia, journalists, judges and even priests who have investigated the racket have been murdered, and in April 1984, the country's zealous justice minister, Rodrigo Lara Bonilla, was assassinated in his chauffeur-driven car. This was his reward for an anti-drugs campaign that culminated in a raid on a massive processing plant deep in the jungle in the Caqueta Department. In response to the Lara Bonilla slaying, the country's president, Belisario Betancur, ordered more raids, arrests, seizures and purges of corrupt officials. And yet he is said to have left the top figures at large. So big is the trade and so precarious the domestic economy there is now only so much Betancur can do. Colombia is literally dependent like a 'junkie' on the cocaine trade it has learnt to market so well. Cocaine shipments by the ten main families are valued at about $8 billion annually (1984). Coke is the country's biggest export earner. Much of the return is funnelled back into legitimate domestic enterprises such as textiles, real estate, transportation, financial institutions and political groups. Though President Betancur was allowed his head of steam, he was warned by the bosses that unless the campaign slackened they would close down some 1,800 businesses in which they owned a controlling interest. And they would feed arms and dollars to anti-government guerrillas.

While the state machine has fallen victim to the drug traffickers' supreme efficiency, the traffickers themselves have also suffered a penalty. By 1983 oversupply had caused a market glut, the wholesale kilo price plummeted and US street prices halved. It was against this background that the last massive Lara Bonilla raid turned out to be not unhelpful, for by taking out $1.2 billion worth of cocaine and equipment, the kilo price again lifted and some of the old financial equilibrium returned to the system. How long the equilibrium can last with more and more dollar-hungry South American entrepreneurs entering the picture is doubtful. There were even reports in the latter half of '84 that American interests were shaping up to take a bigger share of their domestic market by growing and processing their own coca shrub. Suitable frost-free areas would be Hawaii, Puerto Rico or the US 'client states' of the Philippines and Indonesia. Such moves would simply repeat the pattern established five years earlier when the US began home-growing its marijuana rather than buy from the traditional sources of Mexico, Jamaica and Colombia.

Bolivia

The dislocation in Bolivia probably tops that which Colombia has experienced. This is the country where the left-wing guerilla leader Che Guevara fought and died and which between 1964 and 1982 suffered a series of repressive military dictatorships. It was under the pro-US regime of Hugo

Banzer that the cocaine trade was transformed from an important domestic activity into a world-beating export tool with total growing acreage rising from about 10,000 in 1968 to more than 100,000 today. Banzer's key man in the metamorphosis was believed to be former Gestapo chief of Lyon, Klaus Barbie, aka Altman. During the war, Barbie was responsible for rounding up several thousand French Jews for the death camps, and later was hired by the Americans to track and interrogate communists. The British, apparently, had tried to recruit him for the same purpose. When in the '50s Barbie became a political embarrassment he was packed off to South America with cover and documents provided by US intelligence. He began small-scale dealings between Bolivia and Peru, made some important friends, and in 1971 was appointed Security Adviser to President Banzer with the special task of reorganising the police. Under Barbie's guidance cocaine production was expanded and business concentrated into large units under the military's protection.

He trained and recruited a paramilitary enforcement squad composed of old German Nazis, young Italian Fascists, Bolivian Phalangists and common criminals. Its function, aside from eradicating the small growers, was to cap local political protest and then protect the traffic en route to the Colombian processing labs.

Banzer's regime fell in the late '70s. But by 1980 a new military government, under General Garcia Meza, was installed in La Paz. The Meza coup was entirely financed by cocaine money and shooed in with considerable help from Barbie's personally trained mercenary pack. Within weeks exports of the drug to the US were estimated by the American Drug Enforcement Agency to have more than doubled: General Meza said he would stay in office for as long as it took to exterminate his nation's 'Marxist cancer'. Within two years, however, he was ejected; Barbie was extradited for trial in France for WW2 crimes, and a man labelled the King of Coke – a former government minister – was hiding in the Bolivian jungle issuing diabolically credible threats to the new constitutionally elected government.

To top these severe events the South American producer

countries are experiencing their own cocaine 'epidemics'. But instead of it continuing with the age-old leaf chewing, large sections of the population – particularly the young and educated classes – are smoking the more potent leaf paste. This yields between 40 and 90 per cent pure cocaine.

Trafficking

The pattern of distribution from the growing and processing regions to the consumer has changed substantially since the early '70s. Then, according to Philips and Wynne,[10] it was usual for American freelancers to trek down unannounced, stumble across the right connection and make a purchase. By the early '80s the system was more formalised with US-based South American nationals having squeezed out many of the Americans, especially on the bigger deals. If non-Latins were to be used in future, it was frequently as hired couriers. Expanding into the US market was comparatively easy. In non-Spanish speaking Europe there was the problem of distance as well as the absence of ex-patriate communities with whom to make the link. As a result, no clear profile has emerged as to who is bringing over the principal quantities. In the UK, students, business executives and sailors have been involved. As to the methods: it requires little guile to smuggle in a kilo of cocaine if you're a crew member of a supertanker, especially if that tanker is to be searched by three men and a dog. Landing at Heathrow demands a little more cunning (even though the number of Customs officials is being sliced down due to spending cuts). Known methods include swallowing packed condoms (dangerous because they can break inside the stomach), hiding the stuff in jacket seams, in children's toys, souvenirs, metal cannisters; thrusting it down the gullets of pets and exotic animals; liquidised and sprayed on to clothing; and the two-suitcase trick, as outlined by Philips and Wynne: the drug is packed inside one suitcase containing clothing too big or small for the smuggler. If officials find it the smuggler denies ownership, pointing to an identical case containing his/her correct apparel. Though it is unlikely to kid the inspectors, the authors say it apparently works in court. Another suitcase trick involves simply constructing a container from coke-impregnated cardboard, filling it with clothes and carrying it through 'Nothing to Declare'.

Help

Tip-Off Signs

The habits and disposition of the coke freak are not unlike those of the amphetamine lover. See page 90. Fresh calculation should be made to account for the shorter duration of cocaine's effects and therefore its reduced tendency to cut into sleep.

Coming Off

Again comparisons with amphetamine can be made, although the profound depression that results after quitting heavy amphetamine use is not an inevitability when coke withdrawal is made.

Life-Saving

Should the Casey Jones Reaction take hold of a companion (see page 154) immediately try artificial respiration, and call an ambulance fast.

Notes

1 J. L. Philips & R. D. Wynne, *Cocaine: The Mystique and the Reality*, Avon Books, New York, 1980
2 L. Daltrey, 'Freebase: Can You Smoke Cocaine Without Getting Burnt?', *High Times*, January 1980
3 C. Van Dyke & R. Byck, 'Cocaine', *Scientific American*, April 1982, pp. 109–119

4 Ibid

5 Philips & Wynne, *op. cit.*

6 George Gay, 'You've Come a Long Way, Baby. Coke Time for the New American Lady of the Eighties', *Journal of Psychoactive Drugs*, vol. 13(4) Oct–Dec 1981, pp. 297–318

7 Cox *et al.*, *Drugs and Drug Abuse*, Addiction Research Foundation, Toronto, Canada, 1983, p. 229

8 T. Parssinen, *Secret Passions, Secret Remedies: Narcotic Drugs in British Society, 1820–1930*, Manchester University Press, 1981, p. 121

9 Philips & Wynne, *op. cit.*

10 Ibid

7 HALLUCINOGENS

Intro

THE HALLUCINOGENS are a group of substances of great chemical and structural variance – from the wholly synthetic MDA to nature's fungi – but which have the common ability to shake up the user's internal world. While experiences vary, the typical hallucinogenic trip involves visual and auditory distortions, a muddled sense of time and a slippery grip on external reality as well as the user's own sense of 'self'. Terms like 'muddled' and 'distortion' probably won't appeal to the serious proponents of these drugs since they would consider their effects profoundly revelatory in regard to all things in Humankind and Nature. But such awe-ful regard for the hallucinogens is less fashionable since the mystical late '60s gave way to the more resolute '80s. Now they are more often something done for a straight 'laugh'. In fact, looking back on old Home Office statistics, it would seem some of the studenty-intellectual connotations of these drugs in the early days was a result of false image-making. Arrest figures for 1968 show that those convicted were drawn equally from all castes and classes.

Citizens of the United States probably have the world's broadest choice of hallucinogens, for not only are the Americans rich in naturally-occurring mushrooms, roots, seeds and other psychoactive vegetation, but the US schooling system produces high-grade chemists from whose ranks spring many an unlicensed backstreet druggist. Altogether some two dozen natural, synthetic and semi-synthetic products are in common use.

Here in the UK there is a comparative paucity with just

three items popularly employed. There is LSD, plus one species of psilocybe mushroom together with the red-capped, white-flecked toadstool of fairy tales – *Amanita muscaria*. Another group of domestic hallucinogens are those belonging to the 3,000 strong *Solanaceae* family which includes the common potato. It also numbers some of the most potent and deadly plants in existence. Species of mandrake, henbane and belladonna were all important agents of European sorcerers and witches who used them, depending on dose, for healing or mystical excursions. An ointment rubbed into a receptive mucous membrane, such as the vagina, is said to have produced wild, often sexually ecstatic hallucinations. In more moderate doses these drugs would have been used as medicines, and in slightly higher ones (only slightly higher because the difference between the therapeutic and lethal measure is not great) to despatch enemies.

Just as the mystics were ultimately dealt their mortal blow – killed or forced underground by a rampant Christian orthodoxy – so their favourite preparations fell into disregard. Given their great potential for harm it is probably just as well that mandrake and the rest haven't enjoyed the kind of revival among Western recreational users as have other traditional magical plants.

LSD: What Is It?

Properly called d-lysergic acid diethylamide, LSD is part of a chemical family called the indolealkylamines which bear a structural resemblance to a neurotransmitter substance (5-hydroxytryptamine) found in the brain. Its close relatives include LSA (d-lysergic acid amide, which is found in varieties of morning glory seed) psilocybin (found in certain 'magic' mushrooms) and DMT (dimethyltriptamine).

LSD itself is derived from the fungus ergot, which grows on rye and other grasses. In its unmolested state the ergot has been used for centuries as an aid to childbirth. It constricts the blood vessels in the uterus, so preventing or stopping haemorrhage after delivery. Ergot from infected rye bread was also the likely cause of the medieval affliction, St Anthony's Fire, which periodically struck the inhabitants of European villages where rye bread was a staple. Sufferers developed convulsions and hallucinations as well as black 'charred' limbs that were actually gangrenous. The cure was to desist from eating the ergot and so allow the constricted blood vessels to widen out again. Many sufferers did desist in the course of their pilgrimage to the shrine of St Anthony. Naturally it was St Anthony not their ergot-free diet who took the credit.

The first ergot alkaloid in pure chemical form was isolated in 1918 by the Swiss-based chemist Dr Arthur Stoll. His work was carried forward by his young associate Dr Albert Hofmann who, in the 1920s, began to synthesise a number of compounds closely related to ergot at Sandoz Pharmaceuticals in Basle.

Several of Hofmann's ergot analogues were explored in relation to migraine, obstetrics and geriatrics. The twenty-fifth in his series was d-lysergic acid diethylamide. It was made by mixing the lysergic acid found in ergot with diethylamide and, after freezing, extracting the resulting LSD by distillation or evaporation. Animal tests followed, but it was not until April 1943 that Hofmann himself discovered the drug's almighty mind-altering properties when he accidentally ingested a tiny amount either by breathing in the dust or absorbing it through the pores of his skin. He describes pedalling home on his bike and becoming 'transported into other worlds'. There were several more trips, and of one he wrote:

'I lost all account of time. I noticed with dismay that my environment was undergoing progressive changes. My visual field wavered and everything appeared deformed as in a faulty mirror. I was overcome with fear that I was going out of my mind. Occasionally I felt as if I were out of my body. I thought I had died. My ego seemed suspended somewhere in space from where I saw my dead body lying on the sofa. It was particularly striking how acoustic perceptions such as the noise of water gushing from a tap or the spoken word were transformed into optical illusions. I then fell asleep and awakened the next morning somewhat tired, but otherwise feeling perfectly well.'

Hofmann's experience must have indeed been terrifying, not only for the dry, sure world of pharmacology that was his environment but because in 1943 he was alone with these sensations. Sandoz performed further tests on volunteers, after which it was concluded that what had been discovered was a most powerful psychomimetic – in other words, a drug that could produce a 'model psychosis' whose study might unlock the secrets of schizophrenia and other mental illnesses. The war interrupted distribution of the drug, but by its close it had been sent to numerous psychiatric researchers. Often they worked in large teaching hospitals, which meant LSD could be tried out on both healthy volunteers as well as the sick.

A similar dispersal job was performed in Warsaw Pact countries by Spofa of Prague, Czechoslovakia. An Italian company and then Eli Lilly in the US also manufactured LSD using their own processes. A key attraction of the drug in those early days was the concussive effect it could have on memory. For a repressed neurotic eluding his or her Freudian analyst's attempts to probe at the roots of the disorder, LSD seemed capable of delivering the big bang. The problem, as it later emerged, was what to do with the stream of discordant data that poured forth.

It was LSD's big bang effect that also appealed to the military and intelligence communities. It appears the US army tried it as a possible incapacitator of enemy troops and as a means of reversing the brainwashing of liberated prisoners of the Korean war. The CIA also spent some twenty years looking at the drug – as a disabling, brainwashing device that could be mobilised on behalf of the Free World or (in their nightmares) by its enemies. Public enquiries subsequently revealed much of the CIA's experimentation to be at best inept. Outside the intelligence sphere there were also some dubious applications.

Too often, medical practitioners failed to understand the extraordinary 'violence' of the LSD experience and so would have no qualms about, for instance, attaching electrodes to their subject and then putting him/her through some very icy scrutiny in a setting that was in itself sufficiently bleak to induce a panic. To compound such gaucherie the drug, according to Terence Duquesne and Julian Reeves in their book, *A Handbook of Psychoactive Medicines*,[1] was often administered by injection – a method wholly unsuitable since its slams the user straight into the intense hallucinogenic phase without even the shortish run-up that is provided when swallowing the drug in pill form. Peter Stafford states in his *Psychedelic Encyclopedia*,[2] all manner of doses were tried, from small, cumulative amounts to one-off combustive attacks at around 1,500 microgrammes. It was tried in one-to-one therapy and among whole mental wards. It was also used on prisoners such as black American narcotics addicts who were given escalating doses over a period of some two weeks, cut off dead and then reintroduced with a massive dose that sent them through the prison roof. (From this it was learnt that LSD ceases to have any psychoactive powers when used daily over as little as three or four days. A break is needed for its potency to return.) Many doctors reported patients being cured of debilities such as arthritis, partial paralysis, headaches, hysterical deafness and skin rashes. It was also used enthusiastically on alcoholics, often hard-core 'incurables'. A review of 800 treated in a Canadian LSD programme indicated that 'about one-third remained sober after therapy and another third benefitted.'[3] Where schizophrenics were excluded the results were substantially better than that.

'There are no published papers,' claimed psychiatrist Abram Hoffer in relation to the Canadian programme, 'using psychedelic therapy which show it does not help about 50 per cent of the treated group . . . Even more important is that this can be done very quickly, and therefore economically.'[4] Sceptics weren't so sure: couldn't the success rate also be attributed to the keenness of psychiatrists working with such a chic new tool?

Another important area of LSD research, one tackled by the respected Czech physician Stanislov Grof, was with the terminally ill. Grof found that LSD was not only a more effective pain reliever for cancers than traditional opiates, but that sufferers passed on their way with less anguish. In the US too Dr Eric Kast of Chicago reported better pain relief than from traditional analgesics and, again, an ease of passage. 'It was a common experience', wrote Kast 'for the patient to remark casually on his deadly disease and then comment on the beauty of a certain sensory impression.'[5]

Methodical analyses of LSD's disparate, often unruly early use are few. A classic survey was Cohen's 1960 review of the work of 44 American clinicians.[6] It embraced 5,000 experimental subjects as well as patients who between them ingested 25,000 LSD or mescaline doses. The survey revealed two trip-related suicides and eight psychotic reactions lasting more than 48 hours. As would be expected, the psychiatric patients rather than the healthy volunteers were more prone to upsets.

A similar though clearer report (in that it didn't involve mescaline) was produced for the UK by Nicholas Malleson.[7] It aimed to sum up the experiences of all 74 clinicians who by 1968 had dispensed LSD. This time there were 4,500 recipients who between them had received about 50,000 'therapy sessions'. Three people killed themselves close to their therapy. 'There were 37 cases of psychotic disturbances lasting over 48 hours, ten of which became chronic. Two deaths, a small number of superficial injuries incurred during therapy and the birth of one abnormal child were also noted.'

In response to this study and others like it the government's Advisory Committee on Drug Abuse concluded that, 'there is no proof that LSD is an effective agent in psychiatry. Equally there is no proof that it is an exceptionally hazardous or prohibitively dangerous treatment in clinical use in the hands of responsible experts and subject to appropriate safeguards.'[8]

Nonetheless, by the early '60s, the bulk of the clinical work was finished and in psychiatry its uses were becoming confined to two basic groups of cases: chronic alcoholics and those suffering psycho-sexual problems. This work too was to dry up as recreational use of the drug flourished and the authorities took fright.

Magic Mushrooms: What Are They?

As part of the Old World, the UK is endowed with considerably fewer hallucinogenic plants than the Americas, where some hundred-plus species have so far been identified. And yet these isles do offer a dozen types of mushrooms capable of giving a jolt.

Magic mushrooms can be divided into two distinct groups – one for mushrooms containing the drug psilocybin and the 50 per cent more powerful psilocin, and the other much smaller *Amanita* group which have ibotenic acid and its derivative muscimol as their main psychoactive ingredients.

Psilocybe semilanceata (Liberty Cap)

There are ten native species containing psilocybin and psilocin, but the drug content in most of them varies markedly depending on soil, weather and the age of the fruit. Some lose their potency from the moment they are picked, notes Richard Cooper in his *Guide to British Psiloeybin Mushrooms*.[9] By far the most reliable in that it contains roughly predictable amounts of the two drugs is *Psilocybe semilanceata*. Known as the Liberty Cap, it is also the most readily available and the most appreciated by mushroom heads for the distinct yet measured effects it conjures up.

The lethal dose of Liberty Cap is estimated to be around 8lbs of fresh specimens, but an amount considerably less than that will do damage. Though the drug content of Liberty Cap is comparatively reliable, there is still some variation between different fruits – not least because they vary in size. Working out a suitable dose not only has to account for this, but for additional factors like the user's body weight and contents of the stomach: in a hungry mushroom eater the effects will be greater. They will also be heightened if taken with alcohol. These factors considered, an effective dose usually ranges from ten to thirty mushrooms.

Usually seen growing in groups of long lines, they are a tiny, elegant species with a yellow-brown conical cap that often comes to a sharp point. This cap sits on a wavy, lighter coloured stem which is 4–8 cm tall. But since this is a generalised description and one that can fit others of the UK's 230-odd common fungi, it is vital for anyone who decides to eat this or any other species to establish its identity beyond question. This can be done by taking along a mushroom guide and then studying the fungi – once it has been brought home – against a checklist of clues. Important signs are found in the type of gills, spores and the presence of a volva, a veil or a ring. The government-supported drug advice agency, Release, recommends Richard Cooper's book and the standard pocket companion to all types of British fungi, *Collin's Guide to Mushrooms and Toadstools*. At the very least, any mushroom hunter should be able to recognise the dangerous specimens.

Amanita muscaria (Fly Agaric)

The Amanita genus is the most feared of any fungi native to Britain because it includes the Death Cap (*A. phalloides*) and Destroying Angel (*A. virosa*). Both these lethal fungi should be noted well. Like most of their relatives they grow through a 'cracked egg' volva and bear a skirt-like ring on the stem just beneath the cap. *A. phalloides* is 8–12 cm tall with a 6–12 cm cap that ranges from white to olive green and is to be found in a range of habitats, but mostly in oak or beech woods. *A. virosa* has roughly the same height and cap width, and has a similar bag-like volva and skirted ring at the top of a shaggy stem. But it is disturbingly, enticingly white. Both have white spores, and between them are responsible for 90 per cent of all UK mushroom deaths. These mushrooms are really efficient killers: 50 per cent of those who eat them will die.

Cooper identifies two other members of the domestic Amanita genus that deliver a psychoactive punch. One (*A. pantherina*) is so rare that the Collins guide doesn't include it. Cooper warns of its high toxicity.

The other major Amanita species mushroom eaters go for is *A. muscaria*, known commonly as Fly Agaric. This is the toadstool of gnomic fairytales and the most visually extraordinary of all the British fungi. It is 10–22 cm tall and sports a bright red cap speckled with white warty spots. As it ages the cap widens to about 22 cm, fades to an amber colour, and the warts begin to vanish. It has a ring at the top of the stem, but not a volva. It is found principally with birch, and can be seen growing directly beneath the trees either alone or in scattered groups. Because of its proximity to trees, any user has to consider the possibility that a dog might have lifted a leg on the specimen s/he is about to pick. Its fruiting season starts in late July and ends in early December.

Amanita muscaria should not be consumed raw, but either cooked in a low oven or hung up to dry. A maximum of three mushrooms is usually the 'recommended' upper limit.

The first Western reports of Fly Agaric's intoxicant effects came from eighteenth century visitors to Siberia who noted its use among the tribesfolk. These 'primitives' were nothing if not thrifty; knowing that the mushroom's active alkaloid was quickly shed from the body – unmetabolised – via the urine, they made a habit of drinking their own or another's urine in order to extend the period of the high. (Vodka has since taken over as the favourite intoxicant in that part of the world.) But these hardy souls stopped short of drinking their reindeer's waste, even though these creatures are believed to be partial to the fungi.

Other Hallucinogens

LSD, Liberty Cap and Fly Agaric are the clear UK market leaders, but there is a host of other synthetic and organic substances capable of producing bizarre effects and which sometimes show up domestically. The most well known but rarely tried is the peyote cactus (*Lophophora williamssi*) together with its alkaloid derivative, mescaline. Native to Mexico, peyote's hallucinogenic properties were discovered in the late nineteenth century by raiding parties of northern Mescalero Apaches who transported it back to their American homelands, employing it there in religious and healing rites. A cult grew up around the drug. This cult developed into a formalised church, and after several court battles the

US Federal government finally upheld its members' right to use peyote. Mescaline – recognisable as a white crystalline powder – is obtained from the spineless 'buttons' that range across the head of the peyote cactus. It can additionally be synthesised in a laboratory.

An important enthusiast for the mescaline experience was the writer Aldous Huxley, who described its mystical and 'cleansing' qualities in his 1954 work, *The Doors of Perception*. US demand for the drug (and for its organic parent) was further stimulated by the writings of Carlos Castaneda who, in a series of enigmatic books, set adrift a young white novice among some crafty Indian shamans. Here in the UK many people know of the drug, but few have experienced it first hand. Bogus mescaline, however, is in fairly plentiful supply.

Other domestic hallucinogens occasionally employed are as commonplace as nutmeg, mace and morning glory seeds (only some species are psychoactive and beware of eating chemically treated types from a plant nursery). Then there are those produced through lab synthesis and scarcely known in this country: DMT, TMA, PMA, DOM, PCP. This last is better known as *angel dust* or *peace pill* and is massively popular in the States. MDA is a stimulant/hallucinogen that in powdered form has some currency among young British night-clubbers.

A much hyped variable of MDA is MDMA (also a member of the phenylethylamine family) which, like the former, goes to work on the neurotransmitters in the central nervous system creating enhanced appreciation of colour and sound as well as empathy for others. Originally an esoteric psychiatric tool for use with warring marriage partners and even for cocaine withdrawal, it has reached the streets in the last couple of years where, known as Adam, XTC or Ecstasy, it has developed a fabulous reputation. The trip, lasting several hours, goes through several stages starting with a queasy, paranoic rush. Then comes an LSD/speedy episode, followed by sedation and sleep. The intensity of the sensations is, as usual, dose related, larger amounts usually bringing on more vivid hallucinations. The real significance of Ecstasy, however, lies not in its overblown street status but in its status in law – legal at the time of writing with the US government moving quickly to eradicate it, even from medical circles. This current legality is due to the situation in US law which regards all drugs as licit until specified otherwise. Where there is a medical lobby, as in the States, strongly pushing 'therapeutic' benefits then there can be considerable delay in working out precise prescription, security and penal regulations while evidence is heard. Meanwhile the drug is free floating. And even after the measures have been taken a new variable is easily created by making small adjustments to the molecular structure. The phenomenon of inventing-as-you-go is not a new one, it has been practised for decades by the pharmaceutical industry. But since the '60s illicit back-street chemists have been getting more and more practised at the art of 'Designer Drugs', so that they are now capable of a literally infinite output – each one of which has to be weighted in law.

LSD: Sensations

Whether or not enlightenment is sought from the LSD experience, it is a drug to be treated with care, or else it can produce a miserable, stormy passage known as a 'bad trip'. Just 100 microgrammes are sufficient to provoke the most dramatic effects lasting up to twelve hours. It is the most potent psychoactive, weight for weight, ever known – some four thousand times the strength of mescaline. Most experienced users will establish a comfortable setting free from harassment or unexpected intrusion. Another key to the experience is the user's mental condition. Is s/he able to withstand the inevitable sensory buffeting? Can s/he deal with and steer through the maelstrom of visions and emotions, some of them corresponding to concrete reality, others a figment of the drug's chemistry? Even when mood and setting are right there is still an unfathomable factor that is going to shape what takes place. The drug, in short, is too unpredictable to be contained.

Despite all this, users report that getting a balanced frame of mind in a comfortable place and in the company of a friend who knows the drug will help to avoid a bad trip. This 'guide' should have the maturity and calm, unobtrusive manner to steer the user through any tough spots. S/he sometimes stays drug-free or takes a little dose him/herself to aid the connection.

Effects will usually come on in about forty minutes, but could take as long as two hours. The first sensations will be excitement, perhaps agitation, an awareness of body and its motor functions. Some people start worrying that their body is labouring at its task – the rate of heartbeat, the sluggishness of the lungs. It has been known for surgeons who are used to witnessing the body's throbbing innards to picture in high relief the workings of their own. It is said they can release themselves by relaxing into and through the other side of these impressions.

The external world might now start looking unfamiliar, crooked, misshapen. The room has sludgy coloured walls, though in reality they are white. The absurdity of manufactured style may be noticed – that pompous chair, that guzzling, moaning television set straining to exhibit life, perhaps *is* life. The visions need a backdrop to grow from, something as simple as a square inch of carpet or the grain in a wooden table. They can evolve from almost anything the eyes alight upon. To put a stop to them, the eyes are simply swivelled elsewhere. Although the user's own flesh can look curious to him/herself, like putty or meat, it will appear perfectly normal to everybody else. There will be distortion and heightening of sound, warped reverberations and moments of piercing clarity. Familiar records can sound odd, particularly those with a firm, rhythmic beat. Formless music can sound extraordinarily knowing.

'In almost the same breath,' reports one user, 'you will feel elated, scared, wonderful, ridiculous – part of a universal hoax, and then all these swirling certainties and uncertainties will break into fragments and begin and end again.'

In the early stages – the first two or three hours – events can either move rapidly or hang so motionless the user is put on the edge of panic. Activity is said to help. LSD is not an immobilising drug. The more tasks undertaken, the less opportunity the drug's sensory effects have to entrance. But driving and other mechanical functions are not going to be handled effectively: driving and operating machinery of any kind can be dangerous.

Ego Death

Of this initial period when sensory bombardment is at its strongest, some people talk of the death of the ego. By this it is meant that the experience can be so overpowering that the self is forced to retreat in the face of it. This retreat is not so much a death as the learning of proper humility. The 'self' – the drug seems to instruct – is an invention. Not only is it meagre in the context of the whole of creation, it cannot even withstand the battering afforded by some near invisible grains of rye fungus. And yet this meagre self, together with the bodily organism that houses it, *is* part of the universal whole and fittingly so. This constructive lesson passes many trippers by. They attempt to assert the primacy of their own position by staying rigid and attempting to fight off the drug's effects. They will more than likely come off worse in this war and in doing so suffer the vaunted 'ego death'. This could mean a shattering of inner confidence that might take some time to recover.

The Later Stages

After the early sensory bombardment it is usual to become deeply reflective. Now is the time to sift and sort the experiences of the first hours. Alcoholics treated with LSD frequently achieved the vital 'realisation' at this stage. They saw what their shrivelling lives amounted to and resolved to free themselves. But it is at this stage that other kinds of ideas can get reinforced. Charles Manson and his devotees were LSD adepts and came to believe the divine hand was in their bloody work. And a Nottingham man tells me that he remembers a gang of football terrace hooligans in the early '70s who used to dose up with LSD before stomping their enemies.

In the final stages of the trip it is typical to feel a sense of melancholia. This is emphasised if friends who have been tripping together part abruptly. A favourite album is said to help, while some users turn to cannabis to ease them down.

A long sleep is now in order, following which there will be no hangover, although flashbacks in which an acid vision is thrown up without warning are fairly common. These might return over the next few days or even weeks. Cannabis or some other kind of sensory input might trigger them. The medical profession makes a great fuss about the flashback syndrome, but for the vast majority it seems to be of no consequence and rather than interfering with normal functioning acts as an ironic counterpoint to the formalities of daily life.

Magic Mushrooms: Sensations

The Liberty Cap experience is related to LSD but milder and less frenetic. 'Bad trips' are possible, but are rarer than with LSD as there tends to be less of a pressing psychological dimension to the experience – more one of wonder and a calming euphoria. The effects start within half an hour and pass their peak after three or four hours, after which there is a tailing-off, followed by sleep. The head is clear on awakening.

Not many users care to mess with Fly Agaric more than once due to its tendency to provoke nausea, puking and other untoward effects. Fewer still want anything to do with the more toxic *A. pantherina*. While Liberty Cap is like – as one mushroom head put it – 'sipping wine in a punt with fairy lights, Fly Agaric promotes a drunken feeling, stiffness in the joints, uncoordination.' After the initial immobilising phase a light sleep is common, accompanied by vivid imagery. Upon awakening comes the more psilocybin-like euphoria, a sense of increased mental and physical energy, and self-absorption. Strong doses will produce great animation – perhaps derangement and convulsions. The entire episode lasts anything from two to eight hours (longer if urine is consumed).

LSD: Health Effects

As we've seen, LSD was a very proper product of the vast pharmaceutical company, Sandoz of Switzerland, and was initially taken up by researchers into mental illness. Then the CIA and our own defence establishment saw it as a potential chemical weapon. LSD's journey from new wonder drug to the scourge that ate youth followed the pattern we are witnessing many times over in this book. After the industry's medicine-tent hyperbole and wide dissemination of a substance, there are doubts about safety; meanwhile it has been seized on by an illicit class of user which prompts restrictions and legal penalties. LSD is distinguishable because the switch from good to bad was that much quicker and more definitive than usual. The drug is now virtually impossible to acquire, even through licit research channels.

Early Scares

Of all the early scares associated with LSD, the one that caused the most worry was the drug's apparent ability to inflict genetic damage and thus give rise to deformed offspring. Similar fears surface with the introduction of every new drug, but they were particularly strong in relation to LSD and got a special booster from a 1967 article in the US journal, *Science*, which reported that human blood cells, when exposed to LSD, showed some chromosomal breakage. This 'finding' was soon translated by the US pop media to mean LSD equals malformed babies of the sort that were then being born to thalidomide mothers. But the *Science* article was hardly solid. It was built in large part around the observations made on one middle-aged schizophrenic who had been given LSD 15 times while in hospital, and according to British author and doctor Michael Gossop[10] had also been given the tranquillising drugs Librium and chlorpromazine. Both these agents, notes Gossop, are known to cause chromosomal breakage just as (other researchers report) similar changes can be caused by caffeine, aspirin, X-rays, fever and viral infections. But the true flaw in the LSD monster-baby thesis is that no one really knows what such chromosomal damage adds up to – only that these structured bundles of genes play a part in fashioning new life.

By 1971 *Science* had a new angle on LSD, obtained from its own analysis of 68 studies of case reports, most of them US government funded. Its view was now that: 'LSD does not damage chromosomes *in vivo*, does not cause detectable genetic damage and is not a teratogen or carcinogen in man.' Presumably women were included too. To these assurances might be added that exclusive use of LSD has not so far been reported to have caused a human death from overdose,[11] although the psychiatrist Abram Hoffer estimates 14,000 microgrammes would be sufficient to kill half of those who tried such an amount.[12] There are cases where users have jumped out of windows or indulged in bizarre acts of violence. The chances of a healthy individual developing and succumbing to such urges are probably remote, according to research.

Mental Effects

The problems of evaluating LSD's impact on the mind are considerable. In terms of actual 'brain impairment' the Addiction Research Foundation in Toronto reports that psychological and neurological tests 'have failed to reveal any consistent and statistically significant differences between small groups of healthy non-users and regular users of LSD.' It does however warn of 'LSD-precipitated psychoses' that have been experienced by 'some individuals' taking either a single dose or indulging in long-term use. The psychosis might last for several hours or for a protracted period. 'In many respects it resembles paranoid schizophrenia and is characterised by hallucinations, delusional thinking and bizarre behaviour.'

Such a condition sounds remarkably similar to what is known as an 'acid casualty'. But whether or not such a person exists as a medical textbook phenomenon, the 'acid casualty' is a well known creature to the drug laity.

Acid Casualty

The acid casualty is someone who has dosed up on so much LSD s/he has never quite returned from orbit. It's as though a fragment or more of the brain has ceased to function. The processing of sensory data is more difficult and unreliable. There are gaps in logic: a mental lopping-off. The acid casualty might always have been potentiated in this direction and the LSD simply gave extra thrust, or the unhappy condition could be a product, pure and simple, of the drug. No one really knows.

Tolerance

Tolerance of LSD's psychoactive effects builds rapidly so that a normal dose taken three or four days running will by the fourth day produce no 'trip'. Only by abstaining for several days will sensitivity return. Also, a cross tolerance operates with other members of the LSD chemical family – morning glory seeds, LSA, psilocybin and DMT (this last is a product of the laboratory but can be found in plants which have for centuries been used by South American Indians as a hallucinogenic snuff).

The nature of this cross tolerance is that however the LSD family members are interchanged it is not possible to go on a trip using any one of them for more than a handful of days consecutively.

Addiction/Dependence

No true physical addiction for the drug develops whereby the body suffers trauma when deprived. However, psychological dependence, as for many drugs, can occur. It is particularly rare with the LSD family because its members are too mentally combustive to be regular companions.

Magic Mushrooms: Health Effects

Because of psilocybin and psilocin's close chemical relationship with LSD much of what has been written above about LSD's alleged potential for chromosomal damage, its effects on mental stability, tolerance, addiction and so forth can be extended to magic mushrooms. However, there are of course the problems of poisoning by mistake, and other material components of fungi which have so far been little studied.

Avoiding the Killers

As a general rule, mushrooms that emerge from the ground through a volva (like a broken eggshell) should be avoided by the novice. Avoid also those a dog might have pissed on. It is also important to stay away from old, wet, dirty and bug-infested specimens, and not to store any away fresh – particularly not in a plastic bag. The sealed environment encourages them to convert into an extremely unpleasant dark slime.

Dried mushrooms should *never* be bought on the street. The purchaser will have no idea what they are.

Sudden Deaths

Deaths have occasionally resulted from an overdose of Fly Agaric, and more rarely still from *A. pantherina*. A lethal dose triggers delirium, convulsions, coma and heart failure. In terms of Fly Agaric's longer term impact on the body, this has not so far been analysed in any detail.

Addiction/Dependence

Liberty Cap and Fly Agaric are not physically addictive, although like LSD they can give cause to psychological dependence.

Poisoning

If trouble is taken to select healthy specimens of the 'recommended' species in sensible doses there will be no trouble with poisoning. However, mishaps do occur and while relatively few, they are increasing each year with the rising popularity of magic mushroom eating. In 1978 the National Poisons Information Service could trace just 33 cases. By 1981 the figure was 142. Most of these involved quickly resolving symptoms, and there were no fatalities. Mushroom poisoning can mean a quick vomit or it can mean death where the wrong species has been chosen. The longer the symptoms take to appear the more serious the likely outcome, since the toxins will have had time to percolate through the system. Release puts the case straight in its 1979 guide, *Hallucinogenic Mushrooms*: 'If you become ill a day or so after eating the mushroom you should get medical advice at once, even if you begin to feel better after a while. It is characteristic of serious mushroom poisoning that the person affected has periods of recovery but may nevertheless die some days later. Remember, since mushrooms are legal there's no problem about calling a doctor. You won't get busted.'

Many symptoms of mushroom poisoning can be difficult to distinguish from the early effects of a trip on Fly Agaric. They will include vomiting and diarrhea, cramp, watery eyes and mouth, twitching or fits, respiratory problems, a yellow pallor and unconsciousness. Obviously a person in the extreme condition needs emergency treatment. Call an ambulance or get them to the hospital yourself. Take samples of the offending fungi with you and, if available, specimens of your friend's liquid or solid waste. Release offer the following additional tips: if the fungi has been eaten recently and the symptoms are just beginning, help your companion vomit up the poison by feeding him/her hot salty water and then burnt toast to soak up the remaining toxins. But don't try this if they are semi-conscious or spark out. They will choke. If they do pass out lay them on the floor in the coma position – on the side with the knee nearest you bent up and the near elbow and forearm on the floor. Ensure the throat is not obstructed by the tongue or by vomit and check for breathing. If there is none apply artificial respiration.

If a fit or a convulsion starts stick a soft wad of cloth like a hankie in the mouth to prevent chewing or swallowing of the tongue. Lie the victim down in a place free from hard, sharp objects so s/he can thrash without risk of injury.

Attitudes

It is the association of hallucinogens with 'paganism', whether expressed by the red tribes of America or white witches of Europe, that caused such a rending of the statute books when the new hallucinogenic era came to pass. When those LSD-ingesting '60s youths began reporting mystical visions, linking them with profoundly anti-establishment sentiments, the tremor felt within the establishment must have been of the variety experienced by the *Conquistadors* when they first encountered the mushroom-eating Aztecs of the fourteenth century. There was less circumspection in those days. The Spanish simply banned the mushroom and slaughtered its advocates.

When the US, followed by other governments, moved to crush the diabolical LSD manifestation of the '60s they took the judicial route. New legal powers were introduced that placed LSD in the same 'most serious' category as heroin and injectable amphetamine, while the media fell upon stories of LSD-inspired suicides, insanity, deformed fetuses and de-formed sexual practices, not to mention persons struck blind while staring zombie-like at the sun. That the uptake of LSD by a cross-section of young people happened to coincide with a shift in attitudes seemed to be missed by many at the time. They saw the drug as the *thing* on which the perceived social disintegration could be pinned.

Leary & Co.

The former Harvard professor Timothy Leary is inevitably cited as the High Priest of the psychedelic era for having broadcast more vehemently than anyone else the alleged spiritual and sensory benefits of LSD. Initially he was for the democratisation of the psychedelic experience – *turn on, tune in and drop out* – but later recanted, calling this exhortation naïve.

'We failed,' he wrote, 'to understand the enormous genetic variation in human neurology. We failed to understand the aristocratic, élite, virtuous self-confidence that pervaded our group. We made our sessions wonderful and expected nothing but wonder and merry discovery.' Not only did Leary recant, he is also alleged to have 'finked' – according to the San Francisco underground paper *Berkeley Barb* – on his former psychedelic cohorts. He appeared as a prosecution witness in a drug case against his own lawyer[13] and is said to have been used by the authorities in their attempt to mount a case against those who actually helped him escape from the prison where he was serving a term in the mid '70s for marijuana possession.

After the authorities were finished with him Leary toured US clubs and halls as a 'stand-up philosopher and comic', and later surfaced in England partnering on stage the man who was in charge of Richard Nixon's dirty tricks department, the man who in the '60s led the raid on Leary's psychedelic idyll: G. Gordon Liddy. Such was the dismal pass the psychedelic movement had come to. But then Leary and his Harvard colleague Richard Alpert, 'Merry Prankster' author Ken Kesey and others of their prestigious ilk were untypical of the average '60s 'tripper' and in the end unessential to the movement. Mostly they were handy protruberances by which media people could haul themselves up (or down) to inspect what for them was a mysterious new generation of long-haired deviants. The idea that there ever was a homogeneous acid-swallowing 'youth culture' is not entirely, but largely, a delusion. It was fed by the adepts themselves because they felt more powerful as a great uniform wave, and by such forces as the music, clothing and film industries which could get all the wealthier if their customers all wanted to look, sound and be like each other. In reality there were the ever-familiar diverse tastes among '60s youth, both within and without the long-haired ranks. The drugs, together with the faddy routines, simply helped to mask the divergencies. Later those homogeneous hippies were to splinter off into drug dealing and computer programming; the notion of communal youth was unmasked as a fraud. Drugs too lost much of their situational context. There are still some drugs that fit better in a certain place among a particular crowd, but come the '80s and we find a lot of people are doing a lot of everything at no appointed hour.

Even after the flower power bubble had burst at the turn of the '70s there was still plenty of high-grade LSD around, particularly in the UK where an illicit multi-limbed manufacturing operation, said to be the world's largest, was established around a former chemistry student called Richard Kemp. In concert with members of the American pseudo-religious and drug dealing group (established by Leary) called The Brotherhood of Eternal Love, Kemp and his cohorts managed to turn out enough LSD for six million tablets. And this was done in just three bumper runs between 1970 and 1973.

These were the high years for Kemp and for acid aficionados. The following year, 1974, the police had obtained his name and those of his associates, and after a laborious undercover operation called Operation Julie, they were all pinched. Several of the accused were still in jail in 1985.

As is the way of the marketplace, the dearth of LSD following the Julie raids didn't so much persuade users to quit their mind juggling as find an alternative to do the job. This alternative, it turned out, was not only free of charge, it was free of those unpredictable adulterants that could be present in any and all drugs trafficked on the streets. They were those members of the *Psilocybin* and *Amanita* mushroom families containing psychoactive acids and alkaloids. They were easily picked, dried or boiled for an experience that, depending on species, could be as profound as LSD. The fungi habit has persisted even after acid stocks were again plentiful from 1982.

Who Takes LSD

While the breadth of mushroom use is considerable it is probably wider still for LSD. Stocks in the second half of 1984 were mostly arriving via Amsterdam. The drug came in *stamp* format – impregnated into pictures of Superman, Snoopy, ET. The quality was high. The Home Office rated the purity of the stocks it had been seizing at almost 100 per cent, which was too much for some. A drugs councillor in the Avon area, who estimates there is more LSD around today than in the '60s, tells me: 'I saw one young punk drop a tab at the Glastonbury festival and ten minutes later he was complaining it wasn't working. [The drug can take up to 45 minutes to bite.] So he took another one, and when the effects of both hit him it turned out to be very strong stuff indeed, with the hallucinations lasting up to twelve hours. So he decided to do some speed to level it all out. He got into a right state.'

Such daft use would confirm Leary's worse élitist suspicions about the fitness of the average modestly equipped individual to make something lasting and transcendent of the LSD experience. Today, in the '80s, people make of the drug what they will. It is no longer the sacrament of a quasi-religious movement because that movement has gone. To illustrate: I asked one 16-year-old youth from a West London suburb whether LSD had made him think about himself, about life, more deeply than usual. His real habit had been glue and aerosols. He also smoked a little cannabis and sniffed speed. His LSD trip had been taken with half a dozen friends in a local park, lying on their backs, staring at a grey, discoloured wall that made a good screen on which to project visions. They giggled a lot, flashing at each other what he called 'coathanger smiles'. The world seemed odd and one of their group, a black boy, panicked and ran away. Did it make him think?

'Yeah, when I got home it made me think. Me mum and dad were still up and I was still tripping like. And I looked at them going on and that and I thought, you know, what a bunch of boring bastards.'

Who Takes Mushrooms

Magic mushrooms have a smallish, though loyal band of adherents, and in many a centrally located wood or heathland during the peak fruiting season you can find a sprinkling of early morning pickers, their backs bent intently, plastic carrier bags plump with little Liberty Caps or, if they're more daring, the red-capped Fly Agaric.

Two or three generations of hippies now eat mushrooms. So do punks and the less extreme bikers (strictly for laughs; no religion). College students, New Gypsies and 'anarchists' eat them, as do those who have been attending the summer festivals in all parts of the UK in recent years. Some of these festivals are devoted, in their title even, to the celebration of magic fungi. Mushroom tea parties are popular. I also noted that Liberty Caps are consumed enthusiastically in the Bogside district of Derry. Mushrooms are also one of a host of drugs taken by a band known collectively as the 'convoy' – a group that has been tagging the aforementioned summer festivals, causing cardiac arrhythmia among the CND set by refusing to pay entrance fees, brandishing weapons and keeping everyone awake at night with their intoxicated howls.

Controls

LSD

In relation to LSD the law is straightforward. It is a Class A drug controlled under the Misuse of Drugs Act 1971, and liable in the case of either manufacture, supply or possession to 14 years in prison and/or an unlimited fine.

Mushrooms

In regard to Fly Agaric mushrooms the law does not intrude. Neither the fungi themselves nor their main active ingredients are controlled under the MDA and so, until established otherwise in court, it would seem that they may be lawfully consumed.

Liberty Cap's active ingredients, psilocybin and psilocin are, however, controlled. Despite this, the authorities have not yet found it legitimate to penalise possession of the mushrooms themselves. To do so would call into question the legality of a host of otherwise innocuous items containing the controlled substances. Among them would be certain species of toad and even the human animal itself. For we too are alive with naturally occurring analgesics, stimulants and hallucinogens. So for an offence to be committed the controlled drug must first be 'separated' from its host. The Misuse of Drugs Act also penalises 'preparations' of these fungi. 'Preparations' has been interpreted to mean (although not fully tested in court) any tea, soup, omelette, cake, etc. But there is still no clarity on the question of dried mushrooms. In a 1981 appeal case, the court upheld a conviction of possession of a Class A drug where the defendant had simply dried and crushed psilocybe mushrooms. Similarly, if the police find a panful of cooked fungi or a line of them strung across a bedroom wall then that would not look too good in court. However, dried mushrooms per se don't rate as a preparation since they could have been collected after drying in the sun.

After separation and preparation the third possible illicit activity is the actual growing of the mushroom. This was tested at Snaresbrook Crown Court in March 1983 when a North London man was charged under the Misuse of Drugs Act with 'producing a product' containing a Class A drug – namely psilocybin. He was arrested in May 1982 when two ounces of fungi were found growing in his flat. The species was *Psilocybe cubensis* whose spores the defendant was said to have bought via the US magazine *High Times*. (Magic mushroom kits are popular in the States.) In answer to an investigating constable who had asked him, 'What's going on here, then?' he said to have replied, 'I am trying to grow a health food. I am trying to make the world a better place.' When asked if his mushrooms were a narcotic he replied, 'No, they are sacred.' And got himself arrested.

The critical ruling by Judge Clive Callman was that despite the paraphernalia 'the production of *Psilocybe cubensis* up to the time they are fresh and free from preparation is outside the scope of the Misuse of Drugs Act 1971.' And with that he ordered the jury to acquit the accused.

Notes

1 T. Duquesne & J. Reeves, *A Handbook of Psychoactive Medicines*, Quartet, London, 1982, p. 328
2 P. Stafford, *Psychedelic Encyclopedia*, J. P. Tarcher Publishing, Los Angeles, 1983, p. 78
3 Ibid, p. 80
4 Ibid
5 Ibid, p. 74
6 'The Amphetamines and LSD', Report by the Advisory Committee on Drug Dependence, HMSO, London, 1970, p. 36
7 'LSD' – Recurrence of a Communal Nightmare', Institute for the Study of Drug Dependence, London, p. 2
8 'The Amphetamines and LSD', *op. cit.*
9 R. Cooper, *A Guide to British Psilocybin Mushrooms*, Hassle Free Press, London, 1977, p. 5
10 M. Gossop, *Living With Drugs*, Temple Smith, London, 1982, p. 142
11 Cox *et al.*, *Drugs and Drug Abuse*, Addiction Research Foundation, Toronto, Canada, 1983, p. 313
12 *Psychedelic Encyclopedia*, *op. cit.*, p. 70
13 D. May & S. Pendler, *The Brotherhood of Eternal Love*, Panther Books, London, 1984, p. 276

8   HEROIN

Intro

THAT SOCIETY is being scared witless by heroin right now is more a result of society's fears about itself than of the intrinsic nature of the drug. We have only to cast back a couple of decades to see that the scare then concerned LSD and cannabis – two drugs that excite the imagination, leading to unorthodox brands of thinking and activity. Given that those were the days of hippies and weirdo lefty students it is not surprising an LSD panic should have seized the nation. Or we could trace back to the US South of the first couple of decades of the present century. It was a time when white reactionaries were trying to roll back the early promise of Reconstruction by indulging in lynchings and crude South African-style segregation. What they feared, in response, was a black backlash, and when young blacks started taking to cocaine – a drug that charges energy and makes the will manifest – the whites naturally feared their day of reckoning was around the corner. And so it was cocaine that got blamed as the drug that made the negroes uppity.

In Britain in the 1980s the panic is not about a drug that fires the imagination, but about a sleepy, stupefying, painkilling substance which originates in the Indian sub-continent. There lies the malaise-cum-nightmare of Britain. We are a nation that wants to kill the pain that comes from the degenerate slide from Imperial 'lustre' into a squalid, squabbling, mean-spirited, fearful, self-serving present. Heroin – when used habitually – is the drug for those who won't look this reality in the eye. It holds out the promise of escape but, for those who return to it too often, it makes matters worse. Or it kills. That it should be coming over from Pakistan is an historical irony. We used to be the major opium grower and trafficker in what is now known as the Third World. It is also an eerie evocation of Bulldog Britisher's most feverish nightmare: degeneration seeping in, courtesy of the non-white foreigner.

Heroin *is* a powerful narcotic, but it is rarely what it is said to be. In many respects it is less dangerous than several other drugs, and most of the problems associated with it result from its status in law and in the minds of a bigoted culture.

What Is It?

Heroin is one of a class of drugs known as narcotic analgesics, narcotic from the Greek *narcotikos* meaning benumbing, and analgesic from the Greek meaning without pain. Heroin itself belongs some way down the line of the family of narcotic analgesics known as the opiates. They are called such because they all derive from the opium poppy (*Papaver somniferum*). The most straightforward extract from the poppy is opium itself, which starts as a milky juice oozing from the poppy's seed pods. A few days after the petals drop a series of shallow incisions are made in the pod. The juice exudes and a day later, when it has turned a gummy brown, it is scraped off and left to dry in a shaded area, all the while darkening and hardening. Once firm it is shaped into bricks ready for the consumer. Getting smoking opium out of these crude bricks requires repeated boiling and sieving until all impurities are removed and a black, sticky paste results at the bottom of the cooking pot. This paste is then dried and smoked. Pharmaceutical opium comes in tablet or injectable form.

Morphine

Within opium are more than a dozen alkaloids, yet only a few of them have any medical value and fewer still are of interest to the recreational user. Principal in both recreational and medical categories is morphine – a product ten times more potent, weight for weight, than its parent opium. In fact morphine is the analgesic against which all others are compared, being one of the few old-wave drugs of vegetable origin that has not been rejected now that medical practice has become so highly tooled up. In its medical state morphine comes as a pill, a suppository, a hydrochloride solution and in an injectable ampoule. The stuff found on the streets is in one of these formats and probably the product of a chemist or hospital break-in; or else it will be pills or powder smuggled in from India, which supplies most of the licit opiates required by the world's pharmaceutical companies. Tasmania is also an important producer of poppies for licit medicines.

Codeine

Another major alkaloid of opium is codeine, used in the main to deal with coughs and mild or moderate pain. Having about one-sixth the kick of morphine, its street value is limited to a hit of last resort or thereabouts. It can be found in countless across-the-counter preparations, often in tiny quantities mixed in with aspirin, ephedrine and the like. In pure formulations it appears as a tablet, linctus and ampoule. Only in this last condition (known as dihydrocodeine) is it subject to controls under the Misuse of Drugs Act.

Heroin

Heroin is something of a bastard child of mother opium and the laboratory chemist. It is made by boiling equal amounts of morphine with acetic anhydride, a colourless heavy liquid used in the manufacture of synthetic fibres and celluloid film. The combination is called heroin base. To get heroin itself, this product then goes through several more stages calling for hydrochloric acid, strychnine, caffeine; much drying and sieving and other processing – depending on the quality of heroin required. In its purest form the drug is three to four times more powerful than morphine. The street substance is coloured beige to white, either as small rocks or a fine powder, varying on the type and place of origin. Medical heroin comes as a white pill, a linctus and as ampoules of liquid or powdered solution. Most commonly known as *smack*, the term is a corruption of the Yiddish 'schmeck', which means to sniff. Also called *skag*, *junk*, *horse*, *H* and *boy*.

Others

Other opium alkaloids with clinical value are papaverine, noscapine and thebaine. These too are used in various combinations to deal with pain, diarrhea, coughs and wayward behaviour of the muscles, but the question of their 'abuse' has rarely arisen.

Synthetics

Heroin and the other drugs listed above fall into the opiate category, in that they are wholly or largely derivatives of the poppy. Close relatives are the opioids – so called because they mimic the opiates in their action, but are made largely from other materials. There are a score of them, but just half a dozen have been adopted in non-medical circles. These are:

Pethidine – a painkiller of shortish action that is made without any recourse to the poppy and which comes as an orange or yellow tablet or ampoule. It is used in obstetrics.

Dextromoramide – a far stronger and longer-lasting analgesic that comes brand-named Palfium, in tablet, amp or suppository format. Again it is a compound without recourse to the poppy.

Dipipanone – comes in tablet form brand-named Diconal and with the addition of an anti-nausea drug called cyclizine hydrochloride. This pukeless element made Diconal popular with hardcore users, and since the tablet is not designed for injection a number of doctors prescribed it with fairly witless abandon. They believed, or chose to, that it would not go into feeding a needle habit. But it did. The dangers of injecting Diconal – rich in chalk and silicon – have now been recognised by the Home Office. It can no longer be prescribed by doctors unless they are specially licensed.

Dihydrocodeine – one of the most widely prescribed pain-killers in the UK, it is judged to fill the slot between the opiates and milder solutions such as paracetamol. Branded DF-118, it comes as a tab, elixir or amp.

Pentazocine – once oversold as a painkiller of morphine's stature, though supposedly with minimal side effects and addictive potential, pentazocine has now shrunk down to modest proportions. Prescribed for mild to moderate pain, it is of comparatively little interest to street users. Comes in tabs, amps, suppositories and carries the brand name Fortral.

Methadone – this is the official state fix for heroin addicts. The clinics hand it out as a substitute for smack and then reduce the dose down to zero. Where this can't be achieved the addict might be maintained short-term on a stable minimum dose, but such maintenance is getting rarer. In the early days the clinics used to make methadone available in injectable form. Now it comes as a yellowy-brown linctus; more commonly as a green 'mixture' which contains a little chloroform, making injection painful. These 'oral' solutions are of moderate intoxicant interest to the addict. They are valued, however, for relieving withdrawal pains, and thus many users attempt to screw as much of the stuff as possible from the clinics or a GP, and with the income buy something more blissful. Injectable methadone is still being manufactured, and it also comes in tablet form. The branded product, made by Burroughs Wellcome, is known as Physeptone.

The above are the most conspicuous opioids, but there is literally an infinite variety potentially available thanks to the 'Designer Drug' phenomenon now taking off in the US, whereby back-street chemists take a controlled substance and, by making tiny adjustments to its molecular structure, produce a high that remains legal until ruled otherwise. Designer drugs of the opioid class are a special favourite of the underground chemists, particularly those like alpha methylphentanyl, which is several hundred times more potent than heroin.

Routes of Admission

There is a well observed pathway to heroin addiction that starts with sniffing or smoking, graduates to skinpopping then on to mainlining, and often back again to skinpopping when all good veins are used up. This is not to say everyone who begins sniffing or smoking will become an addict, or that you can't be an addict unless you inject. Any route of admission can lead to addiction.

Sniffing

Heroine is sniffed in the same manner as cocaine – chopped with a blade on a hard surface, drawn into lines and snorted up one nostril at a time. Because of heroin's bitter flavour many find this method unappealing.

Smoking

Smoking is the method that the majority of younger British users seem to have taken to – at least initially. A dose is placed inside a strip of tin foil and a flame run underneath it. As the heroin heats up it turns black and wriggles like a snake – hence the term, Chasing the Dragon. The rising fumes are sucked up through the nostrils via a tube.

Skinpopping

Skinpopping is the intermediate stage between snorting/smoking and injecting into a vein. A hypodermic syringe is required for this activity, but the idea is merely to pop through the skin, usually into a muscle. The medical term is subcutaneous or intramuscular injection.

Mainlining

Mainlining means targeting the large vein running the length of the inner arm. It is the most thrifty method of disposing of junk and also affords a rush, at least before a big habit builds up. Repeated injections can cause veins to become scarred or thromboid (they get lumpy and collapse) and so others must be sought out in the neck, wrists, feet, etc. The last resort is to return to skinpopping. To prepare powdered heroin for injection it is placed in a teaspoon with a small amount of water, which is first warmed by running a flame underneath. If the heroin is in *base* form, as in the case with some South West Asian, then lemon juice (containing acetic acid) has to be added. Once dissolved the solution is sucked into the syringe and injected. To filter out impurities a dab of cotton wool can be placed in the syringe and the solution drawn through this; obviously not an especially efficient method and one which can result in fragments of fibres being plunged into the bloodstream. Many hungry addicts simply shake up their gear in a bottle containing water and inject the mixture.

By Mouth

This route is seldom used because the drug – which in the stomach is rapidly transformed into morphine – must first pass through the liver before reaching other parts of the body. A great deal of it never reaches other areas, so effective is the liver in breaking the morphine down.

Combinations

Not many heroin users are purists, but will often use other drugs to either heighten its effects or cope in periods of abstinence. In the latter category are alcohol, barbiturates and tranquillisers. But while these three depressants might ease the craving, they are of limited use during the actual crunch period of withdrawal. Stimulants such as speed and coke work as anti-soporifics, and users often pair up their opiate with a stimulant and inject them together. The archetypical combination is heroin plus cocaine – a *speedball*. Methadone and the speed-like Ritalin are popular, and Diconal – taken alone – was a hot favourite among hard-core users due to its reputation for providing a speedball-type effect.

Agonists, Antagonists and Partial Antagonists

Diconal is part of the family of opiates and opiate-type drugs which can be used interchangeably by addicts. Others in the group include heroin, opium, morphine, Palfium, DF-118 and pethidine. As a group they are known as *agonists* because they are compatible with each other – one being able to relieve the misery of withdrawal from the other. A drug which is effective against pain but has no substitute value for opiate addicts during withdrawal is called a *partial antagonist*. Not only is a partial antagonist an ineffective substitute, it might also precipitate withdrawal symptoms. One such is pentazocine, brand-named Fortral. A third category after agonists and partial antagonists is the pure antagonist of which naloxone (Narcan) is an example. This has no painkilling ability and no substitute effect during withdrawal. Its apparent usefulness lies in an ability to reverse the effects of both the agonists and partial antagonists, thus making it effective in cases of overdoses.

Sensations

The effects of heroin are much the same whether snorted, smoked, skinpopped or mainlined. An additional factor provided by the last two methods – especially mainlining – is the rush. As with all drugs the variety of responses to heroin is considerable. Some people get nothing from it, others find it nauseous and repugnant. In fact retching is not unusual for novice users. Practically all who try it must learn how to steer on to a pleasurable track. The experience usually starts seconds after administration (perhaps a minute or so with sniffing) with a warm feeling in the belly which flows throughout the body producing an overall calm, dreamy, self-sufficient feeling. It is not a euphoric drug in the sense that it sticks a grin on the face, but it does place the troubles of the world at some distance. Some users get drowsy, others become garrulous. One user tells me that he used to enjoy a stiff bicycle ride with his club. At higher doses, it is typical to slip into a dreamy, dozing state where the eyes fall shut mid-sentence and the head rolls in a routine known as *gouching-out*. While gouched-out, users are quite capable of accidentally scarring their bodies with lighted cigarettes, because while in the thrall of such a strong narcotic, they'll not be so riveted by pain. Other more physical effects include sweating, itchy skin, a runny nose, extra peeing, constipation, slowed-down breathing and a lower body temperature. Despite this literally rundown state, the heroin user's brain remains clear and active. Some claim that because the mind is uncluttered by regular worries it can go to work – between gouching – more effectively.

Special sensations are claimed to be particular to various members of the opiate and opioid families. Injected Diconal, for instance, is said to be just like cocaine and heroine combined, while pethidine is rated as 'dreamy'; pentazocine and dihydrocodeine are supposed to lead to panic attacks during withdrawal. But though there may be some truth in such claims, many drug observers are convinced that there is little to choose between the family members in terms of the sensations each give and that any difference is a matter of mythology and subjective reaction.

Pain and the Addict

Knowledge of the extremely complex interactions of the body's natural defences against pain is still very much incomplete. In recent years, though, breakthroughs have been made in recognising the nature of pain and the body's own capacity for perceiving and dealing with it. As Duquesne and Reeves explain in their *Handbook of Psychoactive Medicines*: 'The feeling of pain travels along nerve cells from its point of origin to the brain as waves of electrical signals; these are converted to molecular groupings known as neurotransmitters which transmit the sensation to specialised nerve endings. These latter are called receptors.'[1]

Found chiefly in areas of the mid-brain, receptors govern the individual's response to pain by reacting with or binding to natural opiate substances which are located in and released from other parts of the brain. There are believed to be a host of such substances. Those already identified are called enkephalins. Another natural painkiller that binds to the receptor sites is called endorphin, which has been found in the pituitary gland. If this thesis is right it means, in more simple language, that the body has its own chemicals for dealing with pain. They lie in wait, chiefly in diverse parts of the brain, ready to lock onto the site where the experience of pain is registered. As far as opiates are concerned, these too are believed to seek out and lock onto the pain receptor sites. It is currently being surmised that addicts are people with a low volume of natural opiates, and thus an inadequate natural remedy to pain. They therefore seek out narcotics as a solution, but whether the natural pain-relieving stock runs down as a result of opiate use or whether the individual starts out with a low base can only be guessed at.

Having described the apparent action of narcotics on the pain receptor sites we can now go on to the even more hypothetical area of antagonists. These are believed to lock on the very same sites and dislodge any opiate that happens to have got there first. If none are there, but subsequently show up, the repellent effect of the antagonists will cause withdrawal symptoms that are commensurate with the amount of opiate taken. Thus, the antagonists are sometimes used by clinics – though rarely in this country – to judge the size of an addict's habit.

Casual Use

It must be said that heroin use does not automatically equal addiction. The one-hit-and-you're-a-junkie myth is just that.

Some people manage to engage in non-threatening re-creational use for years, but it is also true that virtually every addict started out believing s/he could boss the drug.

Problem Use

It is a vicious irony that the most cost-effective means of taking heroin is by mainlining it into a vein. This is because the needle route takes the drug straight into the bloodstream and on into the brain with no loss in stray smoke or from material sticking to the nasal passages. It is the stomach that is most often given as the centre of the injection experience; the words used to describe how it feels frequently being sexual. For others the analogy is with death. As the drug is pumped in the feeling is so overwhelming it is assumed to be how death must feel. The joy comes from the relief a short while later at being alive. It is these sorts of melodramatic notions: the sense of running with life and death forces, the co-mingling of deprivation and succour, that keep some addicts engrossed in what in reality is a mundane obsession. And it is from such sources that the addict derives his/her sense of mastery. Normal drug-free living is assumed to be too tough, and so a private sensory world is created, in which 'normal' human experiences are received in reverse. For the non-addict joy is effervescence. For the addict joy is the suppression of such feelings: it is the suppression of sex, hunger, physical vitality, even the need to defecate and cough (though not, interest-ingly, to piss). The addict's life clearly does more closely resemble death rather than orgasm, and not surprisingly addicts say of themselves that their habit is a long and deliberate suicide.

Who's Vulnerable

Who then is most likely to launch themselves into problem heroin use? To answer: 'people with an addictive personality' doesn't help much because we don't know if such a personality is born out of factors environmental, social, political, genetic, or a combination of them all. Why, for instance, does one person turn out a 'junkie' and his brother, growing up in the same house, becomes an abstemious success in the City? In no particular order we can credit – luck, the company that is kept, availability of the substance, vulnerability to these influences, ignorance about the likely outcome of certain types of use. Once the virgin user does start succumbing to such influences the drugs have their very own momentum leading towards addiction. The novice will most probably have come to the drug without any specific pain. The odd thing about heroin is that it will soon provide it. (And though some drug professionals reject the idea that pain *is* experienced during withdrawal, preferring terms like discomfort – pain is how addicts usually perceive and describe what they are going through.) Pain, as the writer Richard Lingeman points out,[2] is heroin's antidote. And vice versa. This pain can develop in mild form after just three or four weeks' use. In other words, the body's molecules can be altered to such an extent, in such a short time, that if the supply is cut off, it signals its dismay by ordering pain. If the use has been for a longer period and in larger quantities then the magnitude of discomfort after withdrawal will increase accordingly. Also speeding up will be the onset of these distress signals relative to the time of last taking the drug. The novice will get high for about four or five hours and experience no distress in the aftermath. The veteran won't get high at all, but merely use the drug, perhaps by needle, half a dozen times a day to put the pain at a safe distance. In a real sense the addict gets into the same condition as some terminally ill cancer patients who are also never without pain or distress unless fuelled with an analgesic. One addict put the formula like this: 'Once hooked you're never straight. You're either stoned, or you're ill. I'd say 60 per cent of the time you're sick, 20 per cent of the time you're racing around trying to get the stuff, and the last 20 per cent you sleep.'

How long it takes to get into such a condition varies; someone shooting up 30 mg of pure heroin a day will have acquired a reasonably handsome habit within two or three weeks. A daily snorter or chaser of perhaps a quarter of a gramme will have to work at it longer. More typically, people drift into addiction, taking weeks, months or even years, and thereafter dropping in and out of dependent use. But once caught in the addictive spiral there are formidable obstacles to quitting. The actual physical withdrawal is not especially awesome – although it can appear so from the addict's perspective – and not in the least physically threatening. It is akin to a stiff bout of 'flu, and as with that ailment can be faced out if a good comfortable environment is found with nourishment and rest. Many addicts face it. Many times. The reasons for slipping back are various.

On a *social* level there are the obvious reasons of same old environment, same old drug-using crowd. Perhaps the job prospects are lousy. Family and straight friends have exhausted their patience so there isn't even a warm hearth. Extending from these social factors are a number of political circumstances such as the negligent way the government has set about providing pick-up-and-mend facilities, the failed strategy of the clinics and the continuing persecution through the courts of ordinary users.

On the *psychological* level there is the user's own inate 'defects' of character or those that have been inculcated through the onset of addiction. The individual probably feels weak, scared, lacking substance or perhaps filled with powerful, inadmissible drives. The heroin has provided relief from these feelings by laying a cloak over them. To remove the drug without dealing with them is to invite relapse.

On a *biological* level there is the relationship between pain and the body's store of natural opiates. This is still a new area of study. Does addiction deplete that stock? If so, for how long after quitting are the defences against pain low? Recovering addicts will often experience vague miseries for many years. They also feel the cravings returning when simply passing through an old drug haunt. As the author Lingeman notes,[3] 'The bodily craving has become by now a demanding, autonomous entity, operating irrespective of the addict's conscious will or reason.'

Health

Impact on the Body

Like most of its chemical relatives, heroin does not cause serious physical problems in itself, even when taken for a lifetime. The problems come from unstable patterns of use, from adulterants, from the hypodermic syringe, the company an addict keeps and the general run-down in health caused by poor eating and rest that results from a drug-fixated existence. Regular users often find themselves breathless, constipated and forever coughing up phlegm. They also lose their appetites for food and sex and because there's an increased risk of respiratory problems, this, in turn, can lead to various lung ailments. Friends might recognise growing use by a marked weight loss, a pale or jaundiced complexion, and a constantly dripping nose.

Risks of Injecting

There are health risks common to injectors of any substance and skinpoppers obtain no immunity from most of them. Indeed, popping brings the added dangers of boils and sores through which tetanus bacillus can enter. In New York City, 75 per cent of all tetanus cases during the early '70s were addicts and 50 per cent of these were fatal.[4]

Overdoses

The term overdose simply means the ingestion of a quantity of drug that the body hasn't built up a tolerance to. Once overloaded the body reacts in a number of ways, some of them fatal. The 'classic' overdose that ends lethally takes from one to twelve hours to run its course. It starts with slow, shallow or simply irregular breathing. The pupils reduce to a pinpoint, the skin turns blue, blood pressure is severely diminished; then comes coma. Pure antagonists (see page 204) can immediately reverse these effects, but since they set off potentially dangerous withdrawal symptoms they should

never be taken without medical supervision. Death, when it does occur, usually results from respiratory failure and complications in the region of the heart.

Why ODs Happen

Over-indulgence by an addict who is insecure about supplies is a common cause of ODs. Another pitfall is where tolerance to the drug's respiratory depressant effects is allowed to fall as a result of a period of not using. When the old high dose is suddenly administered the body can't cope. Addicts who have gone into hospital are particularly vulnerable to this fate when they return to old levels of consumption. A third OD cause is the use of street heroin purer than the user anticipated.

Sudden Deaths

A more dramatic outcome that is often called an OD is where the user dies with the works still hanging from his/her arm. Why such deaths happen isn't known. The bodies of the victims don't always show a high drug count, nor is it necessarily the fault of an adulterant. Some doctors put it down to shock, others to 'acute allergic reaction'.

Pulmonary Oedema

This is a particularly disgusting way of perishing. The victim more or less drowns from bodily fluids that surge into the lungs. The problems start with heart failure, causing the pulmonary arteries (those leading to the lungs) to become congested with blood. As pressure builds and the heart can no longer pump away the blood, fluid is forced out of the capillaries (tiny blood vessels) straight into the lungs.

Suffocation

This happens because of blockages to the air passages by (most commonly) vomit that under normal circumstances would be sicked up. OD victims who have also been drinking are especially prone to this sometimes fatal complication.

With Other Drugs

The simultaneous use of heroin and certain other drugs can be problematic. Heroin and alcohol together may cause vomiting – especially dangerous if the combination has caused unconsciousness. Heroin used with any of the central nervous system depressants (barbiturates, major and minor tranquillisers, as well as drink) accentuates respiratory depressant effects.

Serious and sometimes fatal reactions have occurred following the administration of pethidine to patients receiving drugs known as monoamine oxidase inhibitors (MAOIs) (see pages 84–5). Pethidine and related opioids should not be taken within two weeks of stopping MAOI therapy. Indeed all opiate and opioid drugs should be taken with 'extreme caution', say doctors, in conjunction with the MAOIs.

In Association with Medical Conditions

Heroin can also cause problems for individuals with severe respiratory ailments such as those found in asthmatics and cyanosis sufferers; also for those with illnesses related to alcohol problems, hyperthyroidism, head injuries, liver disorders, certain prostate conditions and anyone suffering with obstructed or inflamed bowels.

Heroin and Women

The repeated use of any drug places a strain on the liver, but because women's livers are usually half the size of men's, they are more susceptible to harm. Women are also more prone to contracting tetanus.

Habitual use commonly stops ovulation and a woman may not see a period for several months or even years if her habit continues. The cycle usually returns to normal when the drug is stopped. Other women will not have a period, but ovulation will continue sporadically. This masking of the cycle makes it easier to get pregnant unwittingly. Nearly all the analyses as to the impact of heroin addiction on birth concentrate on the mother as user while ignoring the habits of the child's father, therefore any review of the literature will give a tilted picture. That said, studies[5] show an incidence of abnormalities in the babies of female addicts which is classed in the 'high normal' range. But this incidence may not be meaningful since the women concerned had many other factors that could adversely affect their babies.

There is sharper evidence suggesting that addicts who are not under medical supervision have an increased chance of low-birthweight babies, and that the child's size is related to the drug rather than to lack of care. There also seems to be an increased risk of losing the baby just before, during or shortly after birth – again due to the baby's diminished size.

Junkie Babies

The spectre of junkie babies is a juicy one for the pop media. Such babies do exist as a result of the mother using regularly in the run-up to delivery. They appear normal at birth, but within a day or two get progressively restless and irritable as they go into a withdrawal syndrome. Feeding is difficult. Diarrhea is common. In the past mothers were encouraged to blow opium smoke into the child's mouth to alleviate these withdrawal symptoms. Today, chlorpromazine (the 'liquid cosh' tranquilliser) is commonly used, although some physicians prefer a camphorated tincture of opium, known as paregoric. In rare cases withdrawal symptoms take more than a month to show up. These should be tackled immediately. Once recovered from early hazards, the long-term outlook for babies of heroin-using mothers is generally good.

Health and the Other Opiates

The health hazards described above apply, more or less, to the whole family of opiates and opioids. Where there are special differences they are described below.

Pentazocine (Fortral) – a partial antagonist (see page 204), it is supposed to reverse the effects of regular opiates while also dealing with pain. A minority of addicts use it as their drug of choice. Not one for nodding off on.

Dipipanone (Diconal) – this causes extra problems when injected, and local infections and gangrene can result. Diconal also predisposes users to oedema. The presence of cyclizine usually puts a stop to vomiting.

Dihydrocodeine (DF-118) – this also contains chalk and so carries extra risk when injected.

Pethidine – there are reports that tolerance develops quickly, so doses tend to go up. Withdrawal is also very fast.

Methadone – rarely found in injectable form now. The linctus generally stabilises rather than elevates. It is just as addictive as heroin and the withdrawal is reputed to last longer, up to a week for the peak phase against three days. Although it can't be directly compared with heroin in terms of its effects and the time they last, a rough equivalent of one gramme of street heroin is 80 mg of methadone. The clinics generally believe, however, that 25 to 40 mg daily is enough to reduce the withdrawal symptoms on somebody using half a gramme of heroin a day down to a bearable level. Someone using in excess of half a gramme might be asked to return when they have cut back.

Earliest Use

Opium, the mother plant of both heroin and morphine, has proved a seductive and often scarifying proposition from the time humankind first incised the poppy pod and saw its milky juice ooze out. It is not known exactly when that was, although there are written references to the poppy as the 'joy plant' in Sumerian texts judged to be 6,000 years old. The Sumerians occupied land in what is now Southern Iraq and it seems that most of the peoples of the Middle East were familiar with poppy juice as a balm for both body and spirit.

The first clear-cut reference to the plant's pharmacology is in the third century BC writings of the Greek philosopher and botanist Theophrastus. Contemporaries were already warning about the drug's addictive potential.

Though opium smoking is firmly affixed by folklorists to Chinamen, it was many centuries before the Chinese developed their taste for the drug and they probably hadn't even glimpsed opium until Arab traders brought it to them in the seventh or eighth century AD. It was used by the Chinese chiefly as a medicine until the seventeenth century, when a fad developed for warming globs in a candle flame and inhaling the fumes. The practice alarmed the emperor who in 1729 ordered all imports to be stopped (China was manufacturing virtually none of her own) unless under licence. But the decree had little impact and the drug continued to flow into the country, largely via the Portuguese who had a settlement in Macao. The Portuguese did well enough from opium, but it was the British who really stepped up trade and in the process became the world's largest peddlars of the drug. Her stocks came from the newly conquered land of the Bengals in the Indian subcontinent. Her agent was the East India Company who owned the monopoly on the Bengal poppy harvest. Though already selling a portion to the Chinese, under licence, the Company saw the chance to do far better out of China's 300-million population. As Brian Inglis notes in his book, *The Forbidden Game*,[6] there was a snag: foreigners were permitted to trade with China only through Canton. The East India Company enjoyed a monopoly of British trade there. If the company shipped in more opium than allowed under licence, it might lose that monopoly.

The solution was to sell the drug in India to Indian merchants who could then smuggle it into China. That way the British stayed legal. By these means, and ignoring Imperial edicts to cease the trade, the drug had reached deep into the interior by the early 1800s. It reached Peking and into the palace itself, enslaving members of the emperor's bodyguards and his court eunuchs. Back home in England a rumbling started over the correctness of pushing so much of what was now considered a destructive drug. A House of Commons

Committee of Enquiry was set up in 1830 to scrutinise the East India Company's affairs, but this was easily disarmed by lies and bogus moral posturing. The Company line of argument was that it had to retain its opium monopoly in order to ensure prices remained high enough to restrict 'non medical' demand. An even more decisive argument was the economic one. The opium trade with China was worth over £2 million which, as Inglis notes, was almost half the amount it cost annually to service the Crown and the civil service in Britain. If not from opium sales, where would the revenues come? From British taxpayers?

The Company was deprived of some privileges and allowed to retain others so that, in effect, it was the British government itself that emerged with the direct responsibility for future opium trade between India and China. The true impact of that trade on the eighteenth and nineteenth century Chinese is open to argument, but it is believed to have bitten particularly sharply into the army and into the children of the wealthy and powerful. The Chinese emperor himself (Tao-Kwang) is said to have lost his three eldest sons from opium addiction.

So what were the Chinese to do? They tried flogging and the *cangue* (a sort of mobile stocks). They tried exile and capital punishment. They seriously considered, in the late 1830s, legalising the drug so as to abolish any need for the black market, but the legalisation lobby lost the argument, and in its place the emperor went to the root of the problem – or at least as much of that root as was visible. Most traffickers lived in Canton. It would therefore be sensible to arrest them there, send all their ships home and forbid more trade of any kind until opium smuggling ceased completely. The man placed in charge of executing the new policy was one Lin Tse-hsu, and he had barely taken office in 1839 when he ordered British merchants to surrender 20,000 chests containing approximately 140 lbs of opium each. The chests were polluted with salt and lime and flushed into the sea. Lin Tse-hsu had then intended to purge the Customs service, but ran into the kind of blanket resistance anti-dopists have encountered throughout history. The drug was simply too much in demand and the trafficking structure too sensitive for prohibitory moves to make headway. If the authorities lunged at imports, bigger bribes were paid to bent officials to account for their extra risk. The additional margin was acquired from the customer who, if addicted, would pay almost any price and simply turn to crime to get money for new supplies. And if the authorities clamped down with more stringent penalties, the participants would get even more desperate, more likely to kill to hide their traces.

Even as Commissioner Lin Tse-hsu was learning this baneful lesson the British were puffing up about 'the most shameful violence' that was the destruction of their opium stocks. In June 1840 an expeditionary force was despatched, and two years later a miserable capitulation had been extracted from the Chinese, under the Treaty of Nanking. The island of Hong Kong was ceded, trading and residential rights were gained at several more ports and there was an indemnity of £60 million China was obliged to compensate Britain for the loss of her opium and the cost of conducting the war. Within a few years other Western powers moved in to claim their portion and the long-dreaded 'Invasion of the Barbarians' became a reality.

In the decade following the Nanking Treaty, opium trade with China (not all accounted for by the British) doubled. A new emperor made more stout moves to prevent the drug's consumption (beheading for persistent users, their families sent into slavery) but he hadn't the muscle to make it stick, even in friendly parts of the empire. Finally another commissioner was sent to Canton to take up the cudgel once wielded by Lin Tse-hsu. The new man, Yeh Ming-Chen, was more circumspect, but the British were only too determined to be gravely insulted and thus have an excuse to undertake a second military excursion. There were issues beyond opium now. Along with France and America, Britain was unhappy with the level of trade in general that had resulted from concessions under the Nanking Treaty. If more ports could be opened up, she believed, the situation would be righted, and the only way to effect such a rupture was militarily. The pretext came in 1856 when a Chinese-crewed smuggling ship was apprehended off Canton. When Commissioner Yeh Ming-Chen refused to apologise for seizing this 'British' vessel (it ran a British flag in the hopes of deterring searches) the British navy shelled his official residence. Back in England a public row broke out. But when Lord Palmerston called a general election on the issue of the grave Chinese insult to the Crown, he found an electorate boiling up with patriotism and could thus claim a mandate for a second war.

The second opium war opened up eleven more ports to Westerners. In addition, the drug was made legal in return for a modest duty payable to the Chinese authorities. Opium trade rose briskly from about 60,000 chests in 1859 to more than 105,000 in 1880 – most of it derived from British India. The Chinese addict population is said to have been in excess of 15 million.

At this point the Chinese authorities finally absorbed the lesson that it is better to take a yen than a beating. They now permitted, even encouraged, the growing of Chinese opium, to try and reduce the strain on their currency. The British resisted by forcing import duties down in order to make their own Indian supplies more competitive, but within a few decades Chinese home-grown production had outstripped British imports from India. The wheel had turned full circle: the drug Britain and other Western powers had pushed on the Chinese under force of arms was beginning to travel in the reverse direction amid sounds of terrible panic and indignation. The West had long been consuming tinctures of medical opium and later on therapeutic shots of morphine, but this smoking of the drug . . . this was considered a filthy, entirely foreign habit.

The European Experience

Though Europeans are on record as having used opium as far back as the ancient Greeks (who also used to smoke it) it wasn't until the Renaissance that the drug began to saturate most parts of Europe. This development was due largely to a pharmacological breakthrough by the formidable Swiss physician, Bombastus von Hohenheim (1493–1541), better known as Paracelsus. His great feat was to produce a tincture of opium by mixing the drug with alcohol. He named it laudanum and it amounted to the beginning not merely of sedation on a mass scale, but the development of what we now know as pharmacology: 'the search for specific drugs in the treatment of specific diseases.'[7] Successive generations of physicians toyed with Paracelsus' prototype – adding to it sherry and spices – and by the seventeenth century laudanum was regarded as the indispensable tool of medicine. It was the aspirin/Valium of its day, used both to kill pain and sedate. It was considered the answer to diarrhea, coughs, menstrual cramps and the discomfort of colicky and teething babies.

If Paracelsus invented pharmacology, then its modern era was launched in 1805 when the German apothecary Frederick Sertürner isolated morphine from opium. This separation of what was known as the 'active principle' from its parent was also rightly recognised as a brilliant feat; it allowed for the first time the administration of near exact doses. What was curiously missed by Sertürner and those who feted him was the danger of addiction posed by a drug that was ten times more potent than opium – which was by now known to cause dependence. Indeed, by 1825 morphine was being marketed as a cure for opium addiction. That there could be problems from the unguarded use of the new drug didn't click even after the hypodermic syringe came into popular use around 1850. In a strange reversal of today's piece of folk whimsy that says you can't get a heroin habit by smoking – only by injecting, it was then believed you couldn't get a morphine habit by injecting – only by smoking. The majority of physicians still were not aware of the consequences of rampant morphine prescribing even after the American Civil War ended in 1866 and some 45,000 soldiers came home, dependent on their fixes.

There was, of course, a corps of progressive physicians who did recognise the problems of morphine addiction, but almost every attempt to correct the situation failed. For a while cocaine was pushed as the answer – users simply switched to leaning on the newer drug, or on both at the same time. The idea that addiction could be knocked flat by administering a more powerful substance continued with the invention of heroin in 1874. Named from the German word *heroisch* meaning heroic or powerful, it was three to four times more potent than its predecessor, and was marketed as a safe, non-addictive substitute for morphine.

A conspiracy theorist might begin to wonder when we consider that it was a German physician who developed laudanum, a German apothecary who isolated morphine and the Bayer Company in Germany which began commercial production of heroin in 1898. It was also in Germany during World War II that methadone was invented as a 'safe' substitute for heroin. Methadone, we now know, can hold a person by the throat every bit as determinedly as heroin and causes more protracted withdrawal.

Birth of the Junkie

If the abuse of drugs is an inescapable feature of human culture, we don't have to ask: 'When did abuse start?' The answer is easy: 'At the beginning.' Opium was being taken to excess in ancient Greece, and it is clear that more than a decent amount of laudanum was used almost as soon as it was introduced to Britain. But there was no clear distinction between medical and recreational users until the second half of the nineteenth century when doctors and pharmacists began coopting the sole dispensing rights to opium and its derivatives. By so doing they created the beginnings of the 'medical context'. And that meant anything falling outside was necessarily deviant. As the availability of all psychoactive drugs became more and more severely controlled, with possession rather than just sales restricted, so the junkie and his culture was forged.

Alcohol apart, worries about immoderate drug use in the early part of the nineteenth century centred mainly on what was called 'opium eating'. In fact it was the drinking of tinctures. Panic waves are reputed to have been caused by the 1821 publication of Thomas de Quincey's *Confessions of an*

English Opium Eater wherein the essayist writes of the terrors of an addiction gained at Oxford while trying to manage the pain of neuralgia. The working classes were a bigger concern: they favoured a spot of self-medication after long nights in the alehouse, a practice that was perceived as injurious to the social fabric. Reports of such usage aren't especially plentiful but they repeatedly emerge from deepest working-class districts where the factories and ports were located – and also areas like the Fens where women took heartily to the habit.

These fears took on a different shade with the discovery of opium smoking among England's Chinese population. In 1861, according to the historian Virginia Berridge, there were an estimated 167 Chinese people living in the entire country.[8] They lived principally in the Limehouse district in London's East End, and initially had been employed as sailors by that supreme opium peddlar, the East India Company. By 1881 there were still just 665 Chinese, but in those two decades the British public had been alerted to the menace the immigrés and their despicable habit posed. Berridge cites[9] an 1868 article in *London Society Magazine* among the first descriptions of domestic opium smoking. The account reports on a man called Chi Ki and his English wife who kept open house for smokers. The 'den' is described as 'mean and miserable', but not a threatening place. When Charles Dickens got hold of the theme for his unfinished *Mystery of Edwin Drood* (1870), there is an injection of macabre evil – and it was this note that sounded with increasing resonance all through the last years of the century.

A London County Council inspector notes of his visit to one den in 1904: 'Oriental cunning and cruelty . . . was hallmarked on every countenance. Until my visit to the Asiatic Sailors' Home, I had always considered some of the Jewish inhabitants of Whitechapel to be the worst type of humanity I had ever seen.'[10] The LCC tried to put a stop to opium smoking by licensing all seamen's lodging houses. Where the drug was discovered the licence would be removed, and with it the proprietor's livelihood. But the measure failed because of ambiguity over what was a 'seaman', what was a 'lodging house', and the deftness shown by the Chinese in throwing off the inspectors. The search for the 'wretched den' was in any case a hopeless task, for rather than taking place in a specially commissioned pit, smoking, as Berridge notes, was simply something that went on for relaxation in what was akin to a Chinese social club, usually poorly furnished, but no more so than a local pub. However, it didn't matter that serious investigators repeatedly came away from these places without evidence of depravity, the public at large wasn't going to be deprived. It was a time of widespread anti-immigrant sentiment – most of it directed at Jews – but with enough venom left over for other foreigners. Egged on by increasingly lurid newspaper and fictional accounts, the anti-opium-anti-Chinese movement grew.

The American Experience

Precisely the same drift, but on a grander scale, had been taking place in the US. In contrast to the pocketful of Chinese who trickled into Britain during the nineteenth century, from 1850 onwards America received scores of thousands. They came with the specific purpose of working the mines and fields of the West so that they could save a hatful of money and return home. But the passage over encumbered most of them with debts, the cost of food and lodgings were more barriers to saving and few were able to make that triumphal homecoming.[11] The Chinese who remained in America became perpetual transients. They were obliged to remain separate from 'decent' society setting up homes in the dingiest red-light districts where they added opium smoking to the domestic vices of gambling, drinking and prostitution.

'The opium den,' writes Terry Parssinen,[12] became something of a 'rogues' paradise . . . where thieves, pimps, prostitutes and saloon keepers could enjoy conversation and relax over a few pipes in the wee hours of the morning, knowing that the informal code prohibited violence or robbery within the den.'

The smoking went on in relative peace until, in the mid-1870s, one of those cyclical depressions hit the US economy, and the Chinese switched from being a vital source of manpower to an irritating surplus. Inevitably aliens began getting more carefully scrutinised. Newspaper stories spoke about the seduction of young whites as part of a Chinese-led global slave trade. As with all panics the stories weren't entirely divorced from fact: there were indeed daring young whites smoking in Chinatown and there was involvement in prostitution by some Chinese, but it was some jump from there into the deep and fantastical waters that led to America's first anti-narcotic laws. In 1875 San Francisco was the first town to pass an ordinance prohibiting opium smoking. Over the next forty years 27 more states followed suit, but smoking still increased. Data estimates that its popularity tripled. Not until 1909 when import controls forced prices up was the habit curbed.

This isn't to suggest, however, that the taste for drugs was thus dispelled. With the heat on opium young men and boys of the inner-city slums simply switched to drugs that were cheaper, didn't smell and could do more easily hidden. That meant heroin and morphine, and to a lesser extent, cocaine. By 1930 the old-style therapeutic addict was on the way out. In his/her place came the dangerous street-wise runt.

Modern Use and Controls

The international process of organised controls can be traced back to a series of meetings between 1909 and 1914 which established the framework for narcotics legislation worldwide. The first symposium was held in Shanghai and, at the instigation of the Americans, focused on opiate use in the Far East. Britain was cool on this initiative, not (as American commentators have suggested) because of her trading interests in the area, but because she was suspicious of America's gung ho internationalism. She preferred the one-to-one approach and had already established by these means an Anglo-Chinese agreement that limited opium traffic. Also, Britain suspected the US of being more interested in promoting her own influence in the Far East than in doing good for the world.

By the time the first of three Hague Conferences came round in 1911, Britain's position had become less ambivalent. Alarmed at increased drug smuggling to her Asian colonies she demanded the meetings look not just at opium smuggling to the Far East, but morphine and cocaine too in terms of a worldwide system of control. The Americans agreed, but the Germans, who had their own special cocaine interests, threw a proviso into the works: there was no point in the convention pledging itself to fair play, Germany argued, unless a sufficient number of nations agreed to join in the game with them. So while the framework could be sorted out there could be no commitment until there were 35 signatories. This is how the situation was left at the outbreak of the First World War.

For the British authorities the war period brought home just how vulnerable the political health of the nation could be to uncontrolled drugs use. In 1916 the army enacted Regulation 40B of the Defence of the Realm Act (DORA 40B), making it an offence for anyone to supply cocaine or any other drug to a member of the armed forces unless ordered by a doctor through a written prescription which had to be signed, dated and marked not to be repeated. Although this was an unprecedentedly stiff measure, it didn't tackle the general volume of domestic traffic and didn't apply itself at all to the problems of smuggling to the colonies. The next step for the Home Office was to extend DORA 40B to the entire civilian population who, it was argued, faced no less grave a menace from hard drugs. The most detailed restrictions under the civilian extension fixed on cocaine, but raw and powdered opium came in for only marginally less stringent controls. The Home Office had also wanted to bring morphine into line, but because of its more thoroughly medical context, was unable to wade through the opposition. Further legislative controls tightened up imports of cocaine and raw opium products by use of a new licensing system. By now the Home Office had positioned itself firmly in the cockpit of drugs policy, a position it has never yielded and is never likely to.

At the same time there were bolder moves being made on

the global canvas. The Versailles Peace Treaty of 1918 placed responsibility for international narcotics regulations in the hands of the fledgling League of Nations (later it would pass on to the United Nations). Article 295 of the Versailles Peace Pact proclaimed that within one year, what had been agreed at The Hague before the war but left unsigned, would have to be put into action. The pact made it incumbent on individual nations to introduce their own domestic legislation. Britain responded with the Dangerous Drugs Act 1920 (DDA). In effect, the DDA was DORA 40B, but widened to draw in other drugs such as medical opium and morphine. A lot of its nitty-gritty was reserved for the regulations that would follow the Act's passage through parliament. The new Ministry of Health had wanted to impose itself in the formulation of these regulations but was easily beaten back by the Home Office. 'The following four years,'[13] notes Virginia Berridge, 'saw consistent Home Office attempts to impose a policy completely penal in direction.' There were moves to ban maintenance prescribing to addicts. There were moves to concoct a blacklist of doctor-addicts that would be circulated to wholesale druggists; and attempts to reach into the finest detail of prescribing. In short, complained a Streatham pharmacist, the profession was being 'treated as a dangerous body of criminals.'

From these tensions came the Government-appointed Rolleston Committee, under Lord Humphrey Rolleston, President of the Royal College of Physicians. Set up in 1924 and reporting two years later, the main brief for Rolleston's panel was to decide whether or not physicians should be allowed to prescribe narcotics to addicts. In particular there was the question of long-term maintenance where a 'cure' wasn't possible. Rolleston's working party conducted a strange, complacent investigation calling no addicts, hearing chiefly medical witnesses and considering only as an afterthought such lower-class habits as the drinking of Chlorodyne patent medicine. In Rolleston's eyes there was principally one sort of addict: s/he was middle-class, middle-aged, often from the medical profession and invariably an abuser of morphine. About 500 such creatures existed nationwide, and rather than representing a threat they were to be pitied. The recommendations, therefore, were that the UK turn away from the US penal route by allowing the profession a better grip on the problem. Morphine and heroin should continue to be prescribed – long-term if this was thought necessary, and confidentiality had to be retained between patient and doctor, which meant there would be no obligation to notify the Home Office about who was being treated, how and why. In this way, the Home Office got its slapdown and heroin continued to be prescribed in Britain for almost forty years, making the system – the British system – a stark and globally contentious curio. The liberality of Rolleston was taken for granted for years, but recently it has been realised that in the seeds of those recommendations were the makings of a far grimmer regime. The better-deal-for-addicts policy applied only as long as they remained numerically small and decorously middle-class. When a new wave of raggedy-arsed users arrived in the late '50s, UK drugs policy once more revealed its spikier profile and the medical profession its willingness to operate a system at odds with what 'kindly old' Rolleston envisaged. Instead of confidentiality, all addicts were to be notified to the Home Office. Instead of the one-to-one GP arrangement, addicts were to be redirected to special clinics presided over by psychiatrists, with GPs being stripped of their right to prescribe. Heroin would subsequently be withdrawn from the clinics, to be replaced by an opioid substitute. And even this substitute (methadone) would come to be available short-term only for the majory of addicts. There is argument about where the thrust for such measures has come from. Some blame a hawkish Home Office. Others suspect the Home Office is in fact uneasy about heroin-free clinics, and that the impulse comes from psychiatrists and social workers.

The New Clinics

The new clinic system was established in 1968 on the recommendations of another government committee – this time headed by Sir Russell Brain (now Lord Brain). They resulted from Brain's second report; the first, in 1961, more or less repeated Rolleston's recommendations, completely missing the advent of the new-style street addicts. By 1965 their numbers had grown so markedly Brain was called out once more to look at what might be done. He believed the main reason for the '60s addiction problem was the wanton over-prescribing by a coterie of private London doctors. Because there was so much being dispensed, addicts were selling off the surplus to friends, creating more addicts who were in turn over-prescribed, and so on. An apparent answer to this malfunction would have been to penalise the doctors concerned, but by this time a new angle on addiction had developed. It was now considered a disease that threatened not just the individual but the whole of society. To prevent its spread a total defence network had to be established. This would be done by restricting the right to prescribe heroin and cocaine to a limited number of licensed doctors. They would be psychiatrists, all of them working within a hospital context, and mostly based at new Drug Dependency Units. Ordinary GPs would retain the right to prescribe narcotics to non addicts. But for their addicted patients they could only issue a range of synthetic opioids such as Fortral and methadone. Since then the squeeze has tightened further on the GP. Guidelines sent out in late 1984 left them with only the methadone linctus or mixture option for addicts.

The New Addicts

So who were these new addicts that Brain so nearly missed? The majority were English and Nigerian jazz musicians and, later, young Americans and Canadians for whom the British system of prescribing was manna. They believed in being cool in the way it was imagined the great US jazz players were cool, and heroin, for some, was the necessary apparatus.

A surviving example from that era is a man, called Tony R. Now in his late thirties, Tony was the child of a couple who worked as butler and servant to some very grand London families. From the earliest age Tony possessed the three most distinctive characteristics that go into the making of a dependent personality: his father was addicted to drink; he constantly looked outside himself for proof of his worth; and he started out, as he puts it, with the 'self-destruct button firing'. The scene he wanted to join from the age of 14 was the Kingston/Richmond beatniks, comprising jazz clubs and barge parties. He remembers it being peopled with individuals of special talent. There is some justification to such a rose-coloured rear view, since from that corps came the basic components of the British r-n-b scene of the '60s: Jeff Beck, Jimmy Page, Eric Clapton, Long John Baldry, The Rolling Stones, Graham Bond, etc. Tony's dream was to be a great artist, but he imagined then that it was sufficient merely to disport oneself in the appropriate style for it to happen. He knows this about himself now. He knows much about himself now after a 20-year drug career during which a great many of his friends perished. That he survived at all is extraordinary. During low times he tried to shoot himself and cut his head off. He has attacked policemen with a meat cleaver, driven a car through a chemist shop window and suffered the OD death of his own 17-year-old son. He has survived these events and is now in the business of helping other 'druggies'.

The Richmond scene of his youth never really fully embraced heroin, it took its pleasures from booze, hash, purple hearts and speed. Tony got his first smack from a Kingston musician who was being prescribed. He crushed it between two spoons, chopped and sniffed it. His voice dropped to a lazy croak and after twenty minutes he was sick, not a filthy retching, but a fairly pleasant sensation of dispensing with surplus bile. Since there was no hangover and no craving he did it again the next weekend. The use of needles started within weeks because, as he puts it, 'I liked the drug, and I always wanted to do things properly.' He began getting swallowed up. Plans for college were dumped and instead he got a job as an apprentice name-plate artist. He knew he was hooked, he says, the Monday night he came home from work and, being short of a fix, began sweating and aching as though stricken with malaria. When his mother said, 'You've being doing horse, haven't you? How long?' He wept. She took him to a drug specialist that same night and got a standby prescription. The next day he was registered and twice daily went to the Middlesex Hospital for an injection. This was a cold-hearted way to get fixed, so the next step was to acquire his personal drugs doctor who would allow him to administer himself. The drugs doctor was a gynaecologist, a well-intentioned old man, who gave him Methedrine on the side to jazz up the heroin rush. The gynaecologist thought he was lessening the risk of respiratory collapse by handing out speed at the same time. Such was the old man's generosity that although Tony had developed a voluminous habit he still had surplus drugs to sell off on the Piccadilly exchange.

For a while he enjoyed the darting around – the scoring, swapping, even the Sunday panics when the chemists were closed. Then in 1965 the scene, he reports, changed. A swarm of what he regarded as lower-class, artless gluttons descended on Piccadilly and began consuming with all the refinement of a scoop truck. By the time the new drug dependency clinics were established in 1968 he was ready for them, and to leave, if not drugs, behind, then the freak show that went with them. But while on one level the clinics gave him the stability to get and hold down a job for ten years as an addict, on another level they caused a greater hunger in his life by replacing his preferred heroin with the tedium of methadone. The amounts he was taking grew, as did his sense of indifference to his own fortune. Some of his early needle habits are remarkable: he'd drain water from toilet cisterns and jack up using an eyedropper fixed by a cigarette paper to a needle. The volumes he consumed also take some believing: 'The Physeptone (a brand of methadone) used to come in ampoules of one ml. each, but I liked to fix 18 at a time. Since the biggest syringe they supplied was 5 ml., I would flog this off to friends who weren't registered and buy myself 10 ml. syringes which I'd use two at a time. I'd be hitting two veins in one arm and pumping them simultaneously. It was supposed to have been enough to render nine people unconscious.'

His dissatisfaction with Physeptone meant periodically returning to do some trading in Piccadilly. He made a connection with local Chinese drug traders, who by this time could see the value of supplying smack-starved white kids. They used him as a courier, schlepping packages from the East End docks to Chinatown. His reward was a portion of the drugs. The Chinese he found to be impeccably straight in business, though impeccably reserved. 'There was always a terrific amount of money around, and they were heavily political – anti communists. You never asked questions in case you found out too much. Someone I know did that and ended up floating in Amsterdam harbour. That's where the thing was based.'

Corpses cropped up regularly on his daily rounds. Because he cared so little for himself they meant little to him. When encountering a body in the Piccadilly toilets, his first instinct was to go through the pockets to see what drugs were left, and if somebody died in his own place he would consider it a supreme inconvenience – what with the police and all. Dimly recognising what he'd come to, he attempted to quit heroin through hospital detoxification. He tried 15 or 20 times before finally stopping in 1979, whereupon the most drastic problems of his life began. Although he had left junk behind, he had substituted it with tranquillisers and, more critically, alcohol. His travails between 1979 and 1983 when he finally cleaned up entirely with the help of Narcotics Anonymous are almost farcically grim. The drink took him into the gutter. He went on time-looping benders lasting for weeks. He became a park bench 'dosser'. It destroyed his pancreas. Eventually he found himself in a mental hospital where he tried to hang himself. He tried to kill policemen, ambulance men, anyone in uniform. He found religion. He shot himself in the head, jumped off Lambeth bridge, slashed his wrists. He couldn't die and he couldn't live. Then after one particularly savage episode, he was deposited in St Bernard's mental hospial where a doctor told him the only way to tell how 'mad' he was would be to come off everything – booze, tranks, magic mushrooms, the lot. 'It was the first time anyone had ever said this to me in my life.' The idea that addiction cuts across the whole spectrum of drugs was a revelation.

Coming off alcohol was excruciating and in a sense he substituted once more, but this time it was with a fellowship of co-addicts. He still attends Narcotics Anonymous meetings several times a week and is furthering the fellowship's growth by encouraging the setting up of new local chapters.

Tony's love affair with drugs is as old or new as the turning of the moon. His father had it. His own son had it and perished at an early age. It took hold of a young woman whom we'll call Dilys. She was part of that later '60s generation that Tony accuses of dirtying the West End scene. Dilys, however, was not an artless dimwit but the child of a middle-class North London couple. She doesn't spell it out, but there is a sense of her having got too much crushing attention as a child, which left her emotionally enfeebled.

'I had what a lot of addicts start out with – low confidence and emotional immaturity. There is this inability to stand up for yourself and accept responsibility. Instead you run to someone else to look after you, or you run to drugs to sort of block everything out. In the end the drugs become an excuse in themselves for not sorting yourself out. I was smoking dope first of all, but got rather bored with that. At university I got hooked on speed because I found it gave me a lot of confidence. I cut myself off the first time because I felt bad about using so much – you know, the moods I got into and the way it isolated me from other people. My friends didn't like me taking it. I then spent a year being very depressed so I got back on because I always felt I had more confidence and ability when I was using speed.'

But the zip soon warped. She became frantic, paranoid, malnourished. The boy she married was simply someone to flaunt at her family: his problems were bigger than hers. Until the breakdown of her marriage she'd always had an aversion to jacking up heroin or any other drug because the image of the junkie appalled her. She still wanted to 'work, not die.' But now on her own with a young child to care for she moved from coke and speed to shooting up smack. The low point came when she took herself down to Piccadilly for a couple of weeks to run in blurred circles with the rest. She remembers a lot of the kids living in squats or in bad hotels around the main stations. A large number were dabbling in burglary and they could be seen – as today – selling the proceeds on the street;

anything from an LP to their parent's furniture. Most of the traffic centred on pharmaceuticals of the upper/downer variety. Traditionally the dealer sits in a café with, say, 15 ampoules of something, one of which is offered to a young runner if the runner can produce some punters. What the punter gets might be an amp filled with water. 'People were being killed for their scripts [prescriptions]' she says, and had she stayed down Piccadilly she believes she'd have wound up selling her body, then dying from one of a hundred causes.

'I suppose, basically, I had had enough of messing up my life and I was lucky enough to get a social worker I could trust. She put me on to Phoenix House (rehabilitation centre) which I was shit scared about going to. Thankfully I hadn't heard that much bad gossip about the place in those days, but I did know it ran a bit along the lines of Synanon in the States – a tough treatment centre that strips you right down to the basics. Phoenix was hard. It was really hard to face up to things and change. But I stuck it out when I felt like leaving because I knew I had nothing to go out to. I knew I'd be on the street again and I wasn't prepared to be out there.' After Phoenix she worked for a few months in film and advertising jobs to test herself away from the drugs world. But she found that world 'very impersonal and very shitty. I just couldn't relate to people who cared only about their own trips, their cars and mortgages. There's so much isolation with people not really caring about one another.'

As so often happens with recovered addicts, she now works in the field of drugs rehabilitation herself. 'I find people panic,' she says, 'because they've gone to a rehab house and they still can't stop, and they think to themselves "*God, what is there left?*" They don't realise it's they themselves who have to stop using.'

Just as Dilys's generation copied and overtook Tony R's, a sequence of events occurred in the mid-'70s that sucked in fresh waves of users. This was partly to do with availability; partly with the increasingly dismal state of the country. Every age is a troubled one, but the period beginning with the recession of the late '70s found the UK being thrown into an historical lurch equivalent to the late eighteenth century transition from ruralism to industrialism, and where that earlier transitional period was accompanied by the most protracted and sordid drinking binge in our history, heroin seems to be the drug we are taking with us into the microchip epoch: I say 'seems' because it is too easy to overrate heroin in a society where there is a far more voluminous traffic in alcohol and the benzodiazepines. Industrial/social change and the unemployment and uncertainty that goes with it is at the root of the current epidemic – tied, of course, to easy accessibility.

Fashion has also played its part. The discovery by a generation of US and British musicians of cocaine sniffing that kept them awake after gigs and gave them an inflated sense of their talents became more universally popular. From sniffing coke it is a short step to sniffing other white powder drugs such as amphetamine – which was suddenly available everywhere as sulphate. The move to heroin was always going to be more difficult because of the resoundingly poor image the drug had carried since the '20s, but the bad imagery, paradoxically, was the thing that ultimately appealed. In the mid '70s, to be rebelliously cool was to be fully equipped. Rolling Stone Keith Richard was one who embodied these attitudes, and there was many a Richard clone ready to proselytise on his and the drug's behalf.

While rock stars and their camp followers were sniffing heroin there was no particular panic, but when the drug was taken up by working-class youth then the steam did start rising. First signs of an 'epidemic' were announced by a couple of researchers at Glasgow University who published a report, 'The Rapid Increase in Heroin Addiction' in 1981.[14] They pointed to a 388 per cent rise in new clinic cases in six months, plus a quantum leap in pharmacy break-ins. Glasgow, they chimed ominously, was beginning to look like New York. 15- and 16-year-olds from the slab concrete estates were jacking up a range of painkilling solutions, many of them foully adulterated. Where they once got ground-up Victory V lozenges cut with their brown Iranian H, they were now getting talcum powder or strychnine with the new whiter stuff. Because of the increased rewards old-fashioned villains had become involved and were practising old-fashioned blood and extortion methods. One man's hands were broken with a baseball bat because he allegedly owed £150. He was later stabbed to death. My own visit to the city in early 1983 found a worsening situation and reports since suggest a further slide. Estimates of the number of heroin addicts in town were pitched around 10,000, and yet the facilities for helping them were absurdly inadequate. I called at a drop-in centre called St Enochs. It is situated in the Gorbals on a patch of muddy land butting onto huge, dark-faced estate blocks. Each morning 200 addicts gathered for their withdrawal scripts of methadone linctus, then drifted in and out. A clutch of nuns were on hand flashing charitable smiles. Two youths were playing pool and an unhappy mother of three kids complained of stones in her one remaining kidney. She said that thanks to Enochs she was down from a habit of half a gramme of heroin plus 10 methadone tablets a day, to just four tabs of methadone. The doctor at the Southern General Clinic, she said, was a hard cow. Later, the town's drugs squad chief, Charlie Rogers, told me things weren't in fact as hysterically bad as they were painted, and that in comparison to alcohol abuse the heroin problem scarcely existed at all. But some way across town from police chief Charlie's, at a community project I agreed not to name because the people I spoke to there didn't want it dragged through the media gutter any more, there was another perception of drugs, police, and the cankerous, hard-faced system they are asked to defend. Among the area's 16–25-year-olds, I was told, the jobless rate was 75 per cent. Heroin had shown up in force in 1981 and now everything was being tried. Bel Air hairspray was being injected between toes, Beechams powders were diluted and then injected, as was a curious cocktail of methadone and pulped travel sickness pills. It was this combination that had lately killed a local boy on his sixteenth birthday. There was open dealing in pubs with stolen goods being humped in and out. Prostitution among young girls was increasing. Guns were turning up to enforce sectional interests and there had been so much thieving from Provident (loan) collectors that they no longer made the rounds. Credit was therefore drying up. It was a disease, they said, that spread more deprivation and more crime. 'None of the kids here has any political views,' said the project's leader. 'Nothing. And they don't care because they see no future. That's why it doesn't matter to them what the drugs do – whether they're left with a limp or a hump. And we can't do anything about it, not until they're ready. Then we can give them support.'

I found a similar picture in Manchester, except here the drug was being smoked from foil – Chasing the Dragon – rather than injected. The scene was much more furtive. A young man called Norman took me on a tour of the city's Hulme district. He was himself an addict, just out of a psychiatric hospital where he'd undergone detoxification. He went in vomiting blood and weighing seven stone. 'What I really want,' he said without a suggestion of humour, 'is healthier drugs. What they sell around here for heroin is mostly St Ivel's Five Pints. I go only for pharmaceuticals these days. They're purer.'

Norman comes from a smart, middle-class family and got his drug habit from an older brother who was a '60s mod. Private school was supposed to have kept Norman wholesome, but there he developed a ferocious drink problem. A year later he was injecting his brother's morphine, his methedrine, Ritalin, barbiturates, an array of synthetic opiates, including heroin – eventually contracting the inevitable dose of hepatitis. 'People like me have something to fall back on to pay for their drugs, even though, as you see,' he flashed his hands before me, 'I've no rings or watches to sell off any more. These working-class kids from the estates though, they start out with nothing and end up in prison.'

He insisted the clinic scene was also basically middle-class in that the middle-classes were the only ones who knew how to squeeze what they wanted from them. We walked together through Hulme's Bullring, a notorious complex of arcing council blocks that no doubt once looked stunning on the architectural graph sheet. 'Over there,' he said, pointing to a low-rise block, 'is what's called the Shooting Gallery, on account of the number of junkies. I think the council likes to keep them all together. At night the kids come out on the concrete open space and you can hear them smashing their cider bottles. No one else comes out. Funny thing is this used to be a smart area. There's the Henry Royce pub, named after the Rolls Royce man. On that same site was a Rolls workshop. Rolls Royce, think of it. And now look.'

But it wasn't just the scummier areas of Manchester that were suffering the heroin blitz. Smart areas such as Salford – average incomes £8,000 to £15,000 – were also affected.

'In our street we've got just one manual worker,' a Salford fire chief and drugs councillor told me at the end of 1984. 'And yet heroin's as easy to come by here as tobacco. A lot of them are getting into it because of the "dare" thing. On another level this is one of the areas where you've got a heavy student population, so it's cash. If you're using and dealing a little, you've got money. No problems.' The other important factor, he suggests, is that the kids living around him have rejected old-style recreational pursuits like getting tanked up on booze and having a busted head in the morning. Heroin seems to them more sublime and sophisticated. It also couples with the 'forbidden' night – which is when many unemployed kids are doing their living these days. They rise close to noon, limp around until early evening, and then come midnight are jazz dancing in one of the practically free discos. Failing that they're hanging out on street corners. 'Living that life,' says the fire chief, 'it's easy to slip into the drug scene because it relieves the tensions and agonies of mind and makes them relax. My youngest lad can stop bloody well looking for work now. I'm a local councillor and I can't help him. I've even gone in my fire chief's uniform and said, "I'm Councillor Blackburn, this is my son." But there was nothing I could do for him.'

The situation in Liverpool, which is even more under-nourished, is comparable. There is the same distress and confusion as parents find their children getting caught in the revolving door of the streets, the courts, prison and back out on the streets again. There is no shortage of unappetising data for Liverpool. Four out of five school leavers are not expected to find work. 65 per cent of all police incidents are reported to be 'drug related', and in 1983, 12 baby addicts are said to have been born in a single Merseyside hospital.

Another area that has caught the media's attention is the Bermondsey and Rotherhithe area of South London. Stories began circulating in mid-'84 of pushers rolling up in Porsches and young teens falling out of the tower blocks to greet them like it was ice cream time. The kids often didn't know what they were taking, so the story went: they called it *scag* as though it were another substance. And even when they knew it was heroin, they believed that by smoking it from foil they couldn't get addicted. This alleged ignorance of young users is sometimes borne out, but most often not. Many know the score precisely. They use the inherent dangers of junk smoking as a mark of their personal mettle. As in Manchester it was a highly furtive scene, keeping itself separate from the local 'puffers' (cannabis smokers). Though they ganged about as a scaghead clan, the actual smoking was done in splinter groups of twos and threes: girls apart from boys. Crime? Yes, it was up in the area, said a representative from the local Community Drugs Project. But let us not panic, they urged. And let us not imagine that it was unrelated to deeper social turmoil.

The fixation on the new working-class metropolitan 'junkies' came to dissipate slightly by the end of 1984 as evidence continued to mount of the drug being used in all parts of the UK and by every social type. Whether in Brighton or Chester or those little postcard towns of Wiltshire (where much fixing goes on) there seemed no heroin-free zone remaining – except, curiously, Belfast and Derry where, it is rumoured, the Provos are keeping it out. One typically trammelled part of rural England was Camberley in Surrey. Here, a young contact tells me, the drug is used by the 'ultra-modernists' who will soak up anything if it's top ten sharp. Like most other kids in the area they have no job to go to, but on a Saturday night a little 'draw' as heroin is called, gives them an edge. They smoke it openly outside the pubs and are the same sort who traditionally have got insensible on alcohol over the weekend. Not all of them will become addicts (despite the determination of sections of the media to insist heroin automatically equals addiction). Not even most of them. But some will come to grief. A friend of my young contact died after a spell in hospital following an overdose. The break from the drug caused his body's tolerance to slip back. On shooting up the amount he'd become used to prior to the OD, his body packed up.

'Until my friend died no one wanted to own up about what was going on, but it was well known. The needles were coming from porters in hospitals. They were coming out boxes at a time. Or you pretend at the chemist that you're a diabetic. The stuff itself comes down every so often with older-looking guys from London, I think. After they've made a connection with someone local, they state terms and that's that.

'They don't look the using type themselves. One little trick people are up to here is to get a letter from your parents saying you got chucked out of the house and that way you get a cheque for, say, £22 a week rent and £25 for the dole from the DHSS. You might be staying in a squat somewhere or still be at home and pretending. They hardly ever come out and check. Then with the money you can put it into building up a dealing thing.'

Scams

There are many such scams employed by users to keep themselves afloat. Seasoned addicts are among the most resourceful citizens in the land. They will know how to tap a vulnerable doctor the way a class of schoolkids can take apart a supply teacher. They also know how to work over even those who know them best – with tears and promises to do better. One man tells me of his method of forging prescriptions that has served him without mishap for four years. First he Letrasets the name of a Harley Street doctor on Basildon Bond paper. He gives an alternative evening and weekend phone number which is actually the phone number of a public call box. An accomplice goes for the script out of hours while he waits in the phone box to confirm its authenticity to the enquiring pharmacist.

Forgery is a means of supplementing the addict's income. As well as this, the addict will probably also attempt to get signed on with the sort of private GP who'll prescribe generous amounts of different types of drug. It can be expensive working through such physicians, for there are consultation fees involved (ranging from £30 to £50) plus the fee the chemist charges for the drug itself. However, once on the books, there are ways of turning a living. As a recent *Harpers and Queen* article demonstrated,[15] even a non-addict can get registered as an addict and acquire regular prescriptions. With just a modest amount of subterfuge (a scruffy appearance, preferably with cigarette-burnt clothing, displays of scratching and sleepiness) it is possible on a first visit to get a 24-hour supply of Physeptone.

To get a repeat prescription requires giving a urine sample. This is to confirm that the user is indeed junk ridden. A way around this, reports the *Harpers* article, is to have an addict friend turn up at the laboratory instead – or s/he could give a bottle containing his/her own fresh urine which the new candidate keeps warm under a coat. Nobody actually watches as the 'patient' pees. Once the sample is confirmed, the patient will probably get an initial supply of 350 ml. methadone mixture a week. In 1984 this was worth a fairly miserable £35, but if the patient were subsequently to complain that the methadone was having a soporific effect, then a script for a stimulant might be forthcoming. This is worth up to £4 a tablet on the black market. Now there is scope for some business. Such one-off initiatives are sometimes overlaid with group activity. It is the style in parts of Manchester and Liverpool, for instance, to establish cooperative 'scoring' ventures with names like Trogs (as in troglodytes). Traditionally there is little trust among addicts so perhaps these young bands – numbering eight to a dozen – are not so much addicts yet, as living the life. By pooling all resources such as dole cheques and stolen goods and sharing out the proceeds, members of these groups are fairly certain of a hit seven days a week.

By banding together they also have the feeling they are backed up in a tough world. It is additionally a work substitute for a generation who have been delivered the message that they are surplus to industrial requirements.

Heroin and Crime

Anyone using street heroin is engaged in a criminal activity because the state has ruled so. But that aside, the relationship between the drug and crimes involving others does cause worry and is worth examining. It has to be said that smack junkies are not an unduly vicious lot even though the compulsion to score drives them to extreme limits. The drug is overwhelmingly a stupefying one. Such violence as does exist is more likely to come from traffickers (who tend to be non-users) and get directed at the addicts themselves. Those addicts who do spill blood will probably have tended in that direction before addiction. The crimes heavy users do commit have traditionally centred on acquiring liquidity for the next hit, thus they would be petty theft, prostitution, forgery and fraud. The scale of such an incursion into the above-board economy is becoming quite formidable. One experienced drug agency worker put it like this in 1984: 'An addict will use approximately half a gramme of heroin per day, which will cost £35 to £40. There are an estimated 40,000 of these addicts in the UK which means some 20 to 30 kilogrammes are needed daily to support the national habit. If half of these 40,000 support themselves by theft and if the retail value of their stolen goods is 10 per cent of their actual value [which is how the police measure it] then to keep the addicts of the UK going, £15 million worth of goods must be stolen each and every day. And these are conservative figures.' While this is becoming the standard formula for assessing fallout from the UK heroin habit, two researchers at the Drug Indicators Project in North London – Roger Lewis and Richard Hartnoll[16] – argue that the figures are misleading in that they suggest that all heroin users are consuming constantly. This is not the case; most use less than the statistical 'average' habit but get attributed more because of the extra high intake of street dealers who, in fact, are entirely self-financing. The latter are able to maintain their habits of perhaps a gramme a day through dealing. Their customers are probably consuming something like one-eighth of a gramme a day which, at the 1982 prices on which the pair made their calculations, translates into a weekly cash requirement of £87.50. Furthermore, such an amount will not be needed for 52 weeks a year. Because of the vagaries of supply, financing, pledges to quit etc., the sum is only spent for an average of 7½ months. Thus, annual expenditure on heroin for the average consumer would be 'only' £2,800. This amount is acquired from work, DHSS payments, petty dealing, theft and prostitution.

Dealers and Traffickers

The ire of users' loved ones inevitably gets directed at 'the pusher', but it is as well to distinguish between traffickers and dealers. The first are usually non-users engaged in large-scale transactions for monetary gain. They bridge the gap between the producer and the consumer. The second are themselves users who distribute comparatively small amounts to finance their own habit. Virtually all addicts deal at some stage, if only in small portions. It is one way to survive in a system where drugs are costly and illegal.

Lewis and Hartnoll break down the domestic supply network into four basic components. There is the *importer* who thinks in terms of kilogrammes and will probably be offering a drug at 70 per cent purity. Then there is the *wholesaler* who at 1982 prices was paying £20,000 per kilo and diluting it down from 70 per cent to 55 per cent. These diluted kilos will be sold in one-ounce lots at £1,000 apiece to *major retailers* who invariably will be users themselves. These major retailers will dilute down from 55 per cent to 45 per cent and sell off in quarter-ounce lots priced at around £350. These quarter-ounces are purchased once or twice a week by *street retailers* who will use about 40 per cent themselves and cut the remainder down to 35 per cent purity, selling it off in single grammes priced in 1982 at £60. It is the street retailers who also make up the £5 and £10 wraps, or else it is done by even smaller fry who buy from them.

The total amount of imported heroin needed to service the

nation's users is also investigated by Lewis and Hartnoll. Bearing in mind 'cuts' introduced at wholesale and street level, as well as seizures by police and Customs, the total amount directed at the UK annually is put at 920 kg, of which 750 kg successfully reaches the consumers. (This is on the assumption that supply meets demand.) Such a figure is some way short of the 7,300 kg often cited.

As for profits, Lewis and Hartnoll put them at £48 million annually: £10 million made at the import stage, £17 million at the bulk wholesale stage, £14 million at the major retailer stage and just £7 million for the street retailers.

Since 1982 the number of 'addicts' has risen from 40,000 to 75,000 and the price of street heroin from £60 to £70–£80 a gramme. Nonetheless, Lewis and Hartnoll argue that their formulae still hold true.

Trafficking Trends

Large-scale trading in illegal heroin involving the West goes back to the 1930s when the drug was shipped from Europe to the US. The poppy was grown in Turkey and moved as opium or morphine base to the Marseilles area where it was converted into heroin by Corsican chemists. It was smuggled to the States by Italian Mafiosi who apparently had an understanding with the Corsicans that stated: you refine it, we sell it, no cross-over. But eventually the French refined, transported and increasingly sold direct to New York themselves – until 1973 when the 'French Connection' was (temporarily) busted. There was also a coexistence at various times between factions of the Corsican and Italian operations, and elements of the US intelligence community. The Americans had called upon the Sicilian Mafia to facilitate the Allied landings on the island during World War II. They later got Corsican mobsters to act as communist strike breakers on the Marseilles waterfront. As a result of these enterprises the Europeans felt sufficiently emboldened to start large-scale heroin shipments to the States, and it is often alleged that those aforementioned elements of US intelligence ensured a blind eye was turned to the traffic.

The unstated pact is said to have still been in operation in the late '50s when the US moved into the Indochinese vacuum caused by the withdrawal of the French. Here they found opium and morphine permeating every crevice of society – which obliged them to turn another blind eye. They needed to keep happy the locals who were engaged in the manufacture and trafficking of the drug; happy and ready to keep up the war effort against the Vietcong. In those days the US authorities were actually flying opium out of the production zones for processing in Laos. By the late '60s American soldiers in Vietnam were picking up the heroin habit on a grand scale and South East Asian stocks reached the US itself in the early '70s. This followed President Nixon's 'War on Drugs' which in effect debarred Turkish smack from America, thus opening the way principally for Mexican stock, but also for the Golden Triangle product.

Golden Triangle heroin continued to back up Mexican stock, serving America's needs until 1977 when the distribution network broke down due to a couple of bad harvests, gang rivalry and successes by drug enforcement teams. The US void was filled by stocks from the Golden Crescent, which is the blend that presently sweeps across all Europe. Just to excite the picture, however, the Golden Triangle now seems to have recovered and for the first time is making headway into Europe as well. Nonetheless it is the Pakistani product, ranging in appearance from a grainy, powdery beige to almost white, that has taken 80 per cent of the UK market. It first came in via a legion of middle-class Iranians on the run from the Ayatollah. Heroin was to be a currency for them in their new country. For those who were themselves users it was also a guaranteed supply. Iranian heroin turned out to be an exercise in pump priming for the whole European market. For where Iranian had been, heroin from Afghanistan and Pakistan was to follow.

The Golden Crescent

The Frontiers of Iran, Pakistan and Afghanistan have long comprised a virtual no-go area for the central governments concerned. Fealty is strictly to the tribe, while any aggressive move to bring the peoples under rein risks destabilising what is already an extraordinarily sensitive part of the world.

Its political shape has changed beyond recognition since the fateful year of 1979. That was the year the Shah of Iran was overthrown, the Soviets invaded Afghanistan and the West, especially America, began emboldening Pakistan's General Zia ul Haq with weapons and money. Previously an international pariah, now Zia was seen as a front-line warrior in the battle against communism.

In concert with the political turbulence of 1979 the poppy trade also gyrated wildly. It was the year when the Golden Triangle's harvest collapsed and, in response, the Crescent put out almost double its usual quantity of 8,000 tons. There have been moves since that boom to stop the flow, but every failed effort illustrates that there is virtually no thwarting the ancient principle of supply and demand. Each time a cork is thrust into one orifice, another opens. An early move in Zia's war against opium came in 1979 when numerous domestic opium outlets were shut down. The consequence, predictably, was that the people switched to the lighter and less odorous heroin.

With domestic demand for heroin up, traffickers were encouraged to open their own heroin-producing laboratories rather than buy in from Western or Thai chemists. And why stop there? Iranian students fleeing to the West with their substandard product had shown the demand for heroin in Europe. They could hook on to existing drugs distribution networks or establish their own. This would be especially easy in the UK where members of the expatriot Asian community could easily travel without suspicion to and from the sub-continent. In those early days kilos of heroin were going begging for want of established routines. Avoidance tactics were also pretty naïve: one man arrived at Heathrow with his shoes so stuffed with heroin he could scarcely walk unaided. Since those days Pakistan has grown into the world's largest supplier of heroin, accounting for some 80 per cent of stocks seized in the UK and 30 per cent of the American market.

This would seem a curious achievement given the

announced successes of the Pakistani authorities. They say they have managed to slash poppy production from 800 tonnes in 1979 to around 50 in 1983. And while less than 10 kilos of heroin were seized internally in 1980, by 1983 the figure had risen to 1,800 kilos.

Traditionally most of the opium poppies have been grown in the Buner district of the North West Frontier by Pathan tribes. The government says it has put a stop to cultivation there by a combination of force and a substitute crop programme partly financed by the United Nations. But visitors to the area in January 1984[17] insisted that poppies were still being cultivated – some within view of Pakistani military forces who were assumed to be taking a cut from the lucrative trade. Claims about the smashing of scores of labs are also treated with scepticism. By June of 1984 41 were said to have been shut down. When US officials examined them, however, they comprised old buckets and tubs: no sign of refining chemicals, opium or heroin. The important labs were said to be operating on the Afghan side of the border, and this is where much of the poppy growing was also said to be taking place. The product is despatched from there to traffickers in Lahore and Karachi for distribution both internally and westward. Why can't the authorities move against the big traffickers? The answer is the same in Pakistan as in any country where the demand is powerful enough. Traders will simply bribe and fight their way through to the profits.

The likelihood of putting a stop to the Afghan end of the trade is even more remote. Moving against a group of people who are in effect a sandbag against the Russians is bad politics. Heroin and opium are important means by which the tribes people can continue supporting their struggle. We can see then that Zia has reason to undertake his battle against heroin with some ambivalence. On the one hand he must keep sweet with the tribal growers at the borders, which is what the West wants too. But the West also wants him to kill the trade. A more powerful impulse to act against the trade comes from within his own country, which has seen a growth in the heroin-using population that outstrips anything witnessed in the West. Before 1980 there were virtually zero users. By 1983 the number was put at 200,000. Inherent in that figure is an awful lot of crime. The volume of use also distorts Pakistan's economy by causing overdependence by growers on a single crop. Additionally, it robs the legitimate economy of a substantial slice of income.

There has been understandable anger from the West about the quantities of heroin it is receiving from Pakistan, but it must be remembered that it was the European powers who introduced mass production of poppies into that country and the rest of the non-industrialised East, sometimes by force of arms. The West now reaps a portion of that harvest and attempts to stop it by threats, bribes and persuasion. It tries to get the impoverished poppy farmers to switch to other crops, but such schemes will have to be backed up with real money, with irrigation projects and roads. For a farmer in the dusty, mountainous Buner district of North West Pakistan, there can be little incentive for switching from poppies when the next most profitable crop – wheat – will fetch only half as much.

The Golden Triangle

The lives of the hill farmers of the Golden Triangle region of Burmah, Thailand and Laos are less caught up in the production of the opium poppy than those of the Crescent. Nonetheless opium has been used for centuries to alleviate hunger and pain on long journeys, and as an aid to sleep. A labour-intensive crop, notes drugs analyst Roger Lewis,[18] the poppy is frequently harvested by entire families so that children are familiar with the plant and its potential dangers from an early age. Addicts are not so much cast out as considered fools.

The advent of the massive heroin trade is very much the achievement of remnants of the Chinese nationalist army who fled to the area in 1949 following their defeat by Mao Tse Tung's communists. Calling themselves the Third Army of the Koumintang (KMT), the nationalists moved first into Burmah and then into Laos before setting up village bases in the remote regions along Thailand's northern border with Burmah. For some years they launched CIA-backed assaults against mainland China. Then, in an attempt to become self-financing, they hit upon opium. Stocks were acquired from the hill people of the North East of Burmah. The crude opium was moved by mule train to border areas for refining. Then, either as heroin or smoking opium, it was transported through Thailand and on to the West via Hong Kong.

This is the pattern that's still used today, although on a severely truncated scale. A neat justification for their entrée into trafficking came from the late KMT general Tuen Shi-wen: 'We must continue to fight the evil of communism. To fight you must have an army and an army must have guns. To buy guns you must have money and in the mountains the only money is opium.'[19]

The Thais were quick to see the logic, and some of her generals quick at taking a cut in return for expediting the stuff through their country. The Americans also saw the sense in supporting the KMT against the communists. Money and arms were laid on, and US engineers built a road linking the KMT headquarters to a highway – supposedly for military reasons, but in reality to facilitate the opium traffic. Inevitably the KMT began indulging in excesses that even the Thais found indigestible. They brutalised the hill growers – demanding they pay an annual opium tax. They forced farmers who'd abandoned the crop to return to it, and in other instances stole land and forced people to work as slave labourers.

In 1984, Thai forces moved against the KMT and by August had captured 13 villages where its power had been centred. There are reports, however, of KMT men still hiding out in the jungle where they continue to work the opium caravans. Clearly their share of the market is down. Until the Thai offensive some 80 per cent of all Golden Triangle heroin was believed to have passed through their hands. The figure subsequently has been put at one-third. The main beneficiary of the KMT's eclipse is one of their former allies, a half-Mongol, half-Chinese warlord called Khun Sa (pronounced cancer). Khun Sa was another main target of the Thai forces, but although they managed to beat him and his Shan United Army back into Burmah, they were showing no signs of being able to curb his heroin dealings. The Burmese government seems equally impotent.

The situation in South East and South West Asia is very complex, but what it does illustrate in all its bizarre and bloody turns is that heroin for those with fierce beliefs and intentions is a currency. It is used to buy power particularly by those who espouse a high moral position. The Americans as an example, profess to be outraged by the ruin of their young people, and yet have financed those who bring the drug to them.

Getting It Here

In both the Crescent and the Triangle, it should be recognised, the great bulk of the poppy harvest is still used locally as opium. Of the quantity that does get illicitly converted into heroin, an ever-increasing amount is being consumed by Asians themselves. But of the considerable proportions that do reach the West, how is it exported? The answer is more complicated than many commentators suggest. We can see this from the contradictory nature of various flowcharts purportedly indicating which way the traffic moves and by whom it is moved: in one chart it's the Sicilians who run the whole show. In another they're a spent force, and the arrows point in all directions. There are, of course, distinct and powerful blocs, but there are also numerous *ad hoc* groups putting together their own deals of varying magnitude. The situation was particularly muddled in early 1985 because the market found itself in the middle of a glut. Also, for the first time bulk amounts of Golden Triangle stock was beginning to show up in Europe to compete with the Crescent variety. That means the various networks of traffickers who, in the midst of plenty coexisted relatively well, are likely to start bickering in blood.

The Networks

There are two principal features needed to make a first-class trafficking network. The first, as drugs expert Professor Pino

Arlacchi explains,[20] is 'impermeability with regard to police enquiries.' The second is 'a respect for undertakings and verbal agreements.' There are a couple of institutions that measure up excellently to such requirements. One is the blood family, the other is the expatriate ethnic community. Both have done well out of drugs trading.

The Turks

Turkish people have been thoroughly engaged in the heroin business since trade to America picked up in the '50s. In those days she grew opium, converted it into morphine base, and then shipped it to France for refinement into heroin by Corsican gangs. Since illicit growing was controlled in the early '70s the mode of operation has had to switch. Turkish chemists learned to master the conversion process from morphine to heroin itself, and by 1977 their buff-coloured product was on the market. Turkish gangs also bite into the distribution network at a high level. Typically, they will place an order with an agent from the growing country and distribute – via lower-rung dealers – in their particular patch of town.

Sicilian Mafia

Though the Italians of the mainland have been involved since the '40s it wasn't until the early '70s that they took over refining from the French, placing them at the top of the European league. The move, ironically enough, was facilitated by the transfer of hundreds of millions of pounds by the Italian government into the Sicilian economy. Ostensibly the funds were to develop the region; instead they went into transforming the Mafia into a vast multinational company whose heroin dealings are said to be the most formidable in Europe. In the early days of the '70s Euroboom the Mafia got its supplies in the form of morphine base that had been smuggled principally from South West Asia to the Middle East by couriers of various nationalities. Once purchased the base would then be taken to Sicily, refined into heroin, and distributed both to the US and through the European market.

A couple of developments have put paid to this mode of working. The first has been the success of the Italian police in recent years in closing down many of the Sicilian refineries. The second has been the increasing trend of opium growers to produce their own heroin.

Some pundits have talked in terms of the Mafia 'allowing' these native labs to take a bigger share in the production cycle. In reality there is no way of stopping them. The Sicilians are still doing well enough, however. They probably retain the most lucrative end of the business – the financial brokerage of international trade – and they are now reported to have moved into the cocaine trade. End-of-year drug profits for 1983 were reported at $1.2 billion.[21]

Tied, however fractiously, to the Sicilian Mafia is the Neapolitan version of the crime syndicate – the Camorra. In addition to petty shakedowns of local citizenry the Camorra (estimated annual turnover $2 billion) are said to control as much of Italy's internal drugs market as the Sicilians themselves. Like their colleagues further south they too are prone to internecine difficulties. In 1982, some 252 people were gunned down in the streets, stabbed or, in one instance, beheaded as part of the internal battle over profits.[22] The people of Naples became so anguished they came out in a virtually solid two-day strike, joined by the inhabitants of more than a dozen surrounding towns. But rather than be quelled, the Camorra are said to be looking for more to feed on. Like the Sicilians they are developing their share of the cocaine traffic, which has been of some importance to them since the mid 1970s.

The Chinese

The Chinese are perhaps the most sophisticated of all the traffickers due to their ancient custom of reciprocity. This allows a system of payment based entirely on trust with nothing damaging being committed to paper. As Jonathan Steinberg noted in a recent *New Society* article;[23] 'A Mr Wu in Hong Kong writes out a small card which authorises a Mr Lee in San Francisco to pay the bearer a sum of money. Mr Lee does so in due course and gets repaid by the same method. Neither Mr Wu nor Mr Lee are necessarily connected with the trade directly. They act as private bankers using no telephone calls or letters of credit.' While the Italians are now chiefly feeding on Crescent-originated heroin, the Chinese have traditionally dealt in the product of the Golden Triangle of the South East. The route to the West has been through Thailand and Hong Kong, but with recent crackdowns in those countries virtually all the product is now being grown and processed in Burmah (north of the Triangle) then shipped westward via India. A London man who dealt with the Chinese in the early '70s describes them as fair, straight, but tough if crossed.

Pakistan

The big Pakistani syndicates are based in Lahore and Karachi where they can easily evade the attentions of the police. The worldwide communities of Asians offer a natural global network, but it is after the material has landed in this country that distribution problems start. Being new to the trade and having no easy means of penetrating white communities, Pakistanis in this country have had to call upon the experience of Turkish traffickers. The organisational factor built into traditional white criminal gangs is also proving important. In the early '80s, Asian traffickers were vulnerable to extortionate demands from such groups. There are now signs that they have toughened up their business practices – though they have yet to develop a conspicuously physical approach.

Others

The above-mentioned networks are those most relevant to our part of Europe although, as already indicated, new units are continually cropping up. Heroin and morphine laboratories are now being found in all parts of Europe and the Middle East – including one in Britain. The French Connection is believed revived again as chemists move across borders swapping technical data with their less informed brethren.

But where there is fellowship there is also bloodshed. British newspaper readers heard recently of the penalty paid by a New Zealand man who 'cheated an international syndicate by diluting their heroin.[24] Believing he was needed in Scotland to close a fresh drugs deal he flew into the UK from his Singapore home and was met by two bullets in the head. His hands were then hacked off, his head battered and stomach ripped open. The remains were trussed, weighted and dumped in a flooded quarry in Eccleston, Lancs.

Faced with such grim precedents British courts continue to act with astonishing naïvety. Not many months later the leader of a Pakistani heroin gang who was reported to have luxury homes in North London, the South of France and Karachi was given £50,000 bail by Horseferry Road Magistrates Court. Not surprisingly he fled while four other members of the team, said to be part of one of the world's largest drugs rings, were jailed. They were reported to have smuggled heroin worth £5 million into Britain.

Techniques

The methods of carrying the material across national frontiers ranges right from straightforward concealment in luggage to the swallowing of loaded condoms. Since the risk comes from being caught in possession of the drug the really big dealers are unlikely to get within a mile of it. Much of the dangerous handling is done by couriers like Asian seamen, who are told that unless they carry their portion they don't get a berth. Students are also favourite envoys, as are 'diplomats', whose baggage is guaranteed free from molestation under diplomatic immunity. Insofar as traffic to the UK is concerned, this country once had the reputation of being one of the toughest nuts to crack. Since government cutbacks of Customs staff the reputation has been turned on its head.

It was easy enough getting drugs into this country before the 1979 cuts of approximately 1,000 staff. It is now likely, says the Customs union the Society of Public and Civil Servants, that 90 per cent of all drugs brought to the UK get through. At Dover and Heathrow, as few as one passenger in

400 is stopped and questioned. During meal breaks one officer may be the only official in the Green (nothing to declare) Channel with up to 1,000 passengers passing by. And one lone officer may be faced with clearing 200 cars or 50 full coaches. Although the union says it believes coaches are widely used by smugglers, it is now Customs Board policy not to enter a coach for a check 'unless there are strong grounds for suspicion.'

Commercial vehicles are another problem. Of the two million sealed cargo containers that arrive each year in the UK, less than one per cent are checked. The situation is similar for ships. Before 1977 every ship and aircraft arriving from abroad was checked. In some ports the figure of boarded vessels has fallen to 20 per cent. Similarly at Heathrow the routine boarding of aircraft has now been abandoned.

Yachts have always been a special risk because of their ability to land goods in remote places where normal Customs controls don't operate. Though there are (increasingly fewer) sporadic checks, most controls are conducted on a voluntary basis. The person in charge of the vessel is supposed to notify Customs on arriving, and again on departure. They can either ignore the obligation altogether or unload before informing Customs. There used to be patrolling crews watching out for suspicious landings. These, says the union, have been almost stopped.

Based on these developments it is not likely that the rising quantities of heroin seizures reflects anything but the higher volume being shipped. In 1979 40.33 kilos were seized. In 1983 the figure was 201.14. The provisional figure for 1984 was 298.96 kilos. Yet the government has not shown itself impressed by the Union's submissions.

'It wants more bottoms on seats,' a spokesman told the Commons in July 1984. 'To obtain that, it has put out some extremely lurid press releases saying that the presence of 500 more officers would solve the drug importation problem.'

The government did announce what appeared to be an increase in Customs officers watching out for drugs. In fact it was merely a decrease in the number of staff due to be scrapped.

Recognising It

Heroin is not a substance of a given quality. Grades vary according to where in the world it was made, and by whom. 'Pakistani' ranges from beige granules to white powder – the latter registering up to 80 per cent purity when landed. Typical street material is about 50 per cent clean. Sometimes considered the most superior brand is South East Asian No 4 – also a white crystalline powder. It is more commonly known as *Thai*. Lesser grades take on a shading that reflects the dilutants used. There is, for instance, beige *Turkish*, and chunky brown *Iranian*.

The conversion of opium into morphine base and then into heroin occurs on a constantly shifting circuit, and such geographical names should be considered simply as a signal to quality rather than strict reference to place of origin. As to the cuts, these tend to be functional rather than malicious. Some physically resemble heroin (Mannitol, lactose, dextrose in powder form). Quinine is used, particularly in the US, because it looks like heroin, tastes bitter like heroin, and is said to enhance the rush. Barbiturates might also be included because they too are a central nervous system depressant. In the more malicious category is the apparently benign household flour. When injected this can cause blockages in veins.

Help

People choose different methods in their attempt to quit opiate use. Some go through the special clinic regime which involves replacing heroin with methadone, then getting reduced down. Others go into hospital to have themselves purged under a detoxification programme. Such a programme is often reserved for people using more than one drug, some of which would be dangerous to withdraw from unsupervised. Others choose to quit from a home base. This is probably the soundest option providing, *to repeat*, drugs such as barbiturates and tranquillisers are not being used at the same time. Overcoming physical dependence is relatively straightforward even when undertaken abruptly. The peak of withdrawal generally occurs between two and three days after the last dose and usually resembles a bout of 'flu (fever, aching limbs, cough) together with violent yawning, spasms, cramps, diarrhoea and twitches throughout the body. The telling struggle comes when the euphoria at having quit is followed by feelings of alienation and anxiety. These two will pass. If an attempt to come off is made and it fails, the user shouldn't despair. It will have been a lesson for the next time. However, a rapid succession of flops can injure confidence, so it's important to think seriously before stopping. Two questions might be asked: why has drug use become such a problem when plenty of people use without getting addicted? Drugs have probably offered short-term relief from physical and psychic pain; what are the means for coping afterwards?

If after answering these questions the user still wants to make the break, s/he might consider this four-point plan devised by a West London drugs counselling agency:

1. Cut down your daily dose to the minimum possible and resist taking just a little bit more just this one last time. It's difficult, so don't rush.
2. Find somewhere warm, safe and comfortable. You'll need a bed, warmth, fresh air and extras like books, records, etc. You'll be able to concentrate on these after a few days. Eat well. Cope with the fever as you'd deal with an ordinary bout of 'flu – cool baths, cool liquids.
3. If you're working take at least two weeks off, but no more than four or you'll mope. Some people go on holiday, but returning to an unresolved home situation can be worse than staying put.
4. Try to enlist the help of a friend to encourage and check up on you. But *stay away* from other users.

Afterwards it's good policy to remain drug-free for six months even if abstinence isn't the final objective. And it's important once in the clear to watch out for excessive booze or tranquilliser use. Many a 'recovering' opiate addict does a surreptitious switch, all the while believing s/he has licked the Big One. Tranquillisers and alcohol are just as difficult to quit.

Outside Help

Whatever resolve an addict might muster s/he can always benefit from family or friends. But these people first need help themselves to understand the problem before engaging it. The same drug agency that gave the four-point quitting plan sketches these basic principles for friends of the addict:

1. Don't panic. Arm yourself with the legal, medical and pharmacological facts.
2. Don't assume the worst. Most drug use is casual, temporary and leads to no serious problems.
3. Recognise that you might be unable to take on the 'case' yourself. You just might be part of the problem.
4. Recognise that addicts can't be beaten into recovery. They must be willing partners in the process. If your help is rejected, don't get miffed. They might come to you another time.
5. Recognise the problem might not relate to a specific drug, but be part of what the professionals call 'poly drug use'.
6. By way of general tips: don't interrogate; calmly acknowledge your friend's fears instead of dismissing them or over-reacting. Resist pressure such as 'I'll die if you don't give me money.' Treat each request separately, and if you're to help, only give cash for food and other necessities.

Policy and Community

Despite the succulent media coverage, heroin addiction is not high in the league table of society's concerns because it is regarded as affecting the kind of numbers that can be managed through normal control measures. What's more, most of those affected are assumed to be the kind of numbskull working-class fodder for whom there is generally no worthy social niche anyway. Let them puke down their lift shafts. Rarely (at the time of writing) were there media splashes on the upper-bracket sort of users – the fashionable clubland snorters and the well-shod gluttons who in olden days would have pigged up on brandy. But then there is an inducement to simplify the issue. If junk equals addiction equals the rumbunctious working classes, then it is one of those vaguely defined 'social issues' on which the authorities can lay their languid hand at some distantly appropriate time.

For example, in 1982 the Department of Health's Advisory Council on the Misuse of Drugs urgently recommended that the UK's 14 Regional Health Authorities set up drug problem teams. By June 1984 just two had done so.[25] The Council also urged that the Secretary of State write to all health authorities getting them to assess the problem and review existing facilities in their areas. That letter took almost two years to send.[26] And so what facilities do exist?

The government's strategy rests on the 70 hospitals throughout the UK which offer some sort of treatment – invariably in their psychiatric wings – for drug addiction. Nearly all operate a strict catchment area system. Most have a waiting list of several weeks and many require new patients be referred by their GPs. Between them they offer approximately 200 beds for in-patient detoxification, and while the policy on out-patient treatment is superficially at great variance, the general trend is moving away from maintenance towards criminalisation. (A clinic worker in the Brighton area tells me the police frequently hang around her own unit hoping to score a few arrests.) There is now only one recommended drug in the treatment of heroin addiction and that's methadone. A small number of old-time addicts will continue to get it in injectable form but for the rest it's a mixture or linctus – and usually for no more than a few weeks.

Several of the 70 hospitals don't even offer the non-injectable methadone, only 'therapy'. All clinics are supposed to offer 'therapy', but addicts frequently report themselves irked by the cold, pompous lectures of junior social workers, while for their part clinic workers are irked at being regarded as 'prescriptions on legs'. Their patients, they report, are exhausting and infinitely devious. The new no-maintenance direction is substantially in line with the present Tory government's overall strategy of throwing people back on to their private resources. For those that have them this policy can work, but for the addict there are frequently shortages of both the emotional and financial sort. And so the black market beckons – and with it the whole subterranean package.

The no-maintenance strategy actually takes us back to the early 1920s when the Home Office was set on starving addicts of their legal supplies, forcing them either to quit or go criminal. In 1926 the Rolleston Committee established the right of GPs to carry on prescribing for addicts on the understanding that addiction was a 'disease' of personal dimensions. In the '60s a wave of young street addicts encouraged the idea of addiction as a social epidemic and the new clinics were established to hand out enough free drugs so that the black market couldn't flourish – but not so much that new addicts were created under the medical aegis. Events since those days have shown the clinics to have failed on all counts. The black market is enormous. The clinic cure rate is poor, and newer addicts are basically ignoring them.

A second feature of the government care package is GPs. Most don't actually want to know addicts because they are considered time-consuming and scary. GPs are in any case often abysmally ignorant on the subject of recreational drugs, which is a great pity. A good, well-informed GP can be a friend to an addict.

Voluntary Agencies

Among the best work in coping with the human fallout from drug use is being performed by the voluntary street agencies. They offer advice, information, counselling and support, and although some have been going since the '60s, they are still without secure funding. This means for every hour spent working with addicts another will be spent on their knees begging local and central government for cash. They are not only short of liquidity, the government still refuses them any say in developing care strategies, whether at local or national level.

Of equal importance are the friendship groups which are entirely self-supporting on all levels. Narcotics Anonymous, the most notable, is growing at a rapid rate in communities and even prisons throughout the UK. It models itself on Alcoholics Anonymous, acting as a mutual help 'fellowship' whose care is spiritual and social, looking to help the 'whole person' rather than just the addiction.

Residential

Other important care facilities are the various residential centres which also exist on a patchwork quilt of temporary funding. Some, like the Parole Release Scheme, deal with released prisoners. Some, like Chatterton Hey, operate a Christian regime. Others, known as 'concept houses', run residents through a stiff hierarchical structure aimed at teaching self-awareness and the acceptance of personal responsibility.

Self-Help

Throughout the country parents and other interested parties are putting together their own self-help groups. Many are getting cash from local authorities and some, such as the one in Wirral, Merseyside, harbour plans for a residential centre. The argument over such groups is just warming up. Some professionals see them as overheated and lacking expert knowledge. More cynically they are being used by councils as an excuse for not laying on proper statutory services: give them a shop and a phone, so the attitude goes, and that's our bit for the drugs problem. Despite all the opposition, ordinary people have been rising up like old-fashioned cowboy town mobs to confront pushers in cities such as Dublin. As an expression of community feelings it can't be bettered. The dangers of such initiatives degenerating into crude vigilante-ism are obvious, but the more likely outcome is that a response will be drawn from the authorities, and 'the people' in recognising their common anguish, will start to act constructively upon it.

Private

Among the most dubious enterprises to have arisen to meet the new heroin wave are the private withdrawal clinics with their instant psychological reconstruction jobs and bills running, in many cases, to several thousand pounds. This is a growth industry and whether the surroundings are spartan or lush they should be examined sceptically.

Policy Options

Some of the sharp business practices of past and present have already been outlined in this chapter. Similarly we've seen the part prejudice and stupidity play in the deliberations of governments as well as ordinary citizens. Given that it is ingrained in the collective intelligence that heroin is the most dangerous drug in existence, and that this notion can't be easily shifted, there is no point in arguing for it to be freely available in the manner of tobacco or beer. But what about returning to pre-Brain Committee when medical people could prescribe to addicts? This is appealing for several reasons: in *theory* it obviates the need for a black market and all its concomitant crime; it would stabilise the addict on his/her preferred drug and since this would be of a proven quality there would be fewer health problems. Against the idea – apart from public resistance – is that the medical world would have to swill about an awful lot of heroin to put the breaks on underground trafficking. There is also the risk that such generosity could lead to casual users being turned into addicts either by direct prescription or by patients selling off surplus. We would also see the UK become a magnet for addicts from other nations – for which the only solution would be for those other nations to follow suit and introduce prescriptions. The chances of this happening are small to the point of invisibility. There is also something illogical about giving regular doses of a material that, on balance, ends up injuring the recipient. If the 'patient' has the maturity to use heroin in a stable way, avoiding the needle, then s/he may be called a recreational, not compulsive, user, and the arguments against heroin being supplied like beer and fags have already been given. I would also be cutting across one of the central tenets propounded in this book if I suddenly championed 'medical smack': this is that fewer, not more, drugs should be dispensed. Finally, as one clinical psychiatrist points out: 'If we're going to give regular doses of heroin to addicts why not a bottle of vodka per day for alcoholics?' The assumptions that both addictions are 'diseases' that cannot be overcome is unnecessarily defeatist – and one not borne out by the facts.

The remaining policy question relates to what to do with people caught in possession of heroin. At the moment they are being arrested under the Misuse of Drugs Act and getting fairly moderate fines. The court will probably also refer them to a probation officer and/or a clinic. If that person should continue coming before them the court will lose patience and despatch them to prison. When they come out they will probably start using again and go back into prison: the revolving door syndrome. The situation is idiotic enough, but it becomes poisoned when police officers, perhaps in the desire to catch a superior's eye, start arresting tuppenny addicts on the more serious charge of 'offering to supply' or 'supplying' itself. These offences usually carry automatic prison terms.

At the 1981 annual general meeting of the influential Standing Conference On Drug Abuse (SCODA, the umbrella agency for the non-statutory groups) a motion was carried urging that the possession of drugs, any drugs, in small quantities should no longer be treated as a criminal offence. Their reasoning was that the 'crime' of possession has no victim except, possibly, the user him/herself.

This would seem to be a solid position to take up. It does, however, embody a major difficulty: if the intention is to go only for 'traffickers', then how is such a person to be recognised? By the amount in possession? That would brand as traffickers hapless couriers while letting off the hook the shadowy drug bosses who don't get near the stuff. One solution would be to set a maximum quantity, possession in excess of which would constitute 'intention to supply', but waive the supply charge where the person before the court is clearly a patsy. Or the softer option could be taken: no one found in possession of whatever quantity is assumed to be intending to supply unless it is proven otherwise.

Whatever policy options are adopted they will amount to mere tinkering with the machine. The 'solution' to the heroin problem lies in individual self-awareness. And it depends on society taking upon itself some sound information and maturity of purpose.

Notes

1 T. Duquesne & J. Reeves, *A Handbook of Psychoactive Medicines*, Quartet, London, 1982, p. 284

2 R. Lingeman, *Drugs From A–Z*, McGraw Hill, New York, 1974, p. 104

3 Ibid, p. 107

4 Ibid, p. 232

5 P. J. Bolton, ed. D. F. Hawkins, *Drugs and Pregnancy: Human Teratogenesis and Related Problems*, Churchill Livingstone, Edinburgh, 1983, pp. 146–147

6 B. Inglis, *The Forbidder. Game*, Hodder & Stoughton, London, 1975, p. 73

7 'Paracelse', *Encyclopaedia Universalis*, vol. 12

8 V. Berridge, 'East End Opium Dens and Narcotic Use in Britain', *London Journal*, 1978, vol. 4, no. 1, p. 3

9 Ibid, p. 4

10 Ibid, p. 14

11 T. Parssinen, *Secret Passions, Secret Remedies: Narcotic Drugs in British Society, 1920–1930*, Manchester University Press, 1981, p. 212

12 Ibid, p. 213

13 V. Berridge, 'Drugs and Social Policy: The Establishment of Drug Control in Britain, 1900–1930', *British Journal of Addiction*, 1984, vol. 79, no. 1, p. 23

14 J. Ditton & K. Speirits, 'The Rapid Increase of Heroin Addiction in Glasgow during 1981', Background Paper Department of Sociology, Glasgow University, 1981

15 Carey Schofield, *Harpers and Queen*, January 1984

6 R. Hartnoll & R. Lewis, 'The Illicit Heroin Market in Britain: Towards a Preliminary Estimate of National Demand', Drug Indicators Project, London, 1985

7 David K. Willis, *Christian Science Monitor*, 14.1.1984

8 Roger Lewis, *Druglink*, ISDD, Spring 1984

9 Neil Kelly, 'Chinese Humbled in a New Opium War', *The Times*, 6.8.1984

20 P. Arlacchi, *Mafia, Peasants and the Great Estates*, Cambridge University Press, 1984

21 Donald Sasson, *New Statesman*, 12.10.1984

22 Don A. Schanche, *International Herald Tribune*, 31.1.1983

23 Jonathan Steinberg, *New Society*, 3.5.1983

24 Harry King & Trevor Reynolds, *Daily Mirror*, 16.1.1981

25 P. Taylor, 'The Battle Against Heroin: The Growing Menace to the Country's Young', *The Listener*, 28.6.1984

26 Ibid

9 THE NITRITES

Intro

THE NITRITES are close relatives in a family of chemical
derived from nitrous oxide. Known as *poppers* and *snappers*
both are highly volatile and flammable liquids, yellowish in
colour, smelling sweet and fruity when fresh, and of old socks
when stale. Depending on location and expectation, the
experience will differ. Used on the dance floor they are said to
deliver a shaft of dizzy, exciting energy. In lovemaking they
can lower inhibitions, relax the body and prolong – in the
mind at least – orgasm, so that it seems to stretch for minutes
though in fact while the drugs might excite the senses they can
easily dull the organs.

What Is It?

Amyl Nitrite

Amyl nitrite was discovered in 1857. Ten years later it was
introduced into the medical pharmacopoeia as a treatment for
the pain of angina. The relief came through the drug's ability
to open up the vessels delivering blood to the heart. The
format it came in was a small glass capsule known as a
vitrellae, which is enclosed by cotton wool. The vitrellae is
crushed with a pop between thumb and forefinger and the
vapour inhaled. It is this popping noise that gives the recreational nitrites their street names, even though the products used for purposes other than medical do no such thing:
the drugs come in little bottles with screw or plug tops.

In the US the 'abuse' potential of amyl nitrite, first noted among gay communities, was recognised and acted upon in 1969, and they were duly restricted to prescription only. In the UK, the drug is still not rated a substance of abuse and is theoretically freely available across the counter from any chemist. In practice, chemist supplies are scarce; in the treatment of angina the drug has been superseded by longer-acting preparations. In bottled form it is allegedly a room odouriser, and by this absurd subterfuge escapes all official recognition as a drug product.

Butyl Nitrite

Butyl nitrite, despite its close chemical relationship and its similar though moderately less potent effects, never has found its way into medical therapy. It too is retained as an air freshener: 'Remove cap, leave in vacated room for half an hour. Return to an outstandingly fragrant atmosphere.' The same 'cunning' will inevitably be applied to a third variant beginning to show up as a sex enhancer. This is isobutyl alcohol which, like the other nitrites, has first found favour among gays. It is rated one notch down in terms of potency than butyl nitrite.

The Difference

With amyl nitrite strongly controlled in the US as a drug, the big recreational bucks are being made from butyl nitrite. One of the big two bottlers is doing something in excess of $50 million business a year – each dollar of which, they insist, is *odour* and not *sex* related. The American butyls are handsomely packaged with elegant names that suggest masculine prowess. The English amyls often carry no name at all and though priced at around the same level – from £2.50 to £5 – contain substantially more of the volatile liquid. (So volatile are the chemicals of both that with the cap off all will have evaporated within a couple of hours. Kept in a fridge and used occasionally a bottle can last for weeks.)

Medical Effects

Some of the less pleasant side-effects of the nitrites include headache, nausea, coughing and dizziness, although these don't seem to occur frequently. There are no recorded sudden deaths and few emergency room visits for nitrite-related health problems.[1]

A study of twenty men who had inhaled an averge of four ampoules daily for seven years showed their lungs were as healthy as a control group of non-users.[2] But while the possibility of death or serious injury from inhalation of either nitrite seems extremely remote, there has been at least one death after someone swallowed the entire contents of a bottle of butyl and then failed to get prompt treatment.

The AIDS Question

The blackest shadow cast over the nitrites is the alleged part they play in spreading the illness called Acquired Immune Deficiency Syndrome, which destroys its victims' natural defences against disease, causing them to waste away from a variety of opportunistic infections and malignancies. AIDS is frequently referred to as the Gay Plague, with the assumption that it originated during the late '70s in the gay male communities of California and New York. In fact the diease – or one very much like it – has now been traced to Central Africa, with the Western outbreak probably taking root via Haiti. Whether or not tropical Africa was its place of genesis isn't clear at the time of writing, but what is clear is there is nothing inherently 'gay' about the disease. Male and female heterosexuals are also threatened.

The spotlight settled for a while on the nitrites after it was realised that of the first 300 sufferers in the West, 98 per cent of those of them who were male and homosexuals had used the drugs, but nitrite usage was found to be just as prevalent in a control group of gay men not suffering from the disease, thus the fact that there were sufferers who weren't users ruled out nitrites as the specific cause. The current state of research identifies a virus named LAV/HTLV III (related to a virus which is responsible for a certain form of leukaemia) as the possible cause. So far no cure is in sight.

Tolerance

Tolerance does develop to these drugs' ability to carry on dilating blood vessels. The picture isn't clear about tolerance to their stimulant effects.

Dependence

The nitrites can encourage psychological dependence. Symptoms of physical addition – with fully-fledged withdrawal problems – have not so far been widely reported.

Who Uses

In showbiz circles amyl nitrite was popular 30 years ago. Then in the 1960s it became celebrated by US gay males, not least because it relaxed the anal sphincter muscle, making sex less troublesome. From about 1982, by which time the butyl variant was being taken up, it was being used widely in straight circles and finding particular favour in places like Leeds, West Yorkshire and Manchester where it is sold over the counter in pubs and clubs. In the equivalent gay establishments it has long been mandatory; no self-respecting leatherware or novelty shop, for instance, would be without a selection.

Notes

1 T. P. Lowry, 'Uses and Abuses of Amyl and Butyl Nitrites', *British Journal of Sexual Medicine*, September 1982
2 Ibid

10 SOLVENTS

Intro

A LEVEL of panic attaches to the sniffing of glue and the other volatile substances that is exceeded only by the reaction to heroin. Perhaps it is the tender age of the average sniffer that scares adults, and because it appears such a bizarre and sordid occupation. And certainly it is bizarre for mainstream adults, whose idea of relaxation is to take a couple of whiskys, to discover their 12-year-old has had his head in a pot of glue – even though the intoxication factor in the drink and the glue are remarkably similar. Because it is easily compared with alcohol, young sniffers accuse their disapproving elders of hypocrisy, claiming that the toluene found in glue is as good an introduction to intoxication and a means to relieving boredom and tension as any that exist. It is also cheap and legal and represents one in the eye for an adult world which displays such horror at the indulgence. Yet what can't be shaken off by young sniffers is the pallid quality of their scene. Glue and the other volatiles are not even proper drugs. They are commercial products re-routed by thrill seekers. They therefore carry no inbuilt quality control in terms of the impact on a sniffer's health.

In the main, no kudos is attached to long-term sniffers from their own age group, and certainly no glamour. Sniffers are generally considered reckless rather than hard or daring. The scene is without any noticeable patois. Most drugs are consigned half a dozen slangy names, but no one seems to have bothered to invent any for the numerous volatile substances. In fact it is an indulgence alone among those covered in this book for which no elegant justification has been mounted.

Amphetamines, heroin and alcohol all have their advocates, but no one dares speak out on behalf of glue and co. – which places those principally young people who use it in a particularly vulnerable position.

Sniffing for pleasure is rooted in the eighteenth and nineteenth centuries, when the fashion for using nitrous oxide, ether and the more dangerous chloroform became widespread. But sniffing among a whole spectrum of youth is very much a product of the modern age. More than one hundred commercially available products are now used to obtain a 'buzz'. They include glues, rubber cements, typewriter correction fluid, nail polish remover, magic markers, petrol, paint and paint thinners, lighter fuel, cleaning fluids, aerosols, fire extinguishers and even the 'volatile' contents of decorative table lamps.

By far the most popularly used are adhesives containing toluene and acetone. These also seem to be the safest and the great majority who sniff them do so short-term and seem to come to no lasting physical or psychological harm. This is not least because it is the vapour rather than the entire product which is ingested. Indeed, 'sniffing' is never the correct term for the use of glues or the other products, rather they are deeply inhaled through the mouth and/or nose. For those seeking more direct access an amount of paraphernalia can be employed. This gear can be extraordinary and it can be fatal. An 18-year-old Manchester youth, for instance, was found dead having choked on his own vomit. He had been feeding himself butane gas from a refill canister via a plastic tube that was tied with a bootlace to a funnel which he had clamped, broad-end extended, over his mouth. This to be sure, was an extreme case, but like many of the other 31 sniffing-related deaths logged in that year of 1981 (no proper check is kept, so the figure could be higher) there was a suggestion of self-destructiveness rather than simple experimentation. Other melancholy endings that year included a 20-year-old from Gateshead who died in his boarding-house room with a plastic bag over his head and a canister of butane gas by his side. He had been in and out of children's homes as a child. And there was a 16-year-old Belfast boy – jobless, father dead –

asphyxiated by the fumes from trichloroethane found in Dab-It-Off cleaning fluid.

It would be unfair and inaccurate, however, to suggest that sniffing deaths are inevitably the result of a tumultuous background. First-time experimenters also come to grief, particularly when using products such as lighter fuel, aerosols and fire extinguishers. With these the margin for error is narrow.

As to who might be the typical sniffer and how many exist, there has not yet been an adequate UK survey. The picture we do have comes from frequently hysterical news reports or the impressions of police, social workers and medical professionals, most of whose 'clients' tend to be disturbed to one degree or another. How much volatile substance use contributes to the disturbance and how often it works the other way round can't easily be deduced. The consensus is that there are two types of sniffer: the first is the experimental, social sort who seeks to engage the world and generate some bodily excitement. He is usually a male in his early teens, and he'll be trying out 'softer' items like Evostik. He will invariably pass through the episode within a matter of weeks, and unless he lacks proper information or is manifestly reckless, he will avoid the more hazardous substances and practices. The second, much smaller, class of user is also predominantly male, but is more interested in retreating from personal misery than seeking thrills. He might have begun socially, but will then continue to indulge himself alone or together with a hardcore group. The range of products employed might not necessarily be broad – he could settle on a favourite or two – but since the body develops a tolerance to the effects of solvents, he will need to consume an increasing amount to get intoxicated. Thus a pattern of use could develop producing repeated overdoses. Such individuals are not only dangerous to themselves, they might also initiate younger acquaintances into the art.

A Scottish survey[1] showed that those sniffers who require medical attention could usually be classed as solitary types. It noted an absent parent due to divorce, death or separation in 52 per cent of cases, and where both parents were present there was likely to be a history of stormy marriage and/or a father who drank heavily and/or was long-term unemployed. Sniffing was seen in some instances to be mimicking the alcoholism of the father with whom the son strongly identified. But not all surveys support the socially disadvantaged scenario. A US study of 110 'sudden sniffing deaths' occurring during the 1960s found that the victims were mainly young males from suburban middle-income white families. And in Britain too there are signs that sniffing, far from being confined to mad-dog, inner-city skinheads, casuals and punks, is especially popular in the outer suburban ring among the trunk roads and canals; a long way from the city centre throb. A UK investigation of every known death associated with sniffing between 1971 and 1982[2] (140 in all) concluded that 'there was little evidence to associate them with adverse or disadvantaged social or environmental circumstances.' Even so, the death rates were highest in the recession-hit big city areas of Scotland, Northern Ireland and Northern England.

As to how much is used by how many, an interesting though possibly dated survey[3] was carried out among 898 male (only!) pupils in a Glasgow comprehensive school during 1976 following the death of a pupil. It revealed that of the 11 to 16-year-olds canvassed, the most indulgent were the 13 to 15s, that the overall involvement was 10 per cent and the extent of use varied from one try only (50 per cent) to 'regular use' (21.5 per cent). Almost half were introduced to the practice by friends.

More recently Northamptonshire police reported[4] a total of 223 'cases' of solvent abuse coming to their notice during the first seven months of 1983. Often it was the same youths re-offending, and from them came just four bouts of criminal activity: two youths were implicated in a burglary involving the theft of glue; three in a police assault; one in criminal damage; and two were found in disused premises sniffing glue stolen from a hardware shop. 'Whilst the statistics are of concern,' noted the chief constable, 'they must be kept in perspective, as the problem would seem to be far smaller numerically than media publicity sometimes makes it appear.' He then reported that it was the opinion of local social service and education professionals that 'less than one per cent of young people experiment with solvents, and of these only one per cent are likely to suffer harmful effects.'

It seems the recreational use of solvents ebbs and flows. It achieves a sudden wash of popularity in a given area depending on the tastes of the relevant groups, or upon the discovery of a novel high. The discovery by a sensation-hungry media of sniffing 'epidemics' might or might not coincide with a genuine spurt in consumption.

Some critics claim the first glue epidemic to be identified was the result of a feverish media campaign in the *Denver (Colorado) Post* beginning in August 1959. This was at a time when the city seemed to have no cases whatsoever of deliberate intoxication by solvents. Two reporters had discovered that several children had been arrested for sniffing in neighbouring towns, and they then banged out warning stories that gave illustrated directions on how to get high. By 1965 the habit was reported in every US state as well as in Africa, South America, Finland and beyond. In Japan, 161 people were known to have died during 1969. However, this is not to suggest that all this was the *Denver Post*'s fault, but media attention does serve to spread information.

The British authorities in any case decided that maintaining a low profile would be the best way to avoid exciting young appetites, and all departments were instructed accordingly. It wasn't until 1970 that police in Lanarkshire, Scotland, first commented on the existence of a problem here in the UK – stories about Scottish epidemics were instantly wrung from the presses and soon after the indulgence had spread, or at least solvent abuse was 'officially recognised' throughout the whole of the UK.

What Are They?

There are many ways of classifying and rating household and industrial products that can be sniffed. We should start by defining some terms and by stating what gives a product sniffability:

1. It must give off a vapour.
2. The vapour must have an intoxicating effect.

These two features apply to most of the volatile hydrocarbons (chemical compounds of hydrogen and carbon) that derive largely from the oil industry, but also from coal and fermented vegetable matter. Industry is keen on this family of chemicals since – along with other substances – it can deploy them as solvents in products that would otherwise solidify in their containers. The job of a solvent is to keep the product dissolved until it is spread, poured or squirted, and then to evaporate from the product quickly without trace. It is this volatility which gives the hydrocarbons their intoxicating effects.

Impact Adhesives and Other Glues

Adhesive products are easily the most commonly sniffed, with Evostik and Thixofix being the favourites. They also seem to be the least hazardous items, partly because the vapour rather than the whole item is consumed, partly because the vapour drifts off the semi-solid glue rather than being rammed down into the lungs as is the case with pressurised gases, and also because they contain fairly simple hydrocarbons – notably toluene – as opposed to the unassimilable fluorine and chlorine compounds. These last two are members of the halogen family of elements, and products derived from them are found mostly in aerosols. Another solvent generally borne by glue is acetone, whose toxicity is considered less than that of toluene.

The usual method of taking it is to put a blob in the bottom of, say, a crisp packet, and then deeply inhale the fumes half a dozen to twenty times. It is principally a group activity and the bag, like the marijuana joint, is passed from mouth to mouth. More serious sniffers in their search for a denser hit will enclose themselves in a vaporous atmosphere by placing a glue-laden plastic bag or blanket over their heads. Both these enclosure methods are hazardous since the user is cut off from fresh air, and if (as is quite possible) s/he passes out while continuing to draw in the vapours, s/he might well asphyxiate.

Nail Polish and Nail Polish Remover

Like the glues, these are generally conceded as not being powerfully toxic by comparison with other sniffed items. Their principal solvents are acetone or amyl acetate, and are typically used by brushing a cuff or other material with the substance and inhaling from close quarters. Not thought to be extremely popular, although a fairly standard choice among those wanting to try the field.

Rubber Solutions

These contain benzene and hexane – both hydrocarbon compounds – and chloroform (a widely-used lab solvent that has been taken for fun since its discovery in 1831). These products would be sniffed straight from the container.

Petrol

Petrol sniffing was the pastime that preceded the glue and aerosol fads in the US, and was particularly noted among minorities such as Mexicans and Indians. It seems never really to have taken off here, which is as well since UK petrol, unlike the US product, contains tetraethyl lead, a particularly toxic substance for children. Its main solvent is benzene, mixed with other hydrocarbons. Rarely used indoors, it is instead sniffed straight from the car or bike tank. Can also be poured onto a rag and inhaled.

Dyes

Sniffed straight from the container or poured onto a rag and inhaled. Dyes usually contain acetone and the anaesthetic methylene chloride. Again these products seem to be of minority interest. A survey of 400 Scottish sniffers revealed not one dye user.

Gas Lighter Fuel

At the time of writing this was rated as a product of increasing abuse. The most straightforward method is to simply uncap the cannister, clench the nozzle between the teeth and squirt the chilly butane gas down the throat, but it is also used in combination with a plastic bag over the head, the gas being squirted into this enclosed space and inhaled. A Stafford boy who died by this system had been using four to five cans daily, at a cost of about £5. His habit had begun two years earlier and so there are certainly indications that butane sniffing can be a long-running habit as well as the cause of sudden deaths.

Although it is released through a nozzle, lighter fuel is not strictly an aerosol. It contains no special propellant – the gas propels itself out – and no solvent is needed to keep the contents liquid. It is pure liquid butane, packed under pressure and which upon release into the atmosphere turns into a cold gas. Of the 140 UK sniffing-related deaths logged between 1971 and 1981[5] butane was the main substance involved in 38 cases. Of these, 27 derived from lighter fuel, four from Calor gas, three from butane containers and four were 'unspecified'.

Aerosol Products

In this category are perfumes, deodorants, antiperspirants, cleaning agents, paint sprays, hair lacquers, pain-relief sprays and fly killers. All contain three principal elements: the advertised product; a solvent to keep it from solidifying, and pressurised liquid gases to propel it from the can. The solvent could be a number of substances: water (starch products); alcohol (hairspray or perfume); or kerosene (insect sprays). The main buzz factor is the propellant gases which are of two principal types.

Firstly, there are the halogenated hydrocarbons (otherwise known as chlorofluorocarbons). Secondly, there is deodorised butane that also contains some propane used to control the vapour under pressure. It is the first type that represents a special hazard when inhaled, and two in this group

(propellant 11 and propellant 12) are also believed to destro
the ozone layer of the atmosphere, rendering all earthl
life vulnerable to ultraviolet radiation which the ozone norm
ally keeps at bay. Manufacturers are, as a result, looking fo
efficient alternatives that are non-toxic and don't go 'floppy
in the can as it begins to empty. Meanwhile, propellants 1.
and 12 – in fact all the gas propellants – continue injurin
sniffers. Partly this is because of the sudden large doses user
subject themselves to; also because the vapour contains solic
particles of paint, lacquer, etc. The presence of these solid
encourages sniffers to look for products with a high proportion of liquid gas. Included here would be pain-relief spray
and antiperspirants. Users sometimes try to filter out impurities by spraying the product into a balloon, hoping the
concentrates will stick to the sides, or by spraying on to a cloth
and then inhaling the fumes. For those seeking an intense
dose – no matter what solids they might ingest along the way –
plastic bags are placed or even tied over the head, or sniffing
of the unfiltered spray is performed under a blanket. The
method free from all trickery is simply to spray into the
atmosphere and suck.

Aerosols first entered the US market in the '50s, but not
until October 1967 did the abuse issue come alive when the
Du Pont Corporation produced a statement acknowledging at
least seven deaths caused by glass chilling products that were
supposed to be used for prettifying cocktail glasses. The
Federal Trade Commission ordered that in future all such
products should carry a 'Death May Result From . . .' warning, and journalists took up the theme with campaigns offering details on how and what could be sniffed. Educational
programmes were developed by trade associations and literature distributed to schools. By March 1972 some 300 deaths
had been recorded, and though the glass chillers were by now
withdrawn, the variety of aerosols being inhaled had increased and so had the fatalities. It was the experience of the
US authorities that led to the British government adopting its
cool approach; avoiding printed warnings and gauche educational assaults. They believed then and still do believe that
such moves *trigger* interest in substances where none existed.

Cleaning Agents

This category includes domestic and industrial cleaning agents, degreasing materials, plaster remover and typewriter correction fluid. The vapours derive from four main solvents: trichloroethylene, trichloroethane, tetrachloroethylene and carbon tetrachloride. The sniffer inhales straight from the bottle or soaks a cloth or piece of cotton wool and places this pad over the nose and mouth. It is difficult to gauge the popularity of these products, although they figure strongly in the list of 140 UK sniffing deaths between 1971 and 1981.[6] While butane claimed most lives (38) the cleaning solvents took the next highest (36).

Fire Extinguishers

The traditional method is to decant the liquid into an empty beer can or crisp packet and inhale the fumes. Again a piece of material or cotton wool might be soaked and the vapours sucked. A survey of 400 Scottish sniffers who came to the notice of parents or the authorities between 1975 and 1981[7] indicated just four who had experimented with fire extinguishers, and at the time of writing there were no indications of a jump in its popularity. Given, therefore, what we must assume to be its low usage, it also figured prominently in the 140 recorded UK sniffing deaths. Seven of them (5 per cent) were attributed to the main solvent in extinguishers called bromochlorodifluoromethane.

In the above-listed products certain gases, chemicals and solids have been identified as the key psychoactive constituents. And yet much of what else goes into these products remain commercial secrets. There are any amount of additives to improve consistency, or flavourings to entertain the nose, and these also might be absorbed by the sniffer, whatever the filtering precautions. The effect on the body of simple hydrocarbons such as toluene is still not really known. The impact of these unspecified materials is a correspondingly bigger mystery.

Sensations

The inhaled solvent vapours are absorbed through the lungs
and pass rapidly through the blood to the brain. They act on
the central nervous system, sometimes as a stimulant, but
generally as a depressant, putting a clamp on that part of the
brain (the cortex) which 'checks' primitive instincts. The
result is what the professionals call 'disinhibition'. General
body functions like breathing and heart rate are depressed
and there is a 'stoned' feeling lasting from a few minutes to
half an hour. Headaches and sickness are not uncommon,
particularly for novices. The majority of users will stop at this
point. Continued or deep inhalation causes disorientation,
drowsiness, numbness and perhaps unconsciousness – much
like the effects of medical anaesthetics. Recovery is usually
quick, but complications arise if the source of the vapour is
not removed after the person has blacked out. Typically this
would occur if the person is alone and sniffing with his head in
a bag or under blankets.

Despite all kinds of scary possibilities, most sniffing bouts
do not end in grief. The experience is said to be much like that
of being drunk, and as any 'social drinker' knows, having a
few can produce results as varied as euphoria, aggression,
deep melancholy, the giggles and raised libido.

Stoned Behaviour

The key factors are the user's mental state: how is s/he
feeling? What has been eaten? Is s/he alone or in a group, and
does that company elevate or lead him/her into fretting over
problems? Hallucinations are never attributed to alcohol,
except by some heavy-to-chronic users – yet these are often
experienced by sniffers of all kinds of volatile substances.
Some (pain-relief sprays, typewriter correction fluid) are held
to be especially potent triggers to the imagination, and the
hallucinations, which are both visual and auditory, vary.
Users talk of shooting stars, babbling cartoon characters,
angelic music and witches. A Wigan girl reported of one of

her friends: 'He suddenly said there were monkeys all over the floor. He tried to climb up an imaginary tree to catch one, but there was no tree there. He really believed those monkeys were there. He kept trying to pick them up.'

Most individuals will know the difference between a solvent dream and reality. The danger arises when they become so intoxicated that they can no longer be bothered or are unable to take cues from their bodily senses. Among the recent sniffing deaths was a boy who drowned in a canal watched lethargically by his stoned friends. He simply bobbed out of sight. Another was a boy who plunged from a high-rise flat after crawling out on to an unguarded ledge that under normal circumstances he presumably would not have gone near. It is because of such accidents that young users must be discouraged from sniffing in potentially dangerous places.

This raises the question of solvents, violence and other antisocial deeds. Like alcohol, solvents lift inhibitions so that the behavioural tendencies lying beneath are revealed. This could be a secret tenderness and humour that the macho street culture won't permit. Or it'll be the kinds of deeds we see regularly headlined: 'Glue-Mad Skinhead Shoots Teenager' (*Southend Evening Echo*, May 1983), 'Glue Sniffers In Church Rampage' . . . 'Glue Sniffer Left Girl In Empty House Bleeding From 15 Stab Wounds.' This last item described a particularly repulsive assault by a 17-year-old jobless decorator on a 12-year-old.

On a milder though related note I remember getting kicked in the back while working in a youth club by a 14-year-old who had never previously laid a hand or boot on me. His friends excused him, saying he was 'on the glue'. But the aggravation wasn't glue-invented. He was a troubled and aggressive young man who had previously attacked another worker with an iron bar. He despised 'liberal' authority and blamed anyone with a black or brown skin for his personal torment. A few months later he was put away in a detention centre for beating up an Asian shopkeeper. Whether or not he was glued up while putting the boot in I couldn't say.

Sniffing Alone

A distinction can be drawn between the solitary and the group sniffer. Obviously an individual might do both, but it is through solitary use that compulsive habits develop more easily, and the chances of coming to grief are increased. This is true of most drugs. Again, looking at the 140 UK deaths between 1971 and 1981, most occurred alone, at home; the age group most at risk – the 15 to 16-year-olds.

Getting Hooked

Tolerance

A novice glue user is likely to be satisfied with a single experimental blob that will keep him/her 'buzzing' for up to half an hour. The level of subsequent use, if there is to be any, is entirely variable. Those who become regular users will require increasing amounts to achieve the same high and might find themselves in a spiralling pattern of use in which scarcely credible amounts of solvents are consumed: perhaps 25 tubes of model airplane glue a day. It used to be said that it takes a year, getting dosed up several times a week, before proper tolerance develops, but now it is argued it could take a quarter of that time involving just one weekly session.

Addiction

Similarly there are considerable differences of opinion about whether authentic physical addiction can develop for solvents, so that the body suffers when deprived. The answer must be that while chills and pains in the chest, legs and head do occur if use is cut off, there seems to be nothing like the crippling, sometimes fatal, comedowns associated with the unmanaged withdrawal from barbiturates and alcohol.

Psychological Dependence

As with all drugs a psychological dependence can develop. One American study reported a user who had to be tied to his

bed, and there have been confessionals in our own media by
ex-users warning of glue's terrible lure. In Derby's *Evening
Telegraph* (June 1982) a 23-year-old called Russ told of
hallucinations 'so powerful that the person becomes en-
tranced and wants to experience them again and again . . .'
and of 'a kick so strong it ensnares you so that after a time you
fall in love with it.' He had stopped using and was running a
help programme for other users.

Health

Sudden Deaths

While there is plenty of debate in medical circles about the
long-term effects of solvents on the brain, liver, kidneys and
blood system, one clear-cut phenomenon is what are known
as 'sudden sniffing deaths': an individual inhales a volatile
product and his/her heart or respiratory system fails. S/he will
possibly choke on vomit, or the liver and kidneys will pack up.
Many of the sudden sniffing deaths in the UK have been due
to asphyxiation caused by plastic bags over the head or the use
of other paraphernalia such as tubes. This is not to say such
devices are the major cause of sniffing deaths – they are not.
Most are due to the direct toxic effects of the substance used.
But in proportion to the number of times they are used,
plastic bags do present an extreme hazard. The first major
report of sudden sniffing deaths was published in the US in
1970[8] when 110 fatalities 'without plastic bag suffocation'
from the previous decade were analysed. As noted earlier,
the casualties were mainly white youths from suburban,
middle-income families – an 'over-educated, under-
stimulated' segment of youth who have traditionally been
experimenters, and who, in the following decade, dosed up
heavily on Quaaludes (the downer methaqualone). The most
common substances sniffed were the propellant gases from
aerosols (54 per cent) and the main explanation for the deaths
was the condition cardiac arrythmia. This is where the heart is

thrown into severely abnormal rhythms. The presence of the gases made the heart more than usually sensitive to the 'fight or flight' hormone, adrenaline. When a user was under stress then the release of adrenaline into the system proved too much. The UK review[9] of 140 deaths produced a more complicated picture. The authors were looking at people aged between 11 and 63, although obviously the vast majority researched were teenagers. The riskiest years were 15 and 16, and there were 13 times more male deaths than female. 56 of the fatalities could not be attributed directly to the fumes, but were due to what the authors called 'trauma'. These included hanging, drowning and, in 26 cases, from plastic bags. As to the other 86, there were a further 26 where the person had vomited and choked to death; two due to liver/kidney failure and 14 where there was 'no information' (they were working with cases where the data was sometimes skimpy). The 68 remaining deaths were attributed to 'asphyxia', which the Oxford Dictionary terms 'suspended animation due to lack of oxygen in blood . . . suffocation.' Translated to ground-level terms, this means young men and women convulsing, turning blue, lying comatose, vomit trickling from their lips, in a state of sudden collapse with their friends probably standing by astonished and helpless.

Deciding on what substance actually killed the user was not always so clear-cut for the UK team, since cocktails such as butane and aerosol, or barbiturates, petrol and glue were used. Where a 'chief substance' was isolated, it was most often butane (28 per cent). Then comes solvents in adhesives (23 per cent), other solvents such as in cleaning agents (26 per cent), aerosols (15 per cent) and fire extinguishers (5 per cent). The high rating for adhesive solvents is, however, misleading, because far more glue is sniffed than any other product. The figures also show that glue deaths were hitting an older age group, which would suggest long-term and probably heavy use. And of the 32 who did die while using it, 'just' 12 could be pinned exclusively to the toxic effects of the vapours. The official figure during 1984 is 61. This is one person less for 'sniffing deaths' than in the previous year. It is likely, however, that in both these figures there are a number of individuals who perished from causes other than the strict inhalation of fumes.

Long-Term Effects

This is an extremely complicated area, because a large number of different products are used, often containing several volatile substances, each of which interact unpredictably. Additionally these products are peppered with additives, not all of them listed, as well as solid matter. Another problem is in trying to establish what happens to a 'normal' cross-section of recreational sniffers over a period of time. The earliest source of solvent information relates to cases of industrial poisoning: those who unwittingly inhaled fumes long-term at their places of work. A second source has been experiments performed on animals which – apart from being a cruel use of fellow creatures – usually involved such absurdly high doses they made the results of use questionable on any level. Data on recreational sniffers themselves has invariably been gleaned from psychiatric or casualty departments. To make assumptions about what long-term sniffing does by looking at such people would be like going to an alcoholic rehabilitation house to make evaluations on a cross-section of recreational drinkers.

An exception to such compromised data has been work done by the Scottish researcher Joyce Watson. In studying 115 solvent sniffers referred to her clinic during 1975 and 1976, Watson found 'no physical or laboratory abnormalities directly attributable to the abuse of solvents.' In one case 'an abnormality was noted that might have represented toxic damage to bone marrow.' But further investigation couldn't be carried out and therefore no correlation could be made. Watson followed up this study with a review of 400 Scottish cases stretching from 1975–81. Among the referrals, 90 per cent of whom were using adhesives, was an aerosol death, several accidental injuries, temporary kidney/liver damage, but no evidence of lasting harm.

However, even those who are unconvinced about some of the long-term effects claimed for toluene – such as Jasper

Woodcock of the Institute for the Study of Drug Dependence – agree that substances like benzene and the solvents used in cleaning fluids 'may be harmful to the kidney and liver,' and that toluene and benzene 'depress bone marrow and might be expected to produce aplastic anaemia.' But this effect, Woodcock notes, 'has only been reliably observed in a few people who all had a pre-existing disorder of the blood – Sickle Cell Anaemia.' In the ISDD's journal *Druglink*[10] Mike Ashton makes the 'case unproven' point more plainly: 'Somebody somewhere in the UK may be suffering from a solvent misuse induced disease that doesn't clear up once sniffing is stopped, but so far reviewers would be hard pressed to find even a single confirmed case.'

Two recent papers that have caused a stir were produced by a team led by L. Fornazzari of Toronto and by Kenneth Schikler of Louisville, Kentucky. Both claim to have noted lasting brain damage from toluene, but neither has satisfied the more meticulous sceptics. The Fornazzari team looked at 24 long-term solvent users who said they touched neither alcohol nor other drugs, and found what it called, 'cerebellar, cortical and function impairment in toluene abusers.'[11] This was subsequently decoded by Fornazzari in a US specialist newspaper as 'deep grooves developing in the abusers' brains, leaving the brains looking like shrivelled walnuts.' He said that 'memory and coordination can be permanently affected by daily abuse of the solvent within a year.' In the technical paper itself, however, he was careful to add an important rider: the damage discovered bore no clear relationship to the amount and frequency of use, which suggested 'the impairment may be the result of some factor associated with heavy use such as malnutrition or anoxia (a deficiency of oxygen). Or it could be through genetic aspects or because his subjects offered him unreliable information (they could have been feeding on all kinds of other drugs over the years).

The research paper by the Schikler team[12] discussed head scans performed on eleven toluene sniffers who were showing symptoms of tremor, slow speech, impaired thought, partial paralysis and amnesia. Five of the eleven registered normal scans. The remaining six – four of them female – were found to have 'cerebral cortical atrophy' (the cortex is the part of the brain that keeps a check on activities concerned with mood). In four of these damaged six the atrophy (shrinkage or wastage) was 'mild'. In the other two it was reported to be 'mild to moderate'. Two of the subjects also had cerebellar atrophy – the cerebellum being the large cauliflower-like structure at the back of the brain which handles balance and coordination. The six impaired subjects ranged in age from 15 to 31. They had been inhaling toluene for at least ten years and had 'no history of chronic abuse of other substances.' They were of normal weight for their height and there was no tradition of degenerative brain disease in the family. Schikler's tentative conclusion was that there was a 'possible correlation between demonstrable central nervous system atrophy and the continued inhalation of solvents (primarily toluene) for at least ten years.'

Identifying a User

A sniffer without guile will signal use in fairly obvious ways. The odour may cling to clothes, there may be freezer bags, milk bottles, crisp packets, plastic bread bags and other paraphernalia lying around in strange places, possibly with chunks of hardened glue in them. If dry cleaning fluids are being used there may be curious fade stains on sleeves, lapels; or spill marks on bedclothes, window ledges, carpets. There will be physical signs too. A number of them are typical of the teenage years, so beware of making rash assumptions. The most common will be like cold-sore spots around the mouth and nose, cracked lips, a cough, runny nose, watery eyes, a pallid, tired look – reminiscent of the symptoms of a stubborn cold. There may also be weight loss together with listlessness. These symptoms will clear up once sniffing stops, probably in a week to ten days.

Help

It is not helpful to leap up in a panic at young experimentalists, much better to talk calmly with them, discover what and how much they're using and by what method. Set before them the risks, and even if they don't quit they might at least be steered towards safer habits. Try to find out whether the sniffing is for 'fun' or whether it masks deeper problems. Sniffing that goes on for more than six to nine months and which is done without friends and or gluttonously will signal something other than recreational use. Then, clearly, the underlying problem has to be unfolded, and a commitment drawn from the user to quit the habit. How this commitment is achieved will vary, but one of the big obstacles will be a failure to see that alternatives to the habit can possibly exist. Most experienced counsellors recommend old-fashioned healthy pursuits to take the solvent's place. All the while self-confidence should be padded out for the awkward road of solvent 'deprivation' lying ahead. A remarkably sensible document by Manchester drugs expert, Rowdy Yates,[13] offers advice for professional counsellors, but it could equally aid parents and friends of compulsive sniffers. Among his recommendations:

Avoid dwelling on the particulars of solvents and their effects since 'this can often reinforce the self-image that the process is attempting to change.'

Avoid getting into 'yes you are – no I'm not' arguments about when the last sniff was had and what it was. 'Better to acknowledge this is a difficult area and move on to the problems which lie behind the denial – fear, inadequacy, lack of self-respect.' A more honest relationship will develop.

Though there'll be a long-term target (to quit or cut down to a manageable level), also have a series of short-term objectives – no matter that they are slight. These can be celebrated when reached.

Avoid depicting small lapses as grave failures. Rather 'use the experience to develop new strategies to overcome particular difficulties and situations.'

Some habits, clearly, are going to be beyond the wit of the user and his/her family and friends. Experienced help will be needed. Unfortunately there is little of it about. It is reported that few drug crisis centres or detoxification units will accept solvent sniffers because they see them as too young, trivial, or unruly. Some long-term rehabilitation units will take them on and some hospital drug or psychiatric units make out-patient appointments. But an appointment for two months' time is generally useless for someone who, having got up courage to seek help, wants fast attention.

One formidable option is the National Campaign Against Solvent Abuse, headed by Alan Billington and encompassing some 25 local aid groups. NCASA aren't interested in steering users on to safer products, but getting them to quit. It maintains the line that great harm can follow from any level of indulgence; that every sniffer is a potential addict, and few are able to stop by themselves. They say a call to their Mitcham headquarters will result in a local counsellor being despatched. The user can choose the location of the session and although parents needn't be informed, they advise it. There are usually eight to ten visits spread over two months.

The Law

There is no British law banning solvent sniffing although, at the time of writing, there was a Private Member's Bill passing through parliament that will: 'Make it an offence in England and Wales for a person to sell or offer for sale substances to young people under the age of 16 if such person knows or has reasonable grounds for believing that those substances are likely to be inhaled to achieve intoxication.'[14]

That the Bill has the backing of the Home Secretary virtually assures its carriage, and yet who but the most conspicuous peddlars of solvents is it likely to catch? Scotland already has a common law that does the same job, and in December 1983 it snared its first glue retailers when two Glasgow shopkeepers were each sentenced to three years' imprisonment (later reduced on appeal) for their absurdly brazen activities. There had been a public demonstration and threats of arson. There were visits from police, social workers, parents and local councillors, and still the pair dealt volumes of glue, already packed a dollop at a time inside crisp bags. A search revealed eight gallons of the stuff.

Most shopkeepers, however, are going to be more surreptitious than this Scots pair, or they'll be labouring under the naive assumption that their young consumers want the glue to stick together toy airplanes.

Policy

Since the worries over volatile substances first started there have been many irate demands for a total ban on their sale. Government has been accused of being apathetic and no doubt there's a powerful element of this, but resistance is also rooted in a strategy going back to the late '60s which recognises the many pitfalls in trying to police these materials from the culture.

The various control options and their drawback are these: *ban all sales of glue to under-16s.* Apart from being unfair to legitimate young consumers the sniffer is likely to turn to other, probably more harmful substances. S/he can buy them her/himself or get them from under the sink at home. *Use an 'aversive', foul-smelling additive to make the products uninhalable.* Again, pity the ordinary consumer. Every single item capable of being sniffed would have to be so doctored, and finding a suitable aversive substance is in any case extremely difficult. The Ministry of Defence's chemical defence establishment at Porton Down worked on it for some time and failed. The substance must be potent, yet it cannot be flammable, cause allergies or in any way be dangerous to the majority of purchasers. *Put clear warning signs on sniffable items.* This will amount to a 'sniffers guide'.

Given the above drawbacks it is little wonder there is scarcely any support for such controls, whether from the 'caring agencies', the government or police.

Being 'Drunk' on Solvents

There is a comparable lack of enthusiasm for passing laws that make it an offence to be 'drunk' on solvents in a public place.

This might seem foolish, but it is even more so to catch possibly thousands of very young sniffers in the criminal net, particularly if they are committing no separate 'outrage' such as thieving or assault, for which laws already exist. And yet because there is an amount of public anger at the very sight of young people with their heads in crisp packets, swaying and giggling, various laws have been turned against sniffers. Most often it is the Public Order Act 1936, which curbs insulting or threatening behaviour. Local bye-laws have been dusted off, such as in Neath recently when a 16-year-old girl pleaded guilty to contravening a local statute making it an offence to 'cause annoyance or commit a nuisance to public decency or propriety.' A 16-year-old boy was arrested for depositing rubbish – a plastic glue bag – in a public park under the GLC's control. He was remanded for three weeks. And a 15-year-old was prosecuted under a British Railway Board bye-law – generally used for rough-sleeping winos – which makes it an offence to be intoxicated on BR property. Carrying a £200 maximum fine, he was separated from £10. In addition to such strictures, all youngsters found sniffing can be rounded up under the Children and Young Persons Act and taken to a safe place. This would be a police station or their home. Eventually they could be placed in care.

Sniffing and Driving

While solvent sniffing has been ruled not to cause 'drunkenness' and is thus safe from prosecution under the Licensing Act 1872, and the relevant clauses in the Criminal Justice Act 1967, it is a different matter while in charge of a vehicle. Here the act specifies being unfit through 'drink or drugs', and two London High Court judges decided on March 30 1983, that it was 'common sense' to regard solvents as a drug. They were ruling in a Queens Bench Divisional Court which is, in effect, an appeal tribunal for points of law raised in magistrates' courts. So a precedent is now authoritatively established. The case in question related to a man whom police found slumped over the wheel of a parked car on Christmas Eve, 1981. His nose was tucked into a plastic bag and there was a can of Evostik on the car floor. He admitted sniffing.

The Law in Scotland

Scotland is ahead of the rest of the UK on several fronts: they had the first publicised 'epidemic'; the first specialist solvent clinic, the first successful prosecution of glue-kit peddlars, and the first piece of anti-solvent legislation, called the Solvent Abuse (Scotland) Act. While not expressly banning sniffing it adds the practice to the list of conditions whereby a child might be referred to the 'Reporter'. This Reporter then decides whether to inform the parents, ask social services to 'take a look', or refer the child to a Children's Panel which has the power to place the child in residential or non-residential care. There have been uneven reports about the workings of the system in its first year. One of the major complaints is that it has driven more sniffers into unreachable places. It is also said to have discouraged parents from coming forward to existing therapeutic facilities in case this leads to a referral to the panel and a separation.

After its first year of operation 533 young people had been referred to the Reporter, who in turn brough 243 of them before the Children's Panel. Of this number, 24 wound up in residential care and 63 were given special supervision requirements, but left with relatives or friends. As a representative of the Scottish Office noted in October 1984, 'The 1983 Act has done little to increase resources. It does seem geared to getting young people into the system of care rather than doing anything for them.'

Summary

If common sense were applied to the often contradictory expert views outlined above, something like the following would result:

1. Toluene is the solvent most often inhaled and, according

to present research, has demonstrated no lasting harm from moderate, short-term use.

2. Where the vapours are concentrated, as in the use of a plastic bag or blanket over the head, there is a risk of passing out, and if the source of the vapours is not removed, asphyxiation could follow.

3. Butane, found in lighter refills and stove bottles, can cause sudden death from heart failure or suffocation. The same applies to aerosols and fire extinguishers.

4. Tetrachloroethane, which is found in cleaning fluids, is implicated more often in 'sudden deaths' than toluene and, though not proven, has been closely associated with damage to liver, kidneys, lungs and intestines.

5. The use of liquor or other drugs with solvents brings extra risks.

6. Persistent solitary sniffing is usually a tip that the use is problematic.

7. Try not to panic if your child is sniffing.

8. Don't be discouraged if the quitting/cutting back isn't instant or if there are lapses. A 'cure' requires understanding that there are healthy and satisfying alternatives to the fumes.

Notes

1 J. L. Herzberg & N. Wolkind, 'Solvent Sniffing in Perspective', *British Journal of Hospital Medicine*, January 1983

2 H. R. Anderson *et al.*, 'An Investigation of 140 Deaths Associated with Volatile Substance Abuse in the UK (1971–1981)', *Human Toxicology*, vol. 1, pp. 207–221

3 A. W. Ramsay, 'Solvent Abuse: An Educational Perspective', *Human Toxicology*, 1982, vol. 1, pp. 265–270

4 M. Buck, Chief Constable, Northampton Police, Report to Northamptonshire County Council Police Committee, 13.10.1983

5 J. M. Watson, 'Solvent Abuse: Presentation and Clinical Diagnosis', *Human Toxicology*, 1982, vol. 1, pp. 249–256

6 H. R. Anderson *et al.*, *op. cit.*

7 Ibid

8 J. M. Watson, *op. cit.*

9 H. R. Anderson *et al.*, *op. cit.*

10 Mike Ashton, 'Poisons Unit Symposium on Solvent Abuse', Review Article, *Druglink*, ISDD, London, Spring 1983

11 D. A. Fornazzari *et al.*, 'Cerebellar, Cortical and Functional Impairment in Toluene Abusers', *Acta Neurologica Scandinavica*, Copenhagen, 1983, vol. 67, pp. 319–329

12 Kenneth M. Schikler *et al.*, 'Solvent Abuse Associated with Cortical Atrophy', *Journal of Adolescent Health Care*, New York, 1982, vol. 3, pp. 37–39

13 Rowdy Yates, 'Sniffing for Pleasure', Lifeline Project, Manchester

14 Limitation of Sales of Solvents Bill, HMSO, 8.5.1984

11 TOBACCO

Intro

THE ONCE ubiquitous smoking of tobacco is running into tough times. With the number of cigarette smokers dropping by 10 million in the UK during the last decade, it was inevitable that the tobacco industry would try some drastic action to revitalise their profits. One of the most disreputable activities has been taking place in Africa and other under-developed tobacco markets where cigarettes parade under names such as 'Long Life' and 'New Paradise', and where adverts depict the lucky smoker alongside expensive Western motor cars.

Here in the UK the public is also being taken some distance from reality by a campaign that links smoking with 'freedom'. Among the aims of the lobby group FOREST (Freedom Organisation for the Right to Enjoy Smoking Tobacco) are to maintain freedom of choice, counter 'biased allegations' about smoking and health, protect the travelling smoker from unfair discrimination in public transport, make represen-tations to government and, most interestingly, 'maintain the independence of FOREST to express views to this end.' This last ambition is easily the most difficult to uphold since the group admits to getting at least 50 per cent of its funding from the tobacco industry. It also has some fascinating links with the cabinet of Margaret Thatcher through its full-time direc-tor, Stephen Eyres.

The idea for FOREST sprouted from the mind of its chairman, Air Chief Marshall Sir Christopher Foxley-Norris, former Battle of Britain fighter pilot and Commander-in-Chief, RAF Germany. As Peter Taylor describes events in his book *Smoke Ring*,[1] Norris, upon retiring in 1979, determined to continue his freedom crusade on behalf of the 'harassed' smoker. He discussed the idea with two pals, one the chairman of Imperial Tobacco, the other a director of Rothmans, and later met more tobacco company magnates under the auspices of old school chum, Sir James Wilson, who was then chairman of the industry's trade association. Money was forthcoming and on June 18 1979, FOREST was launched at the Union Jack Club in London. It was soon understood, however, that Sir Christopher's company contacts were all very nice, but it was more important to link into government since this is where decisions about taxation and advertising rules were made. Through the PR agency, Good Relations, Stephen Eyres was hired as full-time director. Eyres, according to *Smoke Ring*, was a Tory right winger who once edited *Free Nation*, the newspaper of Norris McWhirter's right wing Freedom Association. He had previously been a resident tutor at Swinton College, the Tory Party's political training centre, and had also done important research for both Nicholas Ridley and Ian Gow. Ridley is now a Cabinet Minister. Gow was Parliamentary Private Secretary to Margaret Thatcher before becoming a minister at the Department of the Environment.

Eyres' own style is new-wave libertarianism – pugnacious, bumptious, full of certainty. Since his recruitment he has busied himself on radio and in print arguing against the new smoking bans and battering at the anti-tobacco lobbyists, whom he characterises as unpatriotic killjoys. The summer 1983 issue of FORESTS' campaigning newspaper even disclosed that when Pope John Paul arrived at Gatwick the previous year he presented 200 cigarettes to his aircraft crew in gratitude for a safe journey. The item was headlined, 'Holy Smoke'.

What Is It?

Manufactured cigarettes have commanded the dominant portion of total tobacco sales since the turn of the century. In

Britain we go for Virginia-type 'blond' mixes which are now beginning to colonise other markets where dark, oriental flavourings have been traditional. The average mass-produced cigarette will contain from half a dozen to thirty varieties of tobacco. It will also be pepped up by a selection from the 150 or so additives that are permitted under UK law, ranging from dwarf pine-needle oil to geranyl isobutyrate.

Yet despite the flavouring options, the average cigarette today contains just half the quantity of tobacco as in the 1930s. This, ironically, results from the public's demand for narrower, longer cigarettes capped by ever-lengthening filter tips. It also results from the switch to low-tar brands, a proportion of whose bulk comprises the normally discarded sweepings and stems. The bulk is further inflated by a 'puffing' technique which usually involves injecting freon, a refrigerated gas that vaporises at room temperature. Some of the rest of the mass comes from air, water and steam, which is pumped in to make the leaf 'more pliable'. As to the smoke that we draw into our lungs, this contains at least a thousand different substances including eight known carcinogens.

Tar

The most important is the dark, treacly tar which forms as the smoke cools and condenses. It is this material which carries the flavour, and although it could be eliminated by breeding special plants and by heavy filtering, the result for the smoker would be a gust of flavourless warm air. Tar-yields per cigarette have actually dropped some 25 per cent in the last decade (to about 17 mg).

Nicotine

Pure nicotine is one of the most lethal substances known – able to kill with a few drops applied to the tongue. In the concentrations found in cigarettes, however, it acts as a mild stimulant producing small increases in heart rate, breathing and other internal activity. It is the nicotine that is usually cited as the reason why smokers continue craving tobacco,

although increasingly ingenious research work tends to con-
fuse the picture. Nicotine is found only in tobacco plants and
is carried into the smoker's body via tiny droplets of tar that
get sucked down with the smoke. A typical cigarette delivers
about 2 mg of the drug, although less than this reaches the
bloodstream. The lethal dose is believed to be about 60 mg
when taken in its pure state. The easiest way to achieve such
levels would be to swallow a portion of the pesticide nicotine
sulphate.

Carbon Monoxide

Carbon monoxide is an inevitable consequence of the combustion that takes place while smoking. The yield per
cigarette depends on how closely packed it is and the kind of
paper used. Tighter cigarettes without 'ventilated' filters and
which are smoked right down to the butt will deliver more of
the gas.

Irritant Substances

These are said to cause coughing and phlegm, and reduce the
lungs' natural protection against dust and particles.

Other Products

Pipe and Cigar Tobaccos

Pipe and cigar tobaccos have a higher tar content then
cigarettes, but because practised smokers don't inhale the
fumes they run comparatively less of a risk. Not so the
reformed cigarette smoker who switches to one of the other
methods and carries on the furious sucking.

Snuff

Snuff is pounded, flavoured tobacco. It delivers as much
nicotine per snort as the typical cigarette, but because there is
no fire there is no tar or carbon monoxide.

Non-Tobacco Smokables

The herbal and other non-tobacco cigarettes are subject to the same laws of combustion as the tobacco sort, and therefore deliver up carbon monoxide and tar. But they contain no nicotine. The same applies to smoked hashish, marijuana, cocaine and heroin.

Sensations

The answer to why people should want to smoke is no closer to being answered now than when the weed was first introduced to European society four hundred years ago. Tobacco produces neither euphoria nor stupefaction and yet smokers return to it over and over with a compulsion that could be said to make a heroin addict look decorous. It is not only rare for a smoker not to light up every day, it is rare for him/her not to light up 10, 15, up to 100 times each day. (The national average is about 18.) What pleasures are forthcoming? There was a fashion a while ago to talk in terms of 'oral gratification', a notion all tied up with early mothering and deformed sexuality. This is now regarded as too psychological. There is also the hit factor as the smoke is sucked into the lungs. For the novice this experience is burning and exalting, and even though the impact gets more modest as the lungs weather, the component remains an important one for many smokers. Then there is 'flavour', nutty and sweet with the darker blends such as Gitane, sappy and bright if it's a Virginian. There is more of it when the cigarette is rated high-tar because it is the tar that carries the taste. Probably the most important of all the components is nicotine. Pharmacologically nicotine acts as a mild stimulant, offering tiny jolts to 'reward centres' deep in the brain. If a smoker were to describe it s/he'd probably use the language employed to convey the impact of a cup of tea: it brings you up when you're feeling low, damps you down when you're too fired up; makes you relax; gets you going; helps you think; takes your mind off your problems.

These states of being are plainly at odds with each other and yet experiments with pure nicotine seem to confirm the drug truly does have this dual ability. Smaller doses stimulate whereas larger ones depress. But then other tests suggest the upping and downing isn't dose-related, but a matter of personality. Still more tests indicate nicotine has practically no bearing on how much people smoke. Subjects given injections of the drug[2] carried on smoking at the same rate and in the same manner as though the injections had never happened.

Health Impact

The health argument over smoking goes back in Britain at least to 1604 when James I published his spirited tirade, 'Counterblaste to Tobacco . . .' In modern times the issue was revived by the Royal College of Physicians who in a 1962 report linked smoking with lung cancer and implored the government to do something about rising consumption. The public itself responded by momentarily cutting back, but a year later it was smoking more than ever. The pattern was duplicated in the US following a report by their own Surgeon General. The masses, it seems, cannot be persuaded from their vices by gore stories alone. (It is probable that the current reductions are more closely related to increased taxes in a period of economic hardship.) So what are these smoking hazards? Since its first landmark report the Royal College has updated its advice three times, but the news for smokers gets no better. The habit, by their estimation, accounts for some 15 to 20 per cent of all British deaths, which means *not less* than 100,000 a year. To put it in more manageable terms, if we take 1,000 young male adults in England and Wales who smoke cigarettes, one will be murdered, six will be killed on the roads and 250 will be killed prematurely by tobacco. But besides death there is all the misery of smoking-related diseases, the financial cost to the sufferer these cause through lost work, and the drain on the NHS by millions of individuals knowingly injuring themselves.

There are three principal ailments with which smoking

has been shown to have a causal rather than coincidental relationship – lung cancer, bronchitis/emphysema and heart diseases.

Lung Cancer

Among the most plausible bits of data linking lung cancer with smoking comes from studying the smoking habits of doctors between 1954 and 1971. The proportion of male physicians smoking cigarettes halved during this period from 43 per cent to 21 per cent, while among all men in England and Wales the number of smokers remained about the same. Lung cancer among doctors during the period fell by 25 per cent, whereas in the general population it rose by 26 per cent.[3] It also appears from this same study that the risk of the disease increases in direct proportion to the number of cigarettes smoked. Those who burn 15 a day were eight times more vulnerable than non-smokers, and 25-a-day-or-more types were 25 times more at risk.

Lung cancer has actually started declining among men under 65 in recent years. This is put down to the decline in smoking and the low-tar filter cigarettes that have been the fashion for the past couple of decades.

For women the incidence is on the increase, and this seems to correlate with a previous sharp rise in the number of female smokers. If lung cancer deaths among British women keep rising at their present rate, the wrecking power of the disease will overtake that of breast cancer by the year 2010. It already has in Scotland.

Since lung cancer is seeded many years before the disease appears, quitting smoking will not instantly eliminate risk, but it will start decreasing to the point where after 10 or 15 years the ex-smoker whose habit was moderate is only at slightly greater risk than someone who has never smoked.

Emphysema/Bronchitis

The new preferred term for these progressively disabling conditions is chronic obstructive lung disease (COLD), which indicates what's going on inside. Fundamentally, the air passages to the lungs are being narrowed and damaged and much of the lung tissue itself destroyed. Onset of the disease is gradual and a good deal of harm will probably already have been done by the time the familiar breathlessness becomes disabling. Though the death rate has been decreasing in recent years the disease still despatched 19,000 people in 1982. Until recently COLD was known as the 'English Disease' and was assumed, quite logically, to be a factor of poverty and the filthy state of the industrial environment. The link with smoking is now also proven beyond reasonable doubt. The death rate among smokers is six times greater than for non-smokers and 25 times as great in consumers of more than 25 a day.

Heart Diseases

The part played by smoking in heart diseases is less clear cut. Though the Department of Health estimates that about a quarter of all cases result from smoking, it is also evident that other factors play a principal role in this most prevalent of all causes of death. Not least there is the heredity factor – also, high blood pressure, lack of exercise, too much stress and consumption of too many fatty foods. In the US, heart diseases have fallen dramatically, which could be as much to do with a switch in eating habits as the cutback in smoking. Nonetheless, middle-aged smokers on 15 or more cigarettes a day seem to be three times more prone to the disease than their non-smoking counterparts. And some studies indicate that the risk of sudden death from heart attack is five times as great in the smoking population. Although women under 65 are much less liable to be felled by heart problems than men, they too are being stricken far more often.

Researchers usually isolate nicotine and carbon monoxide as smoke's ravening factors as far as the heart is concerned. The first increases the organ's workload, while the carbon monoxide denies it the normal supply of oxygen. This may lead to what's called atheroma – deposits of fatty substances in the arterial walls. Smokers often have them in abundance.

Diseases of arteries other than in the heart area are also more common in smokers. 95 per cent of all individuals with serious arterial disease of the legs are regular smokers, and it is this condition which causes more leg amputations than any other.

The whole business of marrying smoking with heart diseases is bound to be replete with error if only for the somewhat cavalier way these conditions are cited as the cause of sudden death when the professional is baffled. One study[4] showed that the condition was wrongly diagnosed as the cause of death in 39 out of every 100 cases.

Other Smoke-Related Diseases

Lung cancer, bronchitis/emphysema and heart diseases might be the Big Three smoking risks, but there are several more ailments with which the habit is linked, sometimes, it has to be said, fairly tenuously. These include cancers of the mouth, throat, oesophagus, bladder, pancreas, kidneys and cervix. There is also what the Royal College of Physicians call a 'well recognised association' with peptic ulcers in the stomach and duodenum.

Women and Smoking

Apart from falling prey more frequently to the 'male diseases' of lung cancer and heart failure other special hazards face women. Those who take the contraceptive pill and also smoke are ten times more likely than non-smoking pill users to have either a coronary attack, stroke or blood clot in the leg veins.[5] Babies of smoking mothers also suffer as a result of their mothers' habit. The various poisons contained in cigarette smoke can pass through the placenta into the baby, causing it to be deprived of oxygen. Typically, this can result in smaller, lighter babies who could continue lagging as they grow older. Tobacco use during pregnancy is also reported to double the risk of spontaneous abortion[6] and to promote more complications such as bleeding and premature detachment of the placenta.[7]

However, the news for women who quit before the 20th

week of pregnancy is good. Their risk of having a low-weight baby will be similar to that of a non-smoker and they will also be less vulnerable to the other risks.

As usual, the interrogation light falls on women when it comes to things going wrong with a couple's newborn. So far the assessment of smoking men and their part in reproduction has tended to settle on whether or not their fertility is affected, but if smoking can induce 'sperm abnormalities', as has been reported in at least one study,[8] then it is surely possible for that deformation to be transmitted to the child. At any rate it is estimated[9] that babies under one year run twice the risk of getting serious chest infections when both parents use tobacco. This is attributed not to genetics, but to the fact that the child has to exist in a haze of smoke: known as 'passive smoking'.

Passive Smoking

Passive smoking has to be *the* most passionately disputed area in the great tobacco debate because if smokers really are injuring innocent bystanders then the 'freedom-to-enjoy' line promoted by the likes of FOREST begins to look shabby. Although more research is needed there have already been some quite telling results. For instance, nicotine can be detected in the blood and urine of non-smokers if they occupy poorly ventilated areas with smokers. More pointedly, a Japanese study[10] claimed that non-smoking wives whose husbands did smoke 20 or more cigarettes daily developed lung cancer at rates twice as high as that of non-smoking women married to non-smoking men. But then other studies have found no such inherited damage. The issue will continue to be steadfastly argued.

Dependence

There is only one universally recognised drug in tobacco – nicotine. Being a mild stimulant, it's possible to build up a tolerance to its stimulative effects, which would necessitate a bigger and bigger dose leading, ultimately, to physical dependence. In practice, most people reach a ceiling well below this dependence level and then even out their consumption. The amount they use from then on fluctuates according to their state of being – which is precisely the way they'll use other drugs. When a craving for tobacco does develop this will generally have a psychological and not a physical basis. And even after years of comparatively heavy smoking people can still quit on the spot, experiencing few if any withdrawal symptoms. There might be some extra edginess, but this is as likely to come from fretful anticipation as any physiological change in body chemistry.

Earliest Use

The origins of tobacco smoking can be traced back to the Maya civilisation of Mexico at around 500 AD. This, though, is a modest assumption about tobacco's pedigree. References to the smoking of various plants have been found in the Vedic scriptures of India dating back a couple of thousand years BC. Tobacco is likely to have been one of the selection that was consumed – the habit probably goes back even before those days. Commercial trading on an international scale began with the arrival in the 'New World' of European interlopers some four hundred years ago. From Chile to Montreal the Indians of the new lands were smoking, chewing and eating the leaves, and drinking the juice of the plant. In the West Indies it was customary for small leaves to be wrapped in larger ones or in a palm leaf, the prototype of the modern cigar. In Mexico they were sniffing through tubes made of tortoise-shell and silver. Further north the pipe was traditional, sometimes made of marble, sometimes of lobster claw. Tobacco arrived in England around 1565, probably via French or Flemish sailors at the behest of English herbalists. For the first couple of decades it was used here strictly medicinally – for purging 'superfluous fleame and other gross humours', as one contemporary account had it. Then in 1586 a great cache of the stuff was brought back to England from the West Indies and, on the instructions of Sir Walter Raleigh,[11] was surveyed and written up. It was thanks to this patronage by Raleigh that smoking now became a social ritual and, increasingly, sold from specialist tobacco shops. By the 1600s public houses were also in on the action, as were grocers, drapers, chandlers and goldsmiths. Virginia in what is now the US was the source and the colony soon became the world's tobacco capital with ever open space in the township employed for the growing of the weed.

Other American colonies followed and cultivation started up in every other part of the world. Though some regions gave the plant a frigid welcome, the Portuguese hit lucky in what was to become Malawi and Zimbabwe, while the Dutch were equally successful in Indonesia where the soil and climate were ideal for producing the thick, juicy leaves that go into producing cigars.

In early seventeenth century England smoking was essentially a pastime for the wealthy, given that it demanded expensive metal pipes and other bits of apparatus. Later, the introduction of clay and wood pipes meant that the lower orders could join in, and yet groups like the London dandies still devised means of setting themselves apart. The fashionable kit required a case of expensive clays, an ivory or metal box to hold the weed, ember tongs to convey a heated coal to light the pipe, a metal stopper to compress the tobacco into the bowl, a pick with which to clear said bowl, a knife to shred the tobacco, and a small scoop in which the tobacco could be dried.[12] Patented methods were devised for in/exhaling the smoke, with names such as the *Gulpe* and the *Whiffe*, and perhaps most exciting of all, the *Cuban Ebolition*, whereby smoke was expelled from the nostrils. The new habit clearly vexed members of the clergy. King James, too, was not pleased with it although his '*Counterblaste to tobacco*' was apparently aimed as much at his political enemy Raleigh as the new drug. He followed this up with a new tax, which has grown steeper ever since. James' lunge at the smoke habit was reasonably restrained compared to what was going on elsewhere. In Switzerland smoking meant the pillory, in Persia suffocation by smoke, in China decapitation and, in Russia, being sent into exile with your nose split open.

By the end of the seventeenth century snuff had jumped up to steal the limelight from pipe smoking, a position it held until the early nineteenth century. Snuffing involved paraphernalia and etiquette even more extraordinary than that for smoking. A gentleman was known by his snuff; he laid it down as he would a cellar of wine. That ladies also took to snuffing is illustrated by the will of one Mrs Margaret Thompson whose coffin in 1776 was filled with unwashed snuff handkerchiefs and her body borne by the six greatest snuff-takers in the parish. Inevitably the habit spread to the lower orders, whereupon the product became more and more adulterated with coal or powdered glass, and was ultimately jettisoned from smart circles. *Hints on Etiquette*, published in 1835, called snuffing 'an idle, dirty habit practised by stupid people in the unavailing endeavour to clear their stolid intellect.' By this time cigars were drawing level. Then cigarette smoking arrived via British troops who had seen their French and Turkish allies doing it during the Crimean War (1854–6).

At first, cigarettes were of the roll-your-own sort and made from any type of paper. Then English manufacturers started turning out handmade varieties consisting chiefly of Turkish and Egyptian leaves. By 1870 the 'bright' Virginian blends were coming over in bulk and London fashion switched back across the Atlantic. Now also came the innovation which opened the way to the great tobacco empires that dominate in our own time: the 'Bonsack' automatic rolling machine, patented in 1881. It could do the work of forty employees. The W. D. & H. O. Wills Company quickly secured 'absolute rights' in the UK, while in America a similar deal was sewn up by James Buchanan Duke, inexhaustible head of the American Tobacco Company. Within a few years 'Daddy' Duke had bought out every one of his US rivals. Then he came gunning for Wills and the other leading dozen British manufacturers. Uniting under the banner of Imperial, the family-owned British companies saw off the Duke's challenge, and even went for a chunk of the US market just to demonstrate how they weren't cowed by the big man. As Peter Taylor notes in *Smoke Ring*, a truce was declared. It was agreed, in 1902, that Imperial should confine itself to the British market, the American Tobacco Company to the US, while a new corporation would be formed called British American Tobacco to handle exports for both companies. The arrangement lasted just nine years before the US Supreme Court, which was out hunting monopolies at the time, ordered that the American Tobacco Company be dismantled in the interests of greater consumer choice.

The rended segment which retained the ATC name later transmogrified into a multinational called American Brands. As to Imperial, they stayed intact here in the UK where they concentrated future business.

The fate of the joint export enterprise, British American Tobacco, was more fascinating: this was floated off as an independent corporation registered in London. Thereafter, through adroit licensing and diversifying schemes, it was able to outstrip both its parents as well as all the new competition. Today it is the largest private sector tobacco corporation in the world. Operating in 180 countries, it claims brand leadership in 36 of them. Turnover runs at about $15 billion, and production of cigarettes is about 550 billion. It is best known globally for the Benson and Hedges and State Express brands, but along with the other tobacco giants, BAT readily shares brand names under deals that recognise the different companies' areas of influence. Thus, one company will market a brand in Holland, another the same name in Malawi with the flavour being fixed not according to established standards, but to suit the domestic market.

The Big Five

There are five tobacco traders which rank as truly global megacorporations. BAT is the largest by some distance.

Second in rank is Philip Morris Inc., whose origins lie in a small Bond Street shop opened by one Philip Morris in 1847. Today it operates from New York as part of the group that also governs Seven Up, the Miller Brewing Company, as well as plastics, paper, packaging materials and property interests. In 1981 Philip Morris bought a substantial interest in Rothmans International, which took it closer to the heels of BAT. Top international brands are Marlboro, Merit and Parliament.

Ranking third is R. J. Reynolds Inc., with headquarters in North Carolina and a league table of top brands including Winston, Camel, Salem, More and Now. Reynolds' roots are in the tobacco belt of the US from where it peddled chewing and smoking tobaccos. Today it operates subsidiaries engaged in transport, oil, gas, food and drinks.

Fourth of the giants is London-based Rothmans International which functions more as a group than a corporate entity. Rothmans, Dunhill and Peter Stuyvesant are its top brands and through them it holds a big share of the duty-free business. Non-smoking interests take in everything from umbrellas to wine.

Number five is American Brands – the '80s version of what survived of Daddy Duke's American Tobacco Company. Registered in New York, it commands a major position by virtue of just three markets – the UK, USA and Holland. Top sellers Stateside are Carlton, Lucky Strike, Pall Mall and Tareyton. Here in the UK, because of its ownership of Gallahers of Northern Ireland, it has Britain's top selling Benson and Hedges, plus Silk Cut, Senior Service, Hamlet cigars, Condor pipe tobacco and Old Holborn rollies.

Imperial Group

Not one of the Big Five, nonetheless Imperial sells the most cigarettes in the UK. Once famed for the Woodbine and Capstan brands, today it leads the fight against stiffening domestic competition with John Player King Size. It bothers little with the international market, preferring to direct more resources into non-tobacco areas. Under the group's control are Golden Wonder Crisps, HP Sauce, Courage and John Smith brews and the American Howard Johnson hotel chain.

Tobacco and the Third World

Imperial can be categorised as a national rather than global tobacco corporation. Many other countries have them too. Some are entirely state-owned, some partly. Some operate as a monopoly with foreign competition all but shut out, while others recognise there is no locking the door on the big London and New York companies, and strike up licensing or franchise deals in return for a share in the new technology. This is what is happening in China, which possesses a state-run tobacco enterprise bigger than anything, public or private, seen anywhere else in the world. Catering for 200 million domestic smokers, it turns out some 1,000 brands that are totally unknown outside her borders. Production, at 750 billion cigarettes a year, is considerably larger than BAT's, and the source for this enormous output is a domestic harvest that is also a world beater – topping that which comes out of the US's famed tobacco belt. But the Chinese are not especially secure. Like state monopolies everywhere it is beginning to suffer from the private sector's slick marketing and manufacturing methods. Everyone now wants the 'international' brands, and so the likes of China must enter into deals that win her state-of-the-art assistance, in return for having a hole punched in the home market through which State Express, Camel *et al.* can enter. The race for Third World markets is getting all the more hysterical as smokers in the West rapidly buck the habit.

The line the companies are pushing is the one manufacturers of all manner of products use – namely, 'our brand equals brain power, muscle power and social success.' For instance, a brand in Pakistan, named K2 after that country's highest mountain peak, shows a boy killing a tiger. Similarly, State Express has been advertised in Malawi's *Daily Times* by lining up a picture of the pack alongside a Jaguar XJ6. Malawi is one of the least developed countries in the world with a per capita income of about £100 per annum.

The whole of Africa seems to be an especially luscious market for Western manufacturers. Over the last ten years tobacco consumption has doubled in Libya and Ethiopia. In

Kenya one is now obliged to smoke or be perceived as representing everything that is backward. Even in the painfully impoverished desert country of Sudan the companies have their designs: during 1980, according to a tobacco trade journal, the world's largest airlift of cigarettes was being dropped on it, courtesy of BAT.

Mike Muller of the charity War On Want has done as much as anyone to expose the activities of the big corporations. Why, he asks,[13] given their immense poverty and disease, do Third World countries allow the burden of smoking to be peddled to their people? The question was rhetorical: 'Bribed by big tax revenues, governments are conned into believing that tobacco is good for them.' They are led to believe it is a 'good cash crop for the farmers, a product which the people want [and] a commodity which the country can export.' In fact the cultivator, consumer and country are getting a uniquely raw deal. Farmers, hooked by the help and advice which the tobacco companies lavish on them, end up growing a crop which takes more labour than any other – for diminishing returns. The smoker is callously, if not criminally, being sold specially branded cigarettes packing twice the punch of cancer-causing tar as that of the rich world's cigarettes. The international brand names are the same, but there are seldom health warnings on the wrapper.

'With the support and encouragement of companies like BAT – and sometimes, inexcusably, aid organisations as well – a hungry world is every year devoting some 10 million person days to growing tobacco crops which are then ceremoniously burnt at considerable risk to life.'

The Declining Western Habit

The battle to arrest declining cigarette sales in the sophisticated West might have been expected to take a different course, but essentially it is the same business of linking the habit with physical and social prowess. Since this cannot be done directly in ads (not in the UK, anyway) the manufacturers have taken to promoting car racing, golf, cricket,

motor cycling, polo as well as smart orchestras and smart ar
for an under-the-counter impact that is all the greater fo
being so covert. The most receptive segments left in the
Western markets are women and children. The latter are
especially important because they represent the companies
futures. These days the firms appear to be doing not especially
badly. According to the Ministry of Health, under-16-year-
olds now spend £60 million a year on cigarettes with more
than a third of fifth formers claiming to be regular smokers.
As to brand choices, they appear to want the ones most
closely linked to sports through sponsorship schemes. For
women the thrust has been towards extremely long, 'luxury'
cigarettes, sometimes mentholated, usually packaged in elegant, creamy colours. They carry names like Kim and More,
and women's right to indulge in their own pleasure is profer-
red with a feminist slant. As a tobacco trade magazine
recently noted,[14] with women back at work in large numbers
for the first time since the Second World War, 'They feel
entitled to spend part of what they earn on themselves.' 'It's
true', the article continues, 'that women have recently been
smoking fewer cigarettes, but their fall-off rate is slower than
men's, so that today they are buying well over half of all
king-size brands and probably 70 per cent of all the luxury
length brands.'

For all smokers the attitude of non-indulgers and public
bodies is getting increasingly hostile. London tubes have
banned it. Art galleries, cinemas and restaurants are going
partially or entirely smoke-free. In California smoking is
prohibited in public places by local statute, and in offices the
employer must 'make accommodations' for the preferences
of both non-smoking and smoking employees, but if the
non-smokers are not satisfied then the firm must prohibit the
practice. Meanwhile in Glasgow a campaign is underway to
make the city the first no-smoke zone in Europe. They will
have to stretch a little to beat a lobby group in Norway whose
target is absolute prohibition by the year 2000.

Giving Up

There are a million schemes for easing people out of their smoking habit. The basis for any successful one is to get the preliminaries right, and that means establishing rationally and emotionally that quitting is the goal. Schemes whereby smokers, as it were, jump out of the bushes and startle themselves out of the habit are almost bound to fail. Having got the mind correctly adjusted, it is then not a bad idea to let the prospect stew for a while. The actual moment of quitting can be arranged to suit temperament and circumstances. It might be done on holiday, at the start of a new year, as a birthday treat. Some people like to shout about it and have bets; others like to hush it up to lessen the pressure. Some like ritual – hanging the last pack on the wall; others want to make it no big deal. Remember, it's easier than most people think. Some people say that it's probably best to avoid extremely elaborate substitution ploys: sucking four packs of mints a day is a constant reminder as to the ex smoker's great 'loss'. A little weight might be put on afterwards. This is because the body is able to absorb more of what's eaten through the newly uncongested gastro-intestinal machinery. This is a major worry for some people during the immediate days and weeks after stopping, but body weight will quickly settle down again.

Another worry is that by quitting there will be a loss of mental and physical edge. This is a particular concern to people in 'creative' activities and was recently voiced by an Oxford professor of modern history, who told the *London Standard* that for him life without smoking would probably mean 'long, slow hours hammering out leaden sentences.' In the same article a 'young beauty and author' also insisted that 'people who are smoking are thinking, while people who are not are just staring into space.' This betrays third-rate thinking. No psychoactive drug can regularly deliver the goods over the long term. Also, the physically debilitating effects of tobacco smoke soon knock off any edge that nicotine might provide.

More bogeyman stories abound concerning an alleged nicotine starvation that is supposed to seize the smoker

particularly fiercely after two months, six months, one year,
five years, and so forth. Except in the tiniest chain-smoking
minority there can be no real nicotine starvation because not
enough of the drug is consumed to work up a substantial
physical relationship. If a person continues to feel vulnerable
to stray plumes of smoke, it indicates that he/she is still
concentrating on old, dead habits. This is why it is not a good
idea to go in for elaborate substitution ploys in the period
after quitting. A case history:

'I smoked for some 20 years, from the days of my early
teens. I would alternate between rollies and manufactured
cigarettes and get through at least 20 a day, sometimes 40.
Having made the decision to stop I let the idea marinade for a
couple of years, not knowing when the right moment would
present itself. Finally it came at the beginning of a holiday in
Wales which required a long car journey. My wife asked me if
I'd mind not smoking to avoid clouding up an already
cramped atmosphere. I agreed and decided I'd lay off for the
rest of that day. After that I managed to desist for the first
week, on the third day of which my lungs purged themselves
of a putrid, sticky material that had me coughing and splutter-
ing for half an hour. I was encouraged to keep off the fags for
the second week.

Abstaining in the hills and valleys of Wales was all very
well, but I anticipated a much graver test back in London,
faced with deadlines and telephone bills. I made no promise
to myself and yet when it did come to writing my first article –
which I considered the first big test – I actually forgot that I
was ever a smoker. A couple of tremors of desire came in the
following months, but nothing of consequence. Now I continually remind myself (nearly five years later) how lucky I am
to be free of such an idiotic habit.'

Policy

Though smoking is evidentially bad for the consumer it is
extremely good for government. In 1982/3 the UK authorities
collected some £4,200 million in tobacco taxes, set against a

here £155 million in visible health costs. It is even quite good financial news when smokers die prematurely. The country can afford the loss of manpower, and better such people expire than linger at a cost to the NHS. There is also something to be said in respect of the 24,000 people employed by the tobacco industry. It is an amount almost one-quarter of the number which tobacco kills each year, and so it is no wonder that UK governments have traditionally been flaccid in their approach to the tobacco menace. Room for manoeuvre is in any case limited. By continuing to increase the tax rate a proportion of softcore smokers will be squeezed out, but the committed cannot be shifted by these means. And if prices get too high it will simply encourage crime. Government could control tobacco under the Medicines Act 1968, which would allow it to fix tar, nicotine and carbon monoxide content, but to put too tight a rein on such a popular drug would simply promote underground networks through which fearsomely potent alternatives to the authorised smoke would be peddled. And yet that part of the Medicines Act which allows control of advertising and sponsorship *is* attractive. If promotion of every sort could be eliminated then demand would in due course fall substantially. Let the old high, low and medium tars be available, but let no one shout about them.

On a parallel note, the British government might also usefully look at UN accusations that some of the tobacco giants are promoting their trade in undeveloped parts of the world by means of large-scale bribery. If true, are London-registered companies involved? Do the British authorities intend investigating the allegations?

Notes

1 P. Taylor, *Smoke Ring*, The Bodley Head, London, 1984, p. 24
2 M. Gossop, *Living With Drugs*, Temple Smith, London, 1982, p. 96

3 'Health or Smoking?', Follow-up Report of the Royal College o
   Physicians, Pitman, London, 1983, p. 3
4 M. Gossop, *op. cit.*, p. 99
5 *Fact Sheet Eight*, Action on Smoking and Health (ASH)
   London
6 J. Kline *et al*, *New England Journal of Medicine*, 1977, vol. 297
   pp. 793–796
7 ASH Fact Sheet
8 Ibid
9 Ibid
10 Ibid
11 *A History of the Tobacco Trade*, Imperial Group, London, 1979,
    p. 8
12 Ibid, p. 10
13 Mike Mullon, 'Tobacco and the Third World: Tomorrow's
    Epidemic?', War on Want, 1978
14 Edgar Reisman, 'Female Figures', *Tobacco*, March 1984

12 TRANQUILLISERS

Intro

THE TERM tranquilliser is used to refer to drugs from the class of chemicals known as benzodiazepines, which began pouring on to the market 20-odd years ago with the launch of Librium. They have developed little repute as fun street drugs, which is curious given that they are the most frequently prescribed mood altering agents in the world. Each year about one in every five British women will wash down a benzodiazepine for daytime sedation or as a sleeper, and a tenth of all adult males will do the same. A quarter of a million UK adults are known to have used them continuously for at least five years, and it's likely that even more than this number are dependent. This makes benzodiazepines more 'abused' than heroin and all its kindred opiates by a wide margin. Perhaps it is because of such solid usage – the image is of the overwrought housewife; the frazzled minor executive – that young pugs have never much fancied the drugs. Or at least that has been the pattern until recently.

There are signs that the drugs' reputation, and therefore their pattern of use, is now changing in an important way. The benzodiazepines are fast approaching the classic crossroads reached by virtually all earlier psychotropics: having been launched as safe, non-addictive alternatives to their discredited predecessors (the barbiturates) enthusiastic levels of prescribing are followed by groans from researchers about unadvertised dangers: the bubble bursts, at which point the drugs hit the streets (because everybody has been alerted through advertising to their psychoactive horsepower) and the authorities reply by sticking them on the list of controlled substances under the Misuse of Drugs Act. This results in fluctuating street supplies, chemist break-ins etc, – while in the surgeries the drugs don't so much vanish from the medical picture as flatten out to a more modest profile. The whole cycle starts again with the discovery of a miraculous new replacement.

Benzodiazepines have gone part of the way round this circuit but there is some sharp resistance developing. Most of it comes from the drug manufacturers who have billions tied up in these most popular of all drugs, and nothing in the works to replace them. Parallel resistance is coming from a large faction of ordinary GPs who, having supplied 'trank junkies' all these years, are now loath to own up. So while prescription totals appear to have stopped rising, they weren't falling at the time of writing, merely marking their place at around 24 million per annum.

More obstruction has come from the recreational set. It centres on the drugs' low glamour rating which in turn is linked to the belief that no kick can be had from them. Instead they have taken a supportive role on the scene – back-up for heroin users when low on stocks; comfort for buffeting LSD trippers. It is, however, possible to get a buzz from benzodiazepines roughly equivalent to that provided by barbiturates, and the same volatile relationship with alcohol exists. A handful of Valium washed down with strong lager will jerk the recipient quite some distance. Numerous young people have begun to discover this fact, and they won't have to hang around damp street corners to score their supplies. They will be found in the family medicine cabinet. There is often enough lying around the home to sell a quantity to friends, and in this way a thriving little trank scene appears to be developing in schools throughout the UK.

If the dam does burst, if a quantity of benzodiazepines does wash out on to the streets, the pressure will be on to complete the historical cycle. The drugs will be controlled under the Misuse of Drugs Act and the multinationals will be compelled to invent a brave new substitute.

What Are They?

There is plenty of confusion about what constitutes a tranquilliser as opposed to a sedative, and about how these two are different from a sleeping tablet – another name for which is a hypnotic. The answer is that there is no fixed difference. One drug can do all three jobs. The varying terminology relates to the dose given and the way in which the manufacturer selects to market the product. The benzodiazepines are called tranquillisers because the word has less oppressive connotations than sedative – which is the term applied to the now discredited barbiturates. Both drugs, however, have a similar impact on the central nervous system in terms of repressing anxiety. Barbiturates happen to be more toxic at 'therapeutic' doses. As to the hypnotic part of the equation, the same relationship applies: a large dose of a benzodiazepine will send the recipient to sleep just as will a large dose of a barb.

Having got this far through the terminological thicket, another line now has to be drawn between the minor and major tranquillisers. The benzodiazepines are defined as minor tranquillisers. Major tranquillisers are much more potent compounds used principally to manage severe forms of mental illness such as schizophrenia. Important in this group is the compound chlorpromazine which gets marketed as Largactil. These majors are used to calm violent and hyperactive patients without any soporific action, but their pop name among inmates of prisons and mental institutions tells another story – *Liquid Cosh*. It is because of the cosh effect that the majors have virtually no currency value among 'fun' users.

So now we have isolated a class of drug called, because of their action, minor tranquillisers, which are known, when administered at night in bigger doses, as hypnotics. Let us simply call them tranquillisers and recognise that we are talking chiefly about pills derived from a class of chemicals known as benzodiazepines.

There are about twenty fairly well established benzodiazepine derivatives being marketed at the time of writing – each one packaged under a variety of brand names. While

essentially comparable in their chemical make-up, they are
formulated in different potencies and to be effective over
different timespans – long-, medium- and short-acting. Long-
acting benzos are those that are more slowly metabolised and
excreted. They are used for either daytime sedation or as a
sleeper that goes on sedating into the next day. The short-
acting drug would be for people whose anxiety levels fluctuate
and who need a pill to dowse a sudden panic attack. When the
shorts are used for sleeping it would typically be by someone
whose problem is nodding off in a strange or noisy environment. The mediums, naturally, fall midway between the two.

Sensations

The benzodiazepines produce feelings of tranquillity at low to
moderate doses. But whereas the barbiturates travel down
the spinal column at higher doses, making the body sloppy
and numb, benzos tend to confine their activity to the higher
parts, so even with extremely large doses the results will be
more mental than physical. At one end of the spectrum there
is a feeling of calm, a smothering of anxieties. At higher doses
there will be drowsiness, a blurring of intellectual sharpness, a
decreased ability to line up mental intent with physical performance (for instance, driving suffers). Paradoxically, they
can also release inhibitions so that some people become
aggressive, excitable, prone to crazy mood swings. In fact the
result is very much like alcohol, but without the staggering.
At this dose level the simplest thing is to sleep. If that is
resisted brain performance becomes more and more erratic
until stupor sets in. On awakening the size of the hangover
will depend on the kind of benzodiazepine that has been
taken. Those classified long-acting will still be chasing around
the body, leading to sluggish limbs and a fat head. The reverse
is generally true of the short-acting drugs, although there are
several factors complicating this formula. Only with triazolam
(branded Halcion) are hangover effects believed relatively
unlikely.

Of all the benzodiazepines to hit the street it is diazepam

(Valium) that is the most desired because of its alleged superior euphoriant effects. It is reputed to be more rapidly absorbed than any of its equivalents, reaching its highest concentrations in the blood within about one hour, whereas other products can take three times as long. Diazepam users often go for the high by gulping down large quantities with a glass or two of booze. The alcohol substantially sharpens the effects (while also placing the recipient in more danger. Practically the only lethal benzodiazepine overdoses have also featured the simultaneous use of booze).

The Needle

Benzodiazepines – notably diazepam – are beginning to show up in injectable formats, ostensibly to treat acute anxiety, convulsions, and for premedication. Such formulations, however, can be both painful and dangerous due to the presence of a large amount of solvent. The solvent is included because diazepam, like most of its relatives, is impossible to dissolve in water. Possibly the least pleasant formulation is the standard Valium ampoule which contains some 65 per cent propylene glycol. When injected accidentally into an artery this can be extremely hazardous and in other places can lead to thrombosis of the vein in question. Far safer, according to the medical authors, Duquesne and Reeves,[1] is Diazemuls, which contains diazepam in an oil and water emulsion.

Health Impact

Most of the bad effects of benzodiazepines have been judged to be of a behavioural nature (i.e. relating to such things as upset sleep, panic attacks and aggravation of depressive or violent tendencies) but this could be because the drugs are comparatively under-researched in terms of what they might do to the body's physical fabric.

A recent World Health Organisation 'Update' on benzo-diazepines called them 'relatively safe compounds'. It noted that heart and respiratory depression occurred only in special circumstances (particularly when injected or taken with alcohol) and therefore serious injury was relatively rare as a consequence of overdose. It has been argued elsewhere however, that the drug is more dangerous when used by the very young, old and sick, and also by those persons, however healthy, who consume their pills along with any of the CNS depressants (barbiturates, methaqualone, opiates, major tranquillisers). These combinations have resulted in numerous deaths both accidental and suicidal.

Reproduction

Reports that benzopdiazepines increase the risk of babies being born malformed are, to use the words of WHO, 'not confirmed'. But babies are particularly sensitive to respiratory depression if the mother has had high doses immediately prior to delivery. The baby's immature liver may be unable to break it down, and cases have been reported where transfusions have been necessary to remove the drug.

With Other Conditions

Doctors warn against using benzodiazepines where there is severe kidney or liver disease, severe respiratory problems, or hardening of the arteries. Nitrazepam can be problematic where there is chronic obstructive lung disease, and for the elderly because it can encourage hypothermia.

With Other Drugs

Some doctors warn about using these drugs with alcohol, the tricyclic anti-depressants, thyroid hormone replacements and the anti-epileptic drug phenytoin.

Tolerance

Tolerance develops relatively easily to the anxiety-relieving properties of benzodiazepines, so the dose has to be steadily ncreased in order to maintain the desired effects. Without such an increase the pills become psychoactively useless within a few weeks. Even when the dose is repeatedly raised, a ceiling will be reached beyond which the body will not favourably respond. There is a high degree of cross tolerance between benzodiazepines and other CNS depressants. This means that to recover the old sensitivity to the tranks, all other depressants must be cut out of the diet for several weeks.

Dependence

While some British doctors still resist the idea that benzo-diazepines can produce physical dependence, the World Health Organisation believes such dependence has been clearly demonstrated in 'systematic human experiments'. The degree of dependence, as with all drugs, relates to how much is used and how often, together with the physical and mental make-up of the individual concerned. Some people can swallow low doses for many years and not become dependent. However, these will probably be in the minority. As WHO notes, even at therapeutic doses lasting a matter of months people are making themselves vulnerable. The surest sign of an individual who has become dependent is when the pain of withdrawal overcomes them when supplies are for some reason cut off.

The same symptoms – more or less – might also be experienced by long-term users who are still receiving the drug, but no longer in sufficient quantities to allay withdrawal in between doses. In effect, they are constantly coming off and going back on their drug. Many users endure this helter-skelter for years. Some add to the chaos by raising and lowering their dosage, or switching pills in an attempt to ride out the rough passage. Others achieve a dose that gives them an eerie equilibrium. They become emotionally cauterised; nothing especially interests them, neither their families nor themselves. Theirs becomes the classic drug-centred existence more typically identified with heroin junkies. This state could persist for years, even decades.

History

The great benzodiazepines glut dates back to 1960 when the Swiss multinational Hoffman-La Roche released Librium (chlordiazepoxide) on to the market following extensive testing on monkeys and human subjects. Three years later the same company issued, with a bellow of pride, the more powerful Valium (diazepam). The pair's advantages over barbiturates seemed obvious. They were safer, they went to work quicker and in a more precise way on the central nervous system, and best of all the margin between the therapeutic dose and the one that killed was almost incalculably large. As one wit put it: The only way to kill a lab animal with a benzodiazepine was to bury it in the stuff.[2]

Chlordiazepoxide and diazepam have continued to hold a position of primacy despite a market stampeded by other companies whose compounds tend to get progressively more expensive and redundant. Diazepam is the most successful of all. In fact there is no more widely prescribed psychotropic drug on earth. Such success didn't come to Roche from sheepish marketing methods. A former Roche world product manager, Stanley Adams, testifies to that fact in his recently published book,[3] *Roche Versus Adams*. He tells of practices that increasingly alarmed him and which eventually led to a painful and costly break from the company. And where Adams failed to crack what he considered to be unfair trading methods the British government had scarcely more success.

In 1973 the UK Monopolies Commission published a report[4] 'recommending' the company cut the price of Librium by 60 per cent and Valium by 75 per cent. It took this action after discovering a price policy – made possible by the company's dominant market position – that for some years had produced 'excessive profits on a very large scale'. Specifically it noted that Hoffman-La Roche in Basle, Switzerland, was charging the British associate company, Roche Products Ltd, £370 a kilo for the raw powder ingredients of Librium, when they could be bought in Italy for just £9 (in Italy there is no patent protection on medicines, and so no means of keeping prices high). The UK charge for Valium powder was £922 a kilo, as opposed to £20 in Italy. An inordinately large amount was also transferring to the Group operation to cover research and central administration costs. Thus, despite sales between 1966 and 1972 estimated by the Commission to have produced some £24 million profits for the Group, just £3 million was retained by the UK company, representing a substantial loss for the Inland Revenue. Adams, in his book, makes a more elaborate charge.

'If the Roche headquarters in Basle didn't want their subsidiaries to pay too much tax, then they certainly didn't want to pay too much themselves either. To this end, they had set up a company in Montevideo, Uruguay, called Roche International Ltd ('RIL').

'Montevideo is a tax haven and any profits made in Montevideo are untaxed. Roche had no manufacturing facilities in Montevideo, but customers became customers of RIL rather than of Roche, Basle. If the product concerned cost, for instance, £8 a kilo to make, and the world selling price was £20 a kilo, then the customer would pay the £20 to RIL, and if Roche Basle then invoiced RIL at £8.50 a kilo, just over the cost price, that meant that Basle would have made a profit of only £0.50 a kilo, while RIL made the main (*untaxable*) profit of £11.50. This system applied equally to all Roche subsidiaries.'[5]

The scrutiny of such arrangements was outside the brief of the UK Monopolies Commission, but it had seen enough to state that no future pricing policy which it could practically recommend 'could take full account of the excessive profits which have been made on [Librium and Valium] at the expense of the NHS . . .' It therefore called for a repayment in addition to the stringent price cuts. Roche made the cuts, but fought the compensation order, and in an out-of-court settlement reduced it from £12 million to £3.75 million. It was also permitted to once more stick up the prices of Librium and Valium as, in the next couple of years, they went out of patent. The first drug rose by 50 per cent, the second doubled.

By 1980 Roche still held the dominant share of the UK market, but they were no longer making the rest of the field blush with their prices. Whereas 100 capsules of 5 mg Valium cost £1.44 wholesale, 100 10 mg capsules of a similar long acting product called clobazam was being marketed b Hoechst for £5. The Hoechst item was branded Frisium, bu there were by now products with far more alluring names thar that from other companies: Nobrium, Tranxene, Anxon Serenid-D, Hypnovel, Valrelease, Tensium, Evacalm, as well as the hot-selling Ativan which was delivering a short-acting wallop at £1.85 per 100 1 mg capsules. All were more expensive than their barbiturate alternatives, and in some cases nearly three times as much. It is little wonder the manufacturers should argue that the case against benzodiaze-pines as addictive and toxic is not yet proven.

Patterns of Use

The original idea of tranquillisers was that they should be prescribed short-term to people in a stressed or grieving state. For the first few years this was how they were used. In the mid '60s some 58 per cent of prescriptions were for a single course only.[6] Yet only a decade later the position had reversed. Single-course prescriptions had dropped to 16 per cent while those for repeats had jumped to 64 per cent. By 1980 the Committee for the Review of Medicines began warning that there was no evidence that benzodiazepines were effective after continuous use of more than four months, and it also indicated a *possibility* of dependence. In the US the medical community was becoming altogether clearer about the hazards. From a mid-'70s peak of around 60 million prescriptions a year the total had dropped by 1980 to 34 million. In the UK, meanwhile, there was not simply a reluctance to acknowledge the dangers, but something of a backlash situation whereby concern over benzodiazepines was being ridiculed by some doctors as overheated and unscientific.

Of course the GP can always muster in his/her defence such factors as overcrowded surgeries, pressure from drug firms, the complexity of the modern pharmacopoeia, as well as pressure from the patient. Many on their books can only be

lacated by a bottle of pills, and feel they are being short-
hanged by their 'free' national health if they come away with
othing but good advice. But it is also true that most indi-
iduals who've been on benzodiazepines for any length of
me did not know the addiction hazards when they started,
ut simply fell into a state of dependency that their doctors
re now often loath to acknowledge.

There are several typical sets of circumstances that encour-
ge dependence on tranks. When they affect women they
1variably rest on prejudiced notions about the 'special re-
uirements' of the female gender. Women, as one drugs
gency points out, are far more likely to get boxed in when
eeking release from pressures that affect both sexes. Men
nder strain blow off heat down their local pub. This is
onsidered legitimate, even 'manly'. Women, by contrast, are
ncouraged to bottle up (literally) their emotions. Anger and
outs of waywardness simply don't fit with the traditional
oles carved out for women as passive nurturers (this is
hanging to some extent as old roles get chopped about and
oung women turn more to other drugs, as well as to 'male'
rimes such as violence and robbery). With no room to burn
ff her rage a woman starts burning up herself. The disease is
ubelled anxiety. The symptoms might be anything from
iarrhea to palpitations. On presenting these problems to the
iP, the medical solution proposed will be the reliable fire-
uenching tranks.

Once prescribed, a patient is not necessarily hooked.
*lenty abandon them again of their own volition. Nor is it
ypical for patients to go on blowing up the dose to extraordi-
ary amounts. When problems do occur they are likely to be
oticed when prescribed users decide to quit after a year or
wo of moderate-to-high consumption. Perhaps s/he has read
n anti-tranks article and suddenly resents the chemical
rutch. S/he'll go to the doctor and the doctor will probably go
long with the decision to quit by simply cutting off supply. A
weaty, heart-thumping bout of withdrawal follows whose
everity depends on the amount s/he's been taking, plus the
esponse to the symptoms as they arise. The next step,
ypically, is a return to the doctor, who will read the situation

as the old anxieties returning – the ones for which the trank
had been prescribed in the first place. So the message will be
s/he obviously needs the drugs – perhaps a bigger dose and a
change of brand. Maybe an anti-depressant too, or a barbiturate, or even a major anti-psychotic tranquilliser. When the
patient discovers s/he needs *more* not fewer drugs, confidence
will tend to drain away. Far from thinking about the next
attempt at quitting s/he's more likely to develop strategies for
ensuring a constant supply of the drugs s/he now knows to be
life-supporting.

I met seventeen people who'd gone through these hoops at
a November 1984 meeting of the self-help group called
Tranks. The meeting comprised nine men and eight women in
various states of pain and recovery. Among them there was a
young man who worked as a dance hall bouncer; a grey-faced,
middle-aged couple who came to Valium via a booze habit; a
grey-haired lady who looked like the sort they put on the front
of a cake-mix packet; a thin, blank-looking man alone at the
back reading the *Financial Times*; a young woman who in the
middle of describing her unhappiness became engulfed in
tears and had to be led upstairs; and a dapper business
executive who'd been using for twenty years and was there, he
said, not because they'd caused him problems – far from it, he
felt great – but because he'd heard about Tranks on the radio
and thought he might as well drop in. The idea of quitting
appealed to him.

'Do you get cold sweats?' a man asked a woman.

'No, I get hot flushes,' she answered to a peal of laughter.
Others got numb, wobbly mouths, or panic attacks, agora-
phobia, feelings of unreality, floors shifting beneath the feet
and weird noises and lights. Tips for recovery were exchanged: avoid substituting alcohol for tranks ('the booze is a
wet version of the pills') and remember recovery means
eating healthily, and keeping busy . . .

One of the women at the meeting spoke to me at length
about her experiences of tranquillisers. Her name is Anne;
her habit began 24 years ago when she was forty and suffering
the delayed effects of a broken marriage to a man who had
been a violent heavy drinker. There were three children from

he marriage – two were sent into care until they were
eenagers. The third was too young to survive away from
1ome, and so was returned to Anne to be raised in her little
cold-water flat now shared with a new husband. The pills
started after a panic attack on the way to work. She froze,
while her heart raced. A week later it happened again, so
she went to her doctor who gave her a prescription for
the anti-convulsant barbiturate, phenobarbitone. When this
didn't work he prescribed another barb – amylobarbitone,
plus the tranquilliser Librium.

'The Librium didn't actually help a lot,' says Anne,
'although the other one did give me a little confidence. . . .
By now I was getting afraid of everything. Afraid to get on a
bus. Afraid to go anywhere. I was taking two each of the
tablets every day and getting them on a repeat prescription.

It went on like this for ten years, taking one in the
morning as I woke up. There was this hollow feeling in my
stomach and a feeling that I couldn't face the day. Then by
lunchtime I was getting shaky again and I'd take another.
The next lot were taken before bed. Progressively things
got worse. I would get trembly and scared if ever I went out
without Sam [her husband] so that the best I could do alone
was some shopping close to home. This, in effect, made me
housebound; sitting about depressed and crying and just
sort of looking forward to Sam coming home. In 1970 we
moved, but things didn't really change, not at once. My
new doctor kept me on the same prescription until he
retired two years later. The new doctor saw what I was
taking and stopped me all at once. Well, I had terrible
withdrawal symptoms, waking up in a sweat, the shakes.
There was diarrhea and everything because, to be honest, I
was a junkie and I was without my tablets. I thought I was
going mad. I just walked around the house for three weeks
until I went to another doctor who said I should really have
been weened off. And she gave me some new ones. These
were one 15 mg Serenid-D for the morning and one anti-
depressant called Bolvidon, 30 mg, for the night. I still can't
go any distance on my own without getting attacks, but the

doctor says I should take deep breaths or, at the point I fee
an attack coming on, take another Serenid-D. The wors
time is in the early morning when Sam goes out to work.
feel a lot safer in the daylight and when I feel there i
someone I can turn to. But the doctor says I mustn't come
off the tablets because I've been on them so long now.
need them as a crutch. In any case they're much weake
than what I used to take.'

I met many other people who'd gone through similar experiences at this meeting. Except, unlike Anne, most were
committed to a pill-free future. It wasn't going to be easy.

Controls

While there is still great reluctance to recognise benzodiazepines as problem drugs, it's clear from prescription figures
that business has peaked in the UK. Doctors will argue that it
is their responsiveness to new scientific data that has caused
the halt in growth and what they don't require is more
fettering by outside agencies. The drug companies pitch a
similar line, but with more muscularity. The companies
plainly have a good deal less to fear than doctors since there
seems to be neither a domestic nor international authority
capable of fully checking them. Their performance in the
Third World has been particularly grotesque concerning the
shedding of irrelevant items on to nations too politically weak
to resist. Threats of cuts in investment and 'aid' have been
used against countries such as Bangladesh, and yet against the
odds that nation has persisted in its plan to phase out more
than a thousand unwanted items. Its Preferred Drugs List still
remains broadly intact and serves as an inspiration not just to
the poor nations of the Third World, but to the apparently
sophisticated West. Even the sluggardly UK has introduced a
preferred list, and while opponents read the move as yet
another Tory kick at the poor and the National Health
Service, it has to make sense to relieve the state of paying for
useless, sometimes dangerous items.

Benzodiazepines feature prominently in the Thatcher government's proposed weeding-out exercise. At the time of writing the intention was to supply through the National Health seven unbranded derivatives – oxazepam, chlordiazepoxide, triazolam, lorazepam, diazepam, nitrazepam and temazepam. Between them they cover the entire gamut of short, medium and long-acting preparations that have been issued for sedation and sleep.

All the usual delicious brand names will still be available if the scheme goes through, but not via the National Health. Thus comes the complaint of poor bashing. But a bigger complaint from people experienced in the trank addiction field is that the switch from brand names to unbranded (generic) equivalents will cause prolonged distress because of the difficulties in working out equivalent doses. Patients who are trying to reduce down to zero from a particular pill actually resort to shaving off slivers. This makes the reduction relatively painless and therefore less likely to result in relapse. The switch to generics will require some clear explanation from doctors. Better still, it requires a takeaway chart from the NHS.

Withdrawal

The withdrawal symptoms associated with a trank habit arrive at virtually any time after the last pill is taken, but generally start to roll in heavily within three to six days. Their intensity will relate to the magnitude of the habit (although some people suffer disproportionately) and their nature will be the direct reverse of the drug's advertised benefits. Thus, instead of tranquillity and/or sleep there is the prospect of one or more of the following: anxiety, panic attacks, palpitations, poor or nightmarish sleep, nausea, vomiting, visual distortions, weird noises, wobbly legs, wobbly ground, pins and needles, heightened sensitivity to light and sound, reduced coordination and – more rarely – convulsions and psychosis. The question as to how long they might last can't be accurately answered, since psychological problems are entwined with physical ones. Where there is an underlying emotional or practical problem this has to be identified and attempts made to sort it out, or else symptoms are likely to linger. The rough and ready formula which now seems to be emerging is that there will be one month's distress for every year of use. This doesn't mean the profound symptoms will last that long, but nor does it mean there will necessarily be steady improvement over this period.

While psychological factors do play an important part in the withdrawal process, the suggestion that the suffering is simply the old pre-drug anxieties resurfacing has been disproved. The same symptoms keep repeating themselves in different people and they show up in those who were prescribed benzodiazepines for reasons unconnected with their emotional state – i.e. for back pain. Nor can the symptoms be ascribed to 'fearing the worst' since they occur in people who quit naïvely, not knowing what to expect.

Tips

If you are using a short-acting benzodiazepine it will help to substitute a long-acting one before quitting as this is less traumatic to withdraw from.

Come off the drug slowly by reducing down over a period of weeks, even months. Once on the downcurve, avoid relapsing since the jerking up and down of the dose plays havoc with blood sugar levels, causing extra distress.

Watch consumption of alcohol (and other drugs too) both during and after withdrawal. It often goes up to compensate for the trank deprivation. (In fact, alcohol is frequently stepped up *prior* to withdrawal in order to juice up the drug's flagging effects.)

Keep occupied, even with mundane chores. Don't dwell too much on personal misery, and resist the desire to crawl back under the duvet. Exercise such as swimming helps. Yoga and other relaxation methods might also help once anxiety levels drop sufficiently to coordinate the body.

Eat well, not too much fat, sugar, salt – but allow yourself treats too.

Draw in family and friends to what you're going through so that they can begin to understand the process and adapt to the changing you.

Remember that it takes time. Try to dispense with guilt over your rate of progress.

Notes

1 T. Duquesne & J. Reeves, *A Handbook of Psychoactive Medicines*, Quartet, London, 1982, p. 456
2 Ibid, p. 275
3 S. Adams, *Roche Versus Adams*, Jonathan Cape, London, 1984
4 'Chlordiazepoxide and Diazepam', The Monopolies Commission, HMSO, London, 1973
5 S. Adams, *op. cit.*, p. 31
6 J. Melville, *The Tranquilliser Trap*, Fontana, London, 1984, p. 15

13 THE XANTHINES

Intro

Now IS the time to ask a question fundamental to this whole book: what actually constitutes a drug? The answer cannot be given in terms of certain types of substances which have 'x' effect – but the way in which a substance is used. The Fly Agaric mushroom with its brilliant red cap cannot realistically be described as a drug while growing in the November mist beneath a birch or a larch. It is a fungus with its own integrity. But once plucked from the ground, taken home and infused in salt water, the resulting broth can rightly be called a drug because when consumed it will effect a psychoactive change in the consumer. The same goes for the *Cannabis sativa* plant. This can be converted into rope or bird seed, but it is only when the resin is isolated and consumed for its mind-altering effects that the plant is truly in a drug state.

The caffeine phenomenon is more subtle. Caffeine is one of a family of chemical compounds that stimulate the central nervous system, increase the flow of urine and get the stomach churning, so accelerating digestion. While capable of being manufactured in a laboratory (it looks like baking powder) this is an expensive method. Of the sixty-odd plant species naturally containing the drug, the most commercially attractive concentrations show up in the pit of the greeny-brown fruit of the Arabian coffee shrub (*Coffea arabica*). Other important sources are the commercial tea plant (*Camellia sinensis*), cocoa beans, kola nuts and South American maté leaves – from which tea is made. Most of these species additionally contain one or other of two stimulant drugs closely related to caffeine, and these also show up in a variety of common products: tea, cocoa, chocolate and soft drinks. Caffeine's relatives are known as theophylline and theobromine. All three are generally classed as xanthines, signifying that they are methylated versions of the chemical xanthine. The most powerful of the three in terms of stimulating the CNS is caffeine. Theophylline rates second. Theobromine is virtually inactive. On the other hand, theobromine is better able to stimulate the heart and is more effective at increasing urine production. Given that each of them turns up in such a diverse range of consumer products the question arises as to whether the products themselves are to be counted as drugs, and the answer surely has to be that it depends – depends on the quantity, frequency and manner in which the products are consumed. A pot of mocha at the end of a meal among friends can't rightly be compared in drug terms with the imbibing habits of some early morning coffee drinkers, because without their several cups, they are paralysed. Tea is often considered a more timid beverage than its xanthine-rich relative, coffee. But this isn't so. An average cup of tea contains something approaching the amount of caffeine in a cup of instant coffee (some argue it has more) as well as small amounts of theophylline and theobromine. Thus, someone disposing of four cups before catching the morning train could be said to have a relationship with the beverage that is principally to do with digging for its stimulants. Similarly there is a syndrome turning up in the US labelled 'colaholism' whereby people (usually young) are guzzling ten or more cans a day and reporting sleep problems and jitteriness. New York is a particular hot bed of the cola vice.

Nonetheless, when we look at the way the xanthines have been used by our society, comparing the great quantities consumed with the amount of social and physical damage that has resulted, then we could conclude it might have been a good deal worse. Unlike most other drugs looked at in this book they have provoked no great political tumult, at least not in modern times. They have caused no palpable physical harm on anything approaching the scale of tobacco or alcohol. There *is* an amount of mental harm flowing from them – but this is of a comparatively slight nature.

What Is It?

Caffeine is a white crystalline powder that could have devastating effects if taken in its pure state in sufficient quantities, but it is rarely seen as such. The fact that it is invariably buried in among a mass of other ingredients is the secret of its success. Like the other xanthines it is everywhere and yet we barely see it. We even deny that xanthine consumption amounts to drugtaking. Do they actually move us? Perhaps their effects, for most people, are marginal. But then it could be argued that our whole xanthine-drenched world is suffering the clinically defined symptoms of xanthine poisoning – over-stimulation, anxiety, excitement, abnormally increased sensitivity . . .

The Xanthines in Nature

Here, at a glance are the xanthines as they appear in nature and on the supermarket shelves.

Genus, Species	Active Principle	Used to make
Coffea arabica	caffeine	Arabian coffee
Coffea liberica	caffeine	Liberian coffee
Coffea robusta	caffeine	Congo coffee
Camellia sinensis	caffeine, theophylline	tea
Theobroma cacao	caffeine, theobromine	chocolate, cocoa
Cola acuminata	caffeine, theobromine	soft drinks
Ilex paraguariensis	caffeine	maté

Caffeine is also included in various stimulants, painkillers and cold cures, some available across the counter, some prescription only.

Quantities Present

There seems to be no reliable breakdown on the presence of theobromine and theophylline in the various beverages and confections, and quite often the term 'caffeine' will be applied to xanthines in general. So we too must generalise and use the term 'caffeine' when perhaps other substances are present. The following data on 'caffeine content' has been assembled from several sources.

brewed coffee	115 mg per cup via the drip method, 80 mg per cup when percolated
instant coffee	65 mg per cup
decaffeinated coffee	2–4 mg per cup
tea, bagged	65 mg per cup when brewed for 3 or 4 minutes
loose tea	up to 100 mg per cup
typical chocolate bar	25 mg
canned or bottled, drink	40 mg
standard stimulant tablet	200 mg

Sensations

Pure powdered caffeine has an excitory effect similar to cocaine and amphetamine and can sometimes be passed off as such. Moderate use – up to about four consecutive cups of coffee – combats drowsiness and tiredness and helps with both physical and mental performance. Larger doses start working on the lower parts of the brainstem and spinal column, affecting physical coordination, and giving rise to jittery, anxious feelings. As with cocaine and amphetamine, the more that is consumed the more likely it is that these ill feelings will be intensified, producing the possibility of tremors and the experiencing of odd noises and flashes of light. Any dose can affect sleep, and with any dose there will be a physical and mental comedown roughly commensurate with the preceding high. This is why it is inadvisable to drink a lot of coffee or tea at the beginning of a long nighttime drive, and then nothing during the course of the journey. The effect of the initial dose is to plunder the body of its reserves, inviting drowsiness and poor coordination long before they would have been 'organically' due. It is far better to pace consumption, allowing the body to deal with a dose of caffeine before loading in more.

Medical Effects

Toxicity

Deaths from overdoses of caffeine are sometimes reported, and experts have settled on the figure of 10 grammes as the kind of amount likely to lead to fatal convulsions and respiratory failure: 10 grammes is about 100 cups of coffee. The lowest reported lethal dose[1] is 3,200 mg administered intravenously. Children, as always, are vulnerable at lower doses. Stewed tea also brings with it particular dangers due, it's believed, to the high yield of tannic acid. In what is perhaps an apocryphal story, this acid in tea was said to have been the cause of death in a group of labourers who drank from a pot constantly on the brew.[2]

Long-Term Use

Daily use of moderate amounts in healthy adults is generally not considered damaging. But above six or eight cups of coffee (600 mg) a range of insidious effects can take hold – insidious because they are often regarded as normal symptoms of stress for which another cup would be the appropriate treatment. These include upset sleep, depression, anxiety and irritability, malfunctioning bowels and fast, irregular heartbeat.

Internally, what seems to be happening is that a dose of caffeine is instructing the adrenal glands to release energy-giving glucose into the bloodstream as though for a fight-or-flight emergency. When this doesn't occur, rather than having the surplus sugar hang around the blood, glands in the pancreas issue insulin to prompt its uptake into the body cells. The repetition of this routine can, it is believed, lead to insulin over-reaction, causing blood sugar levels to drop too far. This leads to tiredness and the other symptoms described above.

More disturbing findings arose from a study among coffee drinkers in the Boston area undertaken by Harvard University.[3] This has linked coffee drinking to pancreatic cancer – the fourth most common type in the US. The researchers found that the risk of contracting this cancer was doubled in those who consumed as little as two cups a day. They were unable to state, however, that the coffee itself was the causal factor, merely that those who drunk it were at higher risk. (The risk could have been due to another habit prevalent among coffee drinkers, or to the strange modern 'creamers' and sugar products used in their beverage.) The Harvard study has in any case been criticised for concentrating on hospital patients since such people are necessarily unhealthy.

Even less persuasive data links coffee with cancer of the bladder and with blockages of blood supply to the heart.

Data on the potential physical harm of tea and soft drinks is not so forthcoming. But a windfall of research grants could possibly rectify the situation.

Pregnancy

In November 1980 the US Food and Drugs Administration (FDA) recommended that pregnant women should avoid or limit their consumption of caffeine in food and drink after it was found to have caused 'structural abnormalities' in the litters of rats. However, since these abnormalities didn't start showing up until the parent rodents were force-fed a daily dose equivalent to 30 cups of strong coffee, there has been no human panic either Stateside or in the UK – although the rat world can't be happily anticipating more such experiments.

The FDA findings were in any case overtaken by a January 1983 report,[4] which, resting on the analysis of more than 12,000 women, found no 'excess malformations' among coffee drinkers. Nor was there any impact on the birthweight or the length of the pregnancy. In short, 'coffee consumption had a minimal effect, if any, on the outcome of pregnancy.'

With Other Conditions

Since caffeine activates the acids in the stomach it is as well for people with peptic ulcers not to use it excessively. Because it can effect heart rhythm and blood pressure, people suffering hypertension should show caution.

With Other Drugs

The xanthines react badly to the prescription drugs known as monoamine oxidase inhibitors. There are potentially dangerous side effects. See pages 84–5.

Tolerance

Tolerance describes the way in which the body becomes resistant to a drug's effects and therefore requires increasingly large doses to achieve the desired psychoactive changes – that is, until a ceiling is reached beyond which no amount of drug will achieve success, and will more likely act as a poison. There seems to be some slight tolerance towards the stimulant effects of caffeine, although for many people one daily cup of coffee, particularly in the morning, will go on jolting them awake for years. Quite likely a lot of this thrust from a minimal dose is allied to expectation: the signal of aroma, steam and so forth. But by whatever device, the body is able to remain responsive to the effects fo the same unaltered dose.

Dependence

The caffeine habit is not readily acknowledged because it is concealed in the entirely acceptable routine of swallowing cup after cup of the hot or cold brew. Not that dependence refers imply to something done every day – rather to feelings of physical and mental torment that habitual use can lead to. Caffeine is capable of generating a host of such feelings with regular use of about half a dozen cups of tea or coffee a day, and so can be rightly described as a drug of dependence. Typical symptoms of excess use are anxiety, moodiness, headaches, muscle twitches and chronically disturbed sleep. All will clear up once caffeine intake is reduced.

Chocolate encourages a particularly powerful dependence in some people, but this is likely to do with factors other than its comparatively modest xanthine content. Apart from being outstandingly palatable, chocolate is the classic binge food and is invested with connotations of guilty excess. As noted earlier, xanthine-laced soft drinks (Pepsi, Coca Cola, Seven Up, etc.) can also lead to habitual use – 'Coke, after Coke, after Coke . . .' in the words of the US ad campaign. But again, isolating caffeine as the vital draw might be wide of the mark. The impact of chocolate and soft drinks on the user's health has little to do with their xanthine content, and much more to do with the sugar and synthetic additives contained in them.

Earliest Use

Chocolate

The cultivation of the cacao tree (*Theobroma cacao*) for chocolate goes back 3,000 years or more, but is first reliably noted in the realm of the Aztec emperor Montezuma, who, it was believed, guzzled some fifty cups of xocoatl a day. This xocoatl was a hot beverage, not unlike our own unassuming cocoa, but instead of milk and sugar the beverage was laced with pepper. And instead of sending the Aztecs to sleep it aroused their sex drive. The occupying Catholic church didn't approve.

Peppered xocoatl wasn't a tremendous hit in Europe, but with the addition of sugar and milk its fate across the globe was soon sealed. A clue to chocolate's notable lineage is

contained in the name of the tree that it is derived from -
Theobroma. It is a word coined by the eighteenth-century
Swedish botanist, Linnaeus, and means 'food of the
gods'.

Coffee

Coffee is a far more recent concoction than chocolate and,
according to a Persian saga, one of the many miraculous
bequests of Mohammed (570?–632). Once, when the Prophet
of Islam was suffering from a sleepiness verging on stupor,
the Almighty is reported to have commanded the prophet
Gabriel to appear with a deep back beverage – as black as the
celestial Black Stone of the Kaa'ba, that is the holiest object
in all Mecca. The name of this beverage was Kahwa or
Kahveh, and it came from the pit of the fruit borne by the tree
botanists now call *Coffea arabica*. Mohammed was clearly
refreshed by the black drink, for not only was he able to go out
and defeat a host of Arabian enemies, he also set in motion
the Islamic revolution that proved so bothersome to European Christendom. One of the Prophet's strictures, as con-
veyed through a chapter in the Koran called The Table, is that
wine is an evil, not to be touched. It had been the lubricant of
classical culture, an agent of unconsciousness and darkness.
Coffee, by contrast, was the great stimulator that stole wakefulness from sleep, encouraging sharp, disputatious reason
that is the hallmark of traditional Islamic culture with its
geometric   architecture   and   ultra-correct   procedures.
Heinrich Jacob, in his 1935 book, *The Saga of Coffee*,[5]
suggests that there might have been no Moslem civilisation or
the later Empire without the special fuel of coffee.

Jacob reports the Arabs originally got the brew from
Abyssinia and Somaliland. It was shipped over the desert by
camel caravan, then across the Red Sea and on to a further
long land journey. This made it a commodity strictly for the
wealthy who drunk it not as a beverage, but medicinally –
probably for migraine since caffeine constricts the blood
vessels around the brain, causing the pounding to ease.

Once local varieties began getting cultivated prices fell, but consumption didn't increase noticeably until a prohibitionist movement got underway in the Holy City of Mecca. Like the furore that occurred 200 hundred years later around the London coffee houses, the movement was politically based. It was inspired by the appointment in 1551 of a new ruler of Mecca, who took exception to some local coffee-drinking satirists who were making him the butt of their lampoons. The appointee of the Sultan declared a ban on the all-night establishments in which the beverage was drunk, complaining that the din from them 'wounded the night'. The ban caused a riot which was used as an excuse to outlaw coffee itself. Those who persisted in drinking it, says Jacob, were 'bound face to tail on the backs of asses and driven through the town, being flogged the while'. But the appointee was let down in his grand prohibitory moves by the Sultan. There was nothing in the Koran, the sovereign ruled, forbidding the use of coffee. And, besides, how could he and his courtiers manage without it?

Coffee moved swiftly throughout the whole of the Islamic world, then into Christian territories where it became entangled in something of a theosophic contest with wine. Italian churchmen at first condemned the black beverage as an infidel drink, but it was 'Christianised' by Pope Clement VIII and by the mid-seventeenth century had reached most of Europe.

It was introduced to the UK initially as a medicine. Then, with great suddenness, it became the great rage between the years 1680 and 1730. London became filled with coffee houses and the capital consumed more of the beverage than any other city in the world. Jacob suggests it was a kind of massive sobering-up exercise after a long spell of morbid insobriety that began after the Civil War. He argues that it reshaped the native literature and political consciousness, as individuals of discrimination filled the new houses for late-night verbal jousts. The houses became famous as literary resorts, with men such as Sheridan, Dryden, Swift and Hogarth among the aficionados. But in their earliest days they also enjoyed a spell as places of robust political intercourse – places to campaign, recruit and speechify. This ended when the authorities posted a notice ordering the closure of all the capital's coffee establishments 'because in them harm has been done to the King' majesty and to the realm by spreading of malicious and shameful reports.' The powerful brewers had also been complaining of lost business and women's groups were protesting that family life was suffering thanks to the interminable tongue-flapping that the new inns encouraged.

A 'compromise' – suitable to the Crown – was extracted. The houses could reopen, but only if the proprietors forbade the sale of all books, pamphlets and leaflets, as well as political oratory. Nothwithstanding the Crown's efforts, the coffee house fad ended as quickly as it started. Largely it was a matter of commerce. The drive into India was underway in the early eighteenth century. The British were now landlords of a tea-bearing country.

Tea

Tea has a legend that compares very nicely with the discovery of coffee by a sleepy Mohammed. It concerns an apostle called Dharma, the Buddhist son of an Indian monarch. He is said to have travelled to China where he lived the life of an ascetic, vowing never to sleep so that his body might remain in perpetual communion with God. But he did sleep, to his chagrin, and on wakening ripped off his unfaithful eyelids and flung them to the ground.

The next day he noticed that these eyelid skins had struck roots, and from the roots a tea plant (*Thea sinensis*) had sprouted. He took two of its leaves, laid them on his eyes, and according to the legend, two new lids grew. Then he chewed some more leaves which, as Jacob reports, 'immediately gave him a feeling of enhanced liveliness, which passed into tranquil cheerfulness and firm determination.' This seems a perfect description of a cup of 'char' when doing its best. The Chinese were using tea as a substitute for strong drink from as early as the third century AD, and 500 years later it was being harvested commercially. The Dutch East India Company were the first to import it into Europe in around 1600, and England got hers about sixty years later, with the import monopoly being held by the British East India Company until 1834.

British readers need no special instruction on how popular the beverage has become in these isles, but we are not the most voracious guzzlers on earth. That distinction goes to the 100,000 inhabitants of Qatar in the Arabian Gulf, who on average each drink twice our daily four-and-a-bit cups, an amount clocking up the equivalent of 665 mg of caffeine each day.

Decaffeinated Coffee

Caffeine was first extracted from coffee by a German chemist, Ferdinand Runge. The year was 1820, and Runge had apparently obtained his boxful of beans from the poet/dramatist Goethe who, being a wine man, used to publicly assail the coffee beverage. Runge's work meant the drug was now available in high street apothecaries. But it also brought an awareness of just how potent an experience heavy consumption of coffee was liable to be. A clamour grew about the possible deleterious effects. There were condemnations – now extremely familiar – of the speeding-up of modern life in which coffee was said to be a keen accomplice. A breakthrough was needed. It came from a young German-based merchant called Ludwig Roselius, whose own father was a coffee taster and had died from what Ludwig believed to be coffee poisoning (modern tasters spit out their samples).

Roselius' feat, following on from Runge, was to extract the caffeine, or at least the greater proportion of it, while retaining the essential flavour and aroma. This was done by exposing the raw beans first to steam treatment, then to a wash in solvents that worked only upon the caffeine. The resulting product was well received throughout Europe, although whether Roselius's customers were better off with the caffeine intact or the solvent-streaked alternative is debatable. Decaffeinated brands caused worry a few years ago in the US when it was learned that the chemical solvent employed – trichlorethylene (also found in cleaning agents) was a suspected cancer-forming agent. Soon it was banned.

British decaffeinated brands do not use trichlorethylene but they do use other solvents such as methylene chloride ethyl acetate and dichloromethane. As in the Roseliu method, the unroasted bean is fattened with steam, solvent: are flushed through, taking the caffeine with them, and ther washed or steam-flushed to remove any remaining chemical G. R. Lane and the Nestlé Company, who both use thi: method, report[6] that it eliminates all but about five parts pe: million of the solvent. By the time the pit is roasted, dried anc ground, they say, there is 'no trace' remaining.

Consumption Rates

Some 120,000 tonnes of caffeine are consumed worldwide each year (there seem to be no such sums done for theophylline and theobromine) which averages out to the equivalent per day of half a cup of instant coffee for everyone on the planet. We British drink twice that per capita. All told, our caffeine consumption adds up to 6,500 tonnes per year which, when spread evenly throughout the population, is double that which the Americans are consuming. Indeed since 1960, the US has seen a net decline in caffeine use of about 20 per cent. Their coffee consumption is down 36 per cent, tea is up 33 per cent, but soft drinks . . . these have risen by a massive 231 per cent.[7] Most of the soft drink increase seems to be accounted for by the young, while it is the elderly who are showing most fidelity to coffee. We can see then that the xanthines are everywhere, even though we continue to deny that their consumption amounts to drug-taking.

Notes

1 Cox *et al.*, *Drugs and Drug Abuse*, Addiction Research Foundation, Toronto, Canada, 1983, p. 209
2 'What's Wrong with Tea and Coffee' *Here's Health*, December 1981

3 Ibid
4 S. Linn *et al.*, 'No Association Between Coffee Consumption and Adverse Effects in Pregnancy', *New England Journal of Medicine*, January 1982
5 H. Jacob, *The Saga of Coffee*, Unwin Ltd, London, 1935
6 'What's Wrong with Tea and Coffee', *op. cit.*
7 Ibid

APPENDIX I
DRUGS AND THE LAW

Misuse of Drugs Act

THE MISUSE of Drugs Act 1971 is the instrument by which the state prosecutes individuals for possession, supply or manufacture of 'controlled' substances. Consolidating numerous bits of legislation dating back to 1908, the MDA divides the substances into three categories of seriousness and awards penalties accordingly. It does not deal with those most ubiquitous of all recreational drugs – alcohol, tobacco and caffeine, nor does it incorporate amyl and butyl nitrite and, until Januay 1985, also excluded barbiturates.

Class A

The materials drawing the most severe penalties are called Class A drugs. These include: cannabinol (except where contained in cannabis or cannabis resin), coca leaf, cocaine, dextromoramide (e.g. the product Palfium), diamorphine (heroin), dipipanone (Diconal), fentanyl and its derivatives, LSD, mescaline, methadone (Physeptone), morphine, opium, pethidine (Pamergan) and its derivatives, phencyclidine (PCP), poppy straw and concentrate of poppy straw (poppy straw means all parts except the seeds of the opium poppy after mowing. The advice agency Release notes that it is not an offence to possess, supply or produce a poppy straw, but it is one to smoke it. Concentrate of poppy straw means the material produced when the straw's alkaloids are concentrated. Possession, supply and production of this material *is* an offence,) psilocin (as found in 'magic mushrooms'), n,n-dimethyltryptamine (DMT).

Class B

Class B drugs draw mid-range penalties. They include: amphetamine, barbiturates (e.g. Tuinal, Nembutal, Seconal, Soneryl, Amytal), cannabis and cannabis resin, codeine, dexamphetamine, dihydrocodeine (DF-118), methaqualone, methylamphetamine, methylphenidate (Ritalin), phenmetazine (Filon, Preludin).

Class C

Least severe category is Class C, which includes: Benzodiazepine tranquillisers, dextropropoxyphene (Distalgesic, Doloxene) plus other mild amphetamine-type stimulants.

Schedules

The MDA regulations divide controlled drugs into five 'schedules', relating to the handling of the substances by trade and professional people. Drugs in Schedule 1 (such as LSD and cannabis) are the most stringently controlled in that they can only be supplied, possessed or administered in accordance with a Home Office licence. They are not for medical prescription but more usually for research. Schedule 5 preparations are the most casually controlled. These are various dilute, small-dose, non-injectable products that can be sold without prescription over a chemist's counter and all can be possessed with impunity. Technically, once bought, they cannot be supplied to someone else: an injunction that's rarely enforced. The products include cough medicines, anti-diarrhoea agents and mild painkillers. In between come schedules 2 to 4, which cover the majority of controlled drugs. They are available for medical use but must generally be supplied or administered in accordance with a prescription. The exceptions are the benzodiazepine tranquillisers, in schedule 4, which can be legally possessed without a doctor's authority so long as they are in the form of a medicinal product.

An offence is committed if a prescribed person passes on a

part of the prescription to somebody else. The recipient
ironically, would be in the clear since s/he is merely in
possession. The supplier, even if no money changed hands
would be liable to a trafficking prosecution, carrying a
possible five year prison term.

Offences

There are numerous charges brought under the various sections of the MDA, from simple possession to complex issues
like 'assisting in the commission of an offence outside the
UK.' The sentences available to the courts run from a modest
fine to life imprisonment. In summary, with their maximum
penalties indicated, the major offences are as follows.

Possession

The vast majority of offences are for possession, and the great
majority of those relate to cannabis. 'Possession' means the
smallest measurable trace, whether or not it is sufficient to
cause a whisper of intoxication. In each case of alleged
possession the prosecution must prove three major points –
that the substance was in the defendant's possession or control (a verbal admission of past possession is sufficient if
made in front of a police officer); that it is a controlled drug;
and that the defendant knew s/he possessed the drug. If the
evidence for possession results from a blood or urine test, this
alone does not constitute possession. It is also possible for a
defendant to get an acquittal when the drug is found in a
container and where s/he can satisfy the court that s/he neither
knew nor suspected what its contents were. This is difficult.
There are other factors complicating the possession issue,
such as: 'I had just taken it off another person and was on my
way to the police to hand it in.' This would constitute a proper
defence. The advice agency Release have produced an excellent brochure called *Drugs and The Law*, which gives more
clarification. Release themselves can fill in the remaining
blanks.

Sentencing: possession charges can be brought in either magistrates or crown court with far more severe penalties available to the latter authority. In reality the penalties fetched in are considerably less than the maximum available – unless, that is, the person has a history of serious offences, or the current charge involves a large quantity. There is also a great deal of regional variation. In the inner cities, for instance, a fine of about £25 will be usual for a small amount of cannabis, whereas in the Isle of Man and the Channel Islands, first-time possessors of one joint face imprisonment. Laxest of all are rural areas like Northumberland and North Wales where first-time offenders might be dismissed with a caution.

Then again, each type of drug will draw a different judicial response. Cannabis fetches its comparatively mild reaction because it is considered a 'fun' drug without being unduly decadent. Amphetamine and LSD are seen as somewhat degenerate substances. Cocaine has something of the same decadent connotations, but as a 'narcotic' – so called – it is also considered a suitable case for treatment. This treatment reflex also applies to heroin. Anyone found in possession will likely be directed to a probation officer and/or the medical trade. The tendency in the last couple of years has been for the police to press for trafficking prosecutions, even where comparatively small amounts of drugs are involved.

The maximum penalties available to the courts for simple possession are: for Class A drugs dealt with in a magistrate's court – six months, £2,000 fine or both. Cases heard in crown court – seven years, unlimited fine or both. Class B drugs – three months, £500 fine or both (magistrates); five years, unlimited fine or both (crown). Class C – three months, £200 or both (magistrates); two years, unlimited fine or both (crown).

Possession with Intent to Supply

The amount in question is not relevant and it is possible that a small gift to a friend will render a person liable to this charge. Equally, a large amount for personal use might well be construed as proof of intent to supply.

Offering to Supply a Controlled Drug

The offence is complete once an offer is made, whether or no
it is accepted. The prosecution can even succeed if th
material turns out not to be a controlled drug (e.g. an attemp
by person A to 'burn' person B).

Supplying/Producing a Controlled Drug

If one person buys on behalf of a group then this amounts tc
supplying. Cultivation of cannabis rates as production.

Maximum penalties for the above three 'supplying' offences
are: for Class A or B drugs dealt with in a Magistrates court –
six months, £2,000 fine or both. For Class C before Magistrates – three months, £500 fine or both. For Class A drugs
before a Crown Court – life, unlimited fine or both. Class B –
14 years, unlimited fine or both. Class C – five years,
unlimited fine or both.

Import/Export of a Controlled Drug

Maximum penalties: for Class A or B, three times the value of
the goods or £2,000, whichever is the greater; six months
prison or both (magistrates); unlimited fine, life or both
(crown). For Class C – three times the value of the goods or
£500, three months or both (magistrates); unlimited fine, five
years or both (crown).

Assisting in the Commission of an Offence
Outside the UK

A 1975 case illustrated that this charge could be brought
where two people took some speaker cabinets to another
country knowing they would later be used by someone else to
carry cannabis to a third country.

Maximum penalties: for all three classes – six months,
£2,000 or both (magistrates); life, unlimited fine or both
(crown).

Opium Offences

This is a residue from the turn-of-the-century paranoia over Chinese opium smokers. Coming in addition to the other offences applicable to opium as a controlled drug, the prosecution merely has to prove that the defendant smoked opium, frequented a place used for opium smoking or that s/he possessed pipes or other gadgetry used for smoking. The defence can argue that s/he never knew or bothered to find out the place visited was a 'den', but turning a blind eye isn't good enough. Note the stiff crown court sentences as compared with those for possession of other Class A drugs.

Maximum penalties: six months, £2,000 or both (magistrates); 14 years, unlimited fine or both (crown).

Allowing Premises to be Used

This could apply to the occupier or anyone concerned in the management of a private address, squat, pub, club, student hostel, etc. The prosecution must prove the defendant knowingly permitted or suffered production, supply, or the smoking of cannabis or opium (these giving off a detectable odour).

Maximum penalties: for class A and B – six months, £2,000 or both (magistrates); 14 years, unlimited fine or both (crown). For class C – three months, £500 or both (magistrates); five years, unlimited fine or both (crown).

Obstruction

It is an offence to intentionally obstruct a police officer searching for drugs by swallowing or concealing them, or by concealing or failing to produce documents when asked, unless there is a reasonable excuse. But the police must show in court that the obstruction happened after the person learned the search was conducted under the MDA. In other words, a pill swallowed before the police announced they are doing an MDA search is not obstruction.

Maximum penalties: for all classes – six months, £2,000 or both (magistrates); two years, unlimited fine or both (crown).

Incitement, Conspiracy or Attempt to Commit an MDA Offence

In any of these three categories no offence need have bee:
completed. For the first it simply has to be proved tha
persuasion or pressure was brought to bear. For conspirac:
there merely has to be evidence of an agreement with one o
more other persons; while for the third there has only to be th:
intention to commit an offence.

Maximum penalties: the same as those for the offence t:
which the incitement, conspiracy or attempt charge relates.

The Law and Needle Swap Schemes

Drug users turning in syringes containing traces of controlled
drugs at syringe swap schemes are technically liable to prosecution for possession – the traces possibly being used as
evidence of prior possession of the drug. Prosecution is
considered unlikely but not impossible. Those people running
the schemes – particularly government sanctioned projects –
are assumed to be safe.

Drug Trafficking Offences Act

Introduced in January 1987, its declared object is to prevent
major league traffickers from retaining their proceeds after
being apprehended. In this respect, it provides new powers
for tracing, freezing and then confiscating assets presumed to
be drug related. In the run-up to an arrest, bank managers,
solicitors, accountants etc. can be called upon to break their
tradition of confidentiality and provide details of a customer's
transactions. Once charged a defendant can be restrained
from dealing with his/her property. Before sentencing, the
court determines whether the accused has benefited from
drug dealing in any way. That decision will generally rest on
a written statement supplied by detectives (a feature that
especially worries the legal advice agency, Release, which
regards such police evidence as invariably 'unreliable and

ll-informed'). If profit is assumed to have been made then the court makes a confiscation order assessed as being equal to the proceeds from the defendant's entire trafficking career. This could include all the trafficker's current property and everything owned in the previous six years.

The onus is on the defendant to show such items are not from the proceeds of drug sales. A receiver may be appointed to recover the property confiscated and the act provides for lengthy periods of imprisonment for non-payment. The Act includes two other new imprisonable offences: one is for 'laundering', aimed at persons who facilitate another's 'retention, control or investment' of proceeds. The other prohibits a person making any disclosure likely to prejudice an investigation. In both instances the burden of proof is on the defendant to establish their innocence. The editors of the *Criminal Law Review* have criticised the legislation for reversing three 'supposed principles' of English criminal justice: the presumption of innocence until guilt is proven; the principal requiring criminal intent or knowledge of wrongdoing before conviction for a serious offence, and the principle that offenders should be dealt with only for offences before the court.

Cocaine Kits

An additional offence under the Drug Trafficking Offences Act is the selling of cocaine kits and other drug paraphernalia, such as hash pipes and hookahs. Maximum sentence is six months imprisonment. However, because such items have other uses – e.g. ornamental – and because a drug like cocaine is often ingested using ordinary household items such as a razor blade, and mirror, the Crown will have difficulty in successfully prosecuting cases. A shop advertising 'coke kits for sale' would be a strong candidate for court action.

Intoxicating Substances (Supply) Act 1985

Effective from August 1985, it prohibits the supply of solvents or other substances (e.g. glues, typewriter correction fluid) to people under 18 years of age if there is reasonable cause to believe the substances or their fumes will be inhaled to cause intoxication. The actual inhaling or sniffing of solvents is no illegal.

Stop, Search and Arrest

Under the MDA the police have powers to stop, search and detain a person where there is 'reasonable suspicion' of possession of a controlled drug. They can also search a vehicle or vessel, but need a search warrant specifying the suspect's name and address to raid a home – unless they see an offence being committed (e.g. a cannabis plant in a window box or a joint being smoked). Warrants are valid for one month only, but during this time they can drop in as often as they choose and take whatever they think might serve as evidence of an MDA offence, of anything they think indicates any other crime. They may also search anyone on the premises concerned even though they occupy a separate apartment.

The Police and Criminal Evidence Act (PACE) considerably extends police powers to enter and search. They may now call in without a warrant to arrest a named person and can also stop people in the vicinity of a 'serious arrestable offence' and set up road blocks to undertake searches in areas judged by themselves to justify such action.

Detention and Questioning

The advice agency Release warns that the complexities of the drug laws are such that even a relatively innocent statement such as: 'I smoke cannabis sometimes, who doesn't?' can present quite serious problems. Once arrested, they report, you are under no obligation to say anything or to make a statement, and you should resist pressure to offer information about other drug users. You should immediately demand to see a solicitor and not sign the custody sheet waiving that right. Everything said can be used as evidence against you,

rom the moment you first meet up with the police – even
before being formally cautioned. Once charged you have the
right to inform someone of the arrest, unless the police want
to invoke the Police and Criminal Evidence Act, arguing that
you are being held in connection with a 'serious arrestable
offence'. Drug trafficking constitutes such an offence. If
access to a solicitor or relatives is delayed you can ask why and
have the reason recorded on your custody sheet. Release
advise that notes be kept throughout, since these can be used
as evidence on your behalf. If you are held in connection with
a 'serious' offence, you are entitled to access to a solicitor
after 36 hours, although a magistrate may order your continued detention for up to 96 hours. Then you have the right
to be released if not charged.

If you are not suspected of a 'serious' offence you must be
released or charged within 24 hours of detention. Under
PACE it is the duty of police officers to provide a doctor for a
suspect if they 'know or suspect' that the suspect is dependent
on drugs.

Notification

Only doctors with a special Home Office licence can issue
opiates, opioids and cocaine for reasons other than to relieve
pain caused by illness. Where prescriptions are issued to
dependent individuals, that doctor must notify the Home
Office which then adds the name to its central register. In 1986
the Home Office had 8,445 individuals logged as current
addicts – a 27 per cent jump on the previous year. The true
number – most of them depending on imported street heroin –
is believed to be closer to 85,000. Even if the doctor refuses to
take on as a patient a person who shows signs of dependency
and even if s/he refuses to give a one-off prescription, s/he
must still notify the Home Office or risk coming before a
tribunal. The information the Home Office receives includes:
name, address, date of birth, NHS number and 'name of
drugs to which the person is addicted.' With such data maintained centrally on computer the physician need only phone

up the Home Office to check whether the person before
him/her is already logged and receiving scripts from someone
else.

In addition to these checks, the police regularly look into
double scripting and over-generous prescribing by calling in
on chemists and examining what's being prescribed to whom
and by which doctor.

Medicines Act 1968

The other important piece of legislation is the Medicines Act.
This directs itself to all retail and wholesale dealings in
therapeutic medicines, some of which are used recreationally.
Like the MDA, it divides the substances under its control
into three groups. The least stringently governed are in the
General Sale List – laxatives, antacids and so on which can be
sold anywhere. Secondly, there is the Pharmacy Medicines
List, covering those products that don't require a prescription, but can be sold only by chemists. Then come the
Prescription Only drugs, which require medical supervision.
The Act also watches over doctors, specifying maximum
dosages, as well as certain methods of writing, dating and
repeating prescriptions. Other obligations fall upon pharmacists and drug companies. The latter's imports and exports are
governed, as is the information they supply to doctors about
their products.

Tobacco

In contrast to the welter of controls that apply to the MDA
drugs, society's favourite intoxicants get a wide berth. The
only restraints on tobacco are that a tobacco product must
carry a fairly insipid health warning, a note of tar content, and
that advertising must not step beyond certain limits. All these
measures are voluntarily agreed to by the trade. Under the
Protection of Children (Tobacco) Act, all sales of tobacco
products to children under the age of 16 are prohibited. It is

onetheless extremely rare for any tobacconist to be pros-
cuted for selling to minors, even though the government
ates under-age tobacco sales to be worth some £80 million
very year.

Alcohol

Drinking regulations also set out, notionally, to protect
minors, but again are largely ignored. Except with special
authority it is an offence to give intoxicating liquor to any
child under five years of age, even in the home. It is also
forbidden to allow children into a bar, although they may be
allowed into an off-licence or a room in a hotel where drink is
consumed but not sold. Youngsters aged 14 and over may be
allowed into any part of licensed premises providing they do
not drink. Those aged 16 to 18 may drink beer, cider or perry
with a meal in a place specially designated for dining. In
Scotland this age group can also drink wine in such a setting.
No one under the age of 18 can act as a 'messenger' for an
adult unless they are paid to do so or are related to someone
who is employed in selling drinks. The normal adult freedoms
start applying after a person's 18th birthday. A publican is
free to refuse admission to anyone so long as it's not on
grounds of race or sex.

Drunkenness

Technically it is an offence to be plain drunk in a public place,
although an arrest is generally made only if there is some
rowdy or anti-social behaviour going on.

The more serious drink-linked offences come under the
Road Traffic Act (1967), a piece of legislation which also
applies to persons in charge of bicycles, horses or children.
Where there are 'reasonable grounds' for suspecting a driver
is drunk the police may stop him/her and ask that they blow
into a breathalyser bag. If it comes up positive a second test
will be ordered at a police station. Only if the person is
incapable of blowing into the breathalyser or if the readings

are marginal will that person have the right to ask for a bloc
or urine test, to be conducted by a doctor. A prosecution wi
follow if the breath reading exceeds 35 microgrammes per 10
millilitres, or if the blood or urine samples tops 80 mill
grammes of alcohol per 100 millilitres of blood or urine.

APPENDIX II
ADDRESSES

National Organisations

Advice and Information about Services

Standing Conference on Drug Abuse (SCODA)
1–4 Hatton Place
Hatton Garden
London EC1N 8ND
Tel (01) 430 2341 or dial 100 and ask for Freefone Drug
  Problems.
SCODA is the national coordinating body for voluntary
organisations and agencies working in the drugs field. Re-
gional fieldworkers keep in touch with developments and a
newsletter is published regularly.

Library, Information, Research and Education

Institute for the Study of Drug Dependence
1–4 Hatton Place
Hatton Garden
London EC1N 8ND
Tel (01) 430 1991
The Institute publishes material on various aspects of the use
and misuse of drugs and provides an excellent library service
for interested individuals and professionals.

Teacher's Advisory Council on Alcohol and Drug Educati⌐
(TACADE)
3rd Floor
Furness House
Trafford Road
Salford M5 2XJ
Tel (061) 848 0351
Educational consultancy, resources centre and in-servi⌐
training courses for local education authorities, heal⌐
authorities, etc.

The National AIDS Helpline
Tel (0800) 567123

Self-Help Organisations for Relatives and Friends

Families Anonymous
88 Caledonian Road
London N1
Tel (01) 278 8805 (24-hour ansaphone)
Advice and support groups for families and friends of dru⌐
users. Meetings throughout the country. Office hours Mon⌐
Fri 1 p.m.–4.30 p.m.

Organisation for Parents Under Stress (OPUS)
106 Godstone Road
Whyteleafe
Surrey CR3 0EB
Tel (01) 645 0469, Nottingham (0602) 470551 (24-hour crisi⌐
    line).
Umbrella organisation for various parents groups, including
Parents Anonymous, Lifeline, which offer support to parent⌐
under stress throughout the country. Office open Mon–Fr⌐
9 a.m.–5 p.m.

Al-Anon Family Groups
61 Great Dover Street
London SE1 4YF
Tel (01) 403 0888
These self-help groups are for the families and close associ⌐
ates of problem drinkers. The aim is to relieve the pressure of

ving with the drinker by sharing experiences and giving
support. You can join whether or not the problem drinker is
attending an Alcoholics Anonymous group or receiving other
help.

Al-ateen
1 Great Dover Street
London SE1 4YF
Tel (01) 403 0888
Very similar to Al-Anon but for the teenaged children of
problem drinkers who often feel happier with the support of
people their own age and don't always want to share their
experiences with parents or other adults.

Self-Help Organisations for Users

National Association for Mental Health (MIND)
22 Harley Street
London W1N 2ED
Tel (01) 637 0741
Co-ordinates tranquilliser self-help groups throughout the
country.

Narcotics Anonymous,
PO Box 246, c/o 47 Milman Street
London SW10
Tel (01) 351 6794/6066 (24-hour ansaphone)
Self-help groups for people dependent on drugs. Meetings
and contacts in various parts of the country. Office staffed
Mon–Fri 2 p.m.–8 p.m.

Alcoholics Anonymous
PO Box 1
Stonebow House
Stonebow
York YO1 2NJ
Tel (0904) 664026/7/8/9
A fellowship of nearly 2,000 groups in the UK. The aim of
all AA groups is to develop an entirely alcohol-free life.

Members meet to share experiences and help each other solv
common problems. Local groups usually listed in tl
telephone directory.

Drinkwatchers
200 Seagrave Road
London SW6 1RQ
Tel (01) 381 3155
Helps heavy drinkers reduce consumption. Not intended fo
those alcohol dependent and who wish to abstain totally
Twenty UK branches.

Counselling Services

National Association of Young People's Counselling and
   Advisory Services (NAYPCAS)
17–23 Albion Street
Leicester LE1 6GD
Tel (0533) 558763
Information on counselling and advisory services for young
people throughout the country. Letter service only.

British Association for Counselling (BAC)
37a Sheep Street
Rugby CV21 3BX
Tel (0788) 78328/9
Information and referral to individual counsellors and counselling agencies throughout the country. Telephone Mon–Fri
8.45 a.m.–5 p.m., or write enclosing SAE.

The Samaritans
17 Uxbridge Road
Slough
Berkshire SL1 1SN
Tel (0753) 31011
Befriend anyone in crisis, including people distressed by drug
problems. Branches throughout the country.

urning Point
-12 Long Lane
ondon EC1A 9HA
el (01) 606 3947
ounselling, advice and support centres for users, families
id friends. Branches throughout the country.

dvice Information and Campaigning Services

id for Addicts and Family (ADFAM)
DFAM National Office
: George's
ubrey Walk
ondon W8 7JY
el (01) 727 3595
ampaign organisation to educate, advise, train and publicise
rug-related problems, and to improve treatment and advice
icilities. Mon–Fri 9.30 a.m.–4.30 p.m.

lcohol Concern
05 Gray's Inn Road
ondon WC1X 8QF
el (01) 833 3471
A national charity dealing with drink problems and offering
nformation, advice, referral, educational and campaigning
ervices.

Action on Smoking and Health (ASH)
5–11 Mortimer Street
ondon W1N 7RH
Tel (01) 637 9843
nformation, educational and campaigning group on the
dangers of tobacco smoking.

Release
169 Commercial Street
London E1 3BW
Tel (01) 377 5905 or 603 8654 (24-hour emergency service)
Advice, information and referral on legal and drug-related
problems for users, families and friends. Mon–Fri 10 a.m.–
6 p.m.

Residential Services

Cranstoun Projects Ltd
The Pavilion
Priory Lane
Roehampton
London SW15
Tel (01) 398 6956
Residential centres in the south-east.

Phoenix House
84–88 Church Road
London SE19 2EZ
Tel (01) 771 6122
Residential houses in different parts of the country.

Scotland: National Organisations

Advice and Information about Services

Scottish Drugs Forum
266 Clyde Street
Glasgow G1 4JH
Tel (041) 221 1175
Co-ordinating body providing information and advice about services. Monthly news bulletin.

Scottish Council on Alcohol
137–145 Sauchiehall Street
Glasgow G2 3EW
Tel (041) 333 9677
Provides information on help available throughout Scotland.

ASH Scotland
6 Castle Street
Edinburgh EH2 3AT
Tel (031) 225 4725
Information, education and campaigning on the dangers of tobacco smoking.

Northern Ireland: National Organisations

Advice, Information and Counselling

Northern Ireland Regional Unit
Shaftesbury Square Hospital
116–122 Great Victoria Street
Belfast BT2 7BG
Tel (0232) 229808
Information and help available throughout Northern Ireland.

Northern Ireland Council on Alcohol
40 Elmwood Avenue
Belfast BT9 6AZ
Tel (0232) 57848 (24-hour ansaphone)
Provides information on help available throughout Northern
Ireland.

Contact Youth Counselling Service
2a Ribble Street
Newtownards Road
Belfast
Tel (0232) 57848 (24 hour ansaphone)
Drop-in for counselling Mon–Fri 9 a.m.–12 noon. Mon and
Thur 7 p.m.–9.30 p.m.

The Samaritans
Ballymena Tel (0266) 43555
Belfast Tel (0232) 664422
Befriend anyone in crisis – users, families and friends.

Self-Help and Community Groups

Parents' Advice Centre
Belfast
Tel (0232) 238800
24-hour confidential help-line offering support to parents
under stress.

Simon Community
186 Cliftonpark Avenue
Belfast
Tel (0232) 756572
Night shelter for homeless, including those with drug prob
lems.

Northlands – Alcohol and Drug Abuse
Advice Centre
68 Northland Road
Derry
Tel (0504) 263011
Advice, information, daycare and residential facilities. Ca
be contacted 24 hours a day: telephone or drop-in, thoug
appointment preferred. Satellite centres in Limavady and ir
Tyrone and Fermanagh.

Wales: National Organisations

Advice, Information and Counselling

South Wales Association for the Prevention of Addiction
  (SWAPA)
All Wales Freephone
Tel (0222) 383313
24-hour counselling, advice and information service for drug
and solvent abusers, relatives, friends and professionals.

Alcohol Concern Wales
PO Box 2010
Cardiff
Tel (0222) 398791

MIND Regional Office
23 St Mary Street
Cardiff CF1 2AA
Tel (0222) 395123
Information about groups for tranquilliser users.

INDEX

MORE NON-FICTION AVAILABLE FROM
HODDER AND STOUGHTON PAPERBACKS